Recent Results in Cancer Research 170

S. Dresel (Ed.)

PET
in Oncology

With 97 Figures in 225 Separate Illustrations, 97 in Color
and 29 Tables

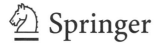 Springer

Professor Dr. med. Stefan Dresel
HELIOS Klinikum Berlin-Buch
Klinik für Nuklearmedizin
Schwanebecker Chaussee 50
13125 Berlin
Germany
stefan.dresel@helios-kliniken.de

Library of Congress Control Number: 2007928442

ISSN 0080-0015
ISBN 978-3-540-31202-4 Springer Berlin Heidelberg New York

Springer is part of Springer Science+Business Media

http//www.springer.com
© Springer-Verlag Berlin Heidelberg 2008
Printed in Germany

Editor: Dr. Ute Heilmann, Heidelberg
Desk Editor: Dörthe Mennecke-Bühler, Heidelberg
Cover-design: Frido Steinen-Broo, eStudio Calamar, Spain
Production & Typesetting: Verlagsservice Teichmann, Mauer
Printed on acid-free paper – 21/3180xq – 5 4 3 2 1 0

Preface

The addition of functional image information to conventional staging procedures, be it through positron emission tomography (PET) as a stand-alone unit or the development of combined PET/CT or by correlation of modalities using software-based image fusion, is striking in several respects.

Not many years ago the use of imaging modalities, particularly in oncology, was generally limited to the search for a tumorous lesion or its metastases followed by immediate surgical or other treatment. Now these therapeutic strategies are changing and the characterization of molecular processes, as has long been delivered by nuclear medicine procedures, has a vital role to play in that development. Just some 20 years ago, students were not taught these innovative approaches, and a highly aggressive therapeutic management was the best means to fight the enemy.

Today modern imaging modalities contribute substantially to the decision of which form of treatment – locally or systemically, surgically or in an interdisciplinary manner – will be most efficient. In some cases, even the watch and wait strategy may be appropriate, even if this approach remains uncomfortable for the clinician. In order to lead to a decision, anatomic and morphological information on the location and texture of a lesion is crucial, including its functional and metabolic description, as is information on the spread of tumors throughout the body. Furthermore, monitoring the response to therapy and diagnostic follow-up to detect recurrent disease require detailed information on the properties of a tumor and its relationship to surrounding tissues. If the information needed to strategically plan therapeutic management can be provided by correlative imaging such as PET and CT or PET/CT, so much the better.

This volume cannot deliver an exhaustive overview of the wide range of applications of combined imaging. For instance, the indications for using PET/CT to stage and monitor lung and colorectal cancer are solidly documented. The first three chapters deal with the use of PET/CT in gynecology, radiation therapy, and urology. In particular for radiation therapy, planning PET in combination with CT increasingly prevails. This not only leads to greater therapy success, but also to a drop in unwanted side effects. This may also convey a change in how we think about the best therapy management, which not only considers the elimination of the tumor but increasingly puts the patient's quality of life and prognosis into the foreground. Innovative imaging modalities contribute enormously to these changes.

Similar results can be achieved – with greater effort – using software-based fusion of different imaging techniques, which is clearly shown in Chap. 4. Even if some educational investment may still be necessary, the use of nuclear medicine modalities in pediatrics has a long tradition. It only makes sense to further explore the possibilities PET offers. In pediatric diagnostic imaging, the application of MRI outweighs the use of CT, which cannot be explained solely by the lack of radiation exposure but by the superior results that can be achieved using MRI for imaging in pediatric oncology. Future developments of combined PET/MRI will be thrilling to follow up.

The next three chapters report on the current use of SPECT/CT with different units. According to some experts, SPECT/CT may not meet the potential of PET/CT; however, these chapters clearly demonstrate that also in conventional nuclear medicine considering the combined imaging results improves the diagnostic accuracy. This becomes impressively apparent in the next chapter on the combination of SPECT and CT in patients suffering from coronary heart disease, possibly the most important application for SPECT/CT. In addition, this contribution conspicuously demonstrates that brain and software fusion as well as interdisciplinary team work may very well lead to superbly comprehensive results.

Consideration of the consequences associated with the use of combined imaging devices with regard to radiation exposure will aid in defining the diagnostic work-up in order to minimize unnecessarily repeated examinations. One of the most important challenges of these new methods may be to encourage cooperation between all disciplines so as to make use of the full potential of these methods and to avoid potential disadvantages. The current issue of *Der Nuklearmediziner* is summarized by a typically witty writing on the general use of combined devices and the consequences that arise for hospital and inpatient as well as outpatient use.

In a recently published issue of another journal on a similar topic, the editors headlined their editorial "1+1=3". This term splendidly conveys the development that can be observed these days in nuclear medicine and radiology. In particular for a nuclear medicine physician, radiology and its integration into the clinical scene may sometimes appear to be a threat. However, from successful cooperation with our radiology colleagues we know that an open discussion and the recommendation of nuclear medicine procedures by the radiologist in clinical conferences will help to communicate the usefulness and accuracy of nuclear medicine examinations. It is evident that radiologists' interest in and understanding of PET are clearly enhanced by the advent of PET/CT. There is even a degree of fascination noticeable. If this leads to additional reporting of the significance of our methods, it will be very helpful for everyone involved, not least of all for clinicians and patients. This will further strengthen the relevance of nuclear medicine in clinical and scientific settings.

Berlin   S. Dresel

Contents

List of Contributors

W. Albinger
Klinikum der Ludwig-Maximilians-Universität
München-Grosshadern
Klinik und Poliklinik für Nuklearmedizin
Marchioninistraße 15
81377 München
Germany

Prof. Dr. med. R. P. Baum
Zentralklinik Bad Berka GmbH
Nuklearmedizinische Klinik
Robert-Koch-Allee 9
99437 Bad Berka
Germany

Dr. rer. nat. Th. Beyer
Klinik und Poliklinik für Nuklearmedizin
Universitätsklinikum Essen
Hufelandstraße 55
45122 Essen
Germany

Prof. Dr. med. Dr. rer. nat. A. Bockisch
Klinik und Poliklinik für Nuklearmedizin
Universitätsklinikum Essen
Hufelandstraße 55
45122 Essen
Germany

Prof. Dr. med. S. Dresel
HELIOS Klinikum Berlin-Buch
Klinik für Nuklearmedizin
Schwanebecker Chaussee 50
13125 Berlin
Germany

Dr. med. W. Eberhardt
Innere Klinik und Poliklinik
(Tumorforschung)
Universitätsklinikum Essen
Hufelandstraße 55
45122 Essen
Germany

Dr. med. L. S. Freudenberg
Klinik und Poliklinik für Nuklearmedizin
Universitätsklinikum Essen
Hufelandstraße 55
45122 Essen
Germany

Prof. Dr. med. A. Frilling
Klinik und Poliklinik für Allgemein-,
Viszeral- und Transplantationschirurgie
Universitätsklinikum Essen
Hufelandstraße 55
45122 Essen
Germany

Prof. Dr. med. C. Grohé
Medizinische Klinik II
des Universitätsklinikums Bonn
Sigmund-Freud-Straße 25
53127 Bonn
Germany

Prof. Dr. med. K. Hahn
Klinikum der Ludwig-Maximilians-Universität
München-Innenstadt
Klinik und Poliklinik für Nuklearmedizin
Ziemssenstraße 1
80336 München
Germany

Dr. med. A. Haug
Klinikum der Ludwig-Maximilians-Universität
München-Grosshadern
Klinik und Poliklinik für Nuklearmedizin
Marchioninistraße 15
81377 München
Germany

PD Dr. med. D. Hörsch
Zentralklinik Bad Berka GmbH
Klinik für Innere Medizin/NET-Zentrum
Robert-Koch-Allee 9
99437 Bad Berka
Germany

Dr. med. M. Hommann
Zentralklinik Bad Berka GmbH
Klinik für Allgemeine Chirurgie/
Viszeralchirurgie
Robert-Koch-Allee 9
99437 Bad Berka
Germany

Prof. Dr. med. Y. Ko
Medizinische Poliklinik
des Universitätsklinikums Bonn
Sigmund-Freud-Straße 25
53127 Bonn
Germany

PD Dr. med. S. Könemann
Universitätsklinikum Münster
Klinik und Poliklinik für
Strahlentherapie und Radioonkologie
Albert-Schweitzer-Straße 33
48129 Münster
Germany

PD Dr. med. F.-W. Kreth
Klinikum der Ludwig-Maximilians-Universität
München-Grosshadern
Neurochirurgische Klinik und Poliklinik
Marchioninistraße 15
81377 München
Germany

PD Dr. med. R. Linke
Nuklearmedizinische Klinik und Poliklinik
Universitätsklinikum Erlangen
Krankenhausstraße 12
91054 Erlangen
Germany

PD Dr. med. F. Lordick
III. Medizinische Klinik
der Technischen Universität München
Klinikum rechts der Isar
Ismaninger Straße 22
81675 München
Germany

Dr. rer. nat. M.-J. Martínez
Nuklearmedizinische Klinik und Poliklinik
der Technischen Universität München
Klinikum rechts der Isar
Ismaninger Straße 22
81675 München
Germany

Dr. rer. nat. R. Michael
Wittenberger Straße 82
01309 Dresden
Germany

PD Dr. med. U. Mueller-Lisse
Klinikum der Ludwig-Maximilians-Universität
München-Grosshadern
Institut für Klinische Radiologie
Marchioninistrasse 15
81377 München
Germany

PD Dr. med. K. Ott
Chirurgische Klinik und Poliklinik
der Technischen Universität München
Klinikum rechts der Isar
Ismaninger Straße 22
81675 München
Germany

Prof. Dr. med. H. Palmedo
Klinik und Poliklinik für Nuklearmedizin
des Universitätsklinikums Bonn
Sigmund-Freud-Straße 25
53127 Bonn
Germany

PD Dr. med. Th. Pfluger
Klinikum der Ludwig-Maximilians-Universität
München-Innenstadt
Klinik und Poliklinik für Nuklearmedizin
Ziemssenstraße 1
80336 München
Germany

PD Dr. med. G. Pöpperl
Klinikum der Ludwig-Maximilians-Universität
München-Grosshadern
Klinik und Poliklinik für Nuklearmedizin
Marchioninistraße 15
81377 München
Germany

Dr. med. V. Prasad
Zentralklinik Bad Berka GmbH
Robert-Koch-Allee 9
99437 Bad Berka
Germany

Prof. Dr. med. M. Reinhardt
Pius-Hospital
Klinik für Nuklearmedizin
Georgstraße 12
26121 Oldenburg
Germany

M. Reiser
Klinikum der Ludwig-Maximilians-Universität
München-Grosshadern
Klinik und Poliklinik für Nuklearmedizin
Marchioninistraße 15
81377 München
Germany

Prof. Dr. med. S. N. Reske
Universitätsklinikum Ulm
Klinik für Nuklearmedizin
Robert-Koch-Straße 8
89081 Ulm
Germany

Dr. Dr. R. Rödel
Klinik und Poliklinik für Nuklearmedizin
des Universitätsklinikums Bonn
Klinik und Poliklinik für Nuklearmedizin
Sigmund-Freud-Straße 25
53127 Bonn
Germany

Dr. med. S. J. Rosenbaum-Krumme
Klinik und Poliklinik für Nuklearmedizin
Universitätsklinikum Essen
Hufelandstraße 55
45122 Essen
Germany

Dr. med. B. Scher
Klinikum der Ludwig-Maximilians-Universität
München-Grosshadern
Klinik und Poliklinik für Nuklearmedizin
Marchioninistraße 15
81377 München
Germany

Prof. Dr. med. Dr. h. c. P. M. Schlag
Robert-Rössle-Klinik
Charité Universitätsmedizin Berlin
Campus Buch
Lindenberger Weg 80
13125 Berlin
Germany

B. Schlenker
Klinikum der Ludwig-Maximilians-Universität
München-Grosshadern
Klinik und Poliklinik für Nuklearmedizin
Marchioninistraße 15
81377 München
Germany

Dr. med. I. Schmid
Dr. von Haunersches Kinderspital der
Ludwig-Maximilians-Universität München
Kinderklinik und Kinderpoliklinik
Lindwurmstraße 4
80337 München
Germany

Dr. med. M. Seitz
Klinikum der Ludwig-Maximilians-Universität
München-Grosshadern
Urologische Klinik
Marchioninistraße 15
81377 München
Germany

Prof. Dr. Dr. med. H. L. Sommer
Klinikum der Ludwig-Maximilians-Universität
München-Grosshadern
Klinik und Poliklinik für
Frauenheilkunde und Geburtshilfe
Maistraße 11
80337 München
Germany

Dr. med. A. Stahl
Institut für Röntgendiagnostik
der Technischen Universität München
Klinikum rechts der Isar
Ismaninger Straße 22
81675 München
Germany

Prof. Dr. med. H. C. Steinert
Universitätsspital Zürich
Department Medizinische Radiologie
Klinik für Nuklearmedizin
Rämistrasse 100
8091 Zürich
Switzerland

Prof. Dr. med. Ch. Stief
Klinikum der Ludwig-Maximilians-Universität
München-Grosshadern
Urologische Klinik
Marchioninistraße 15
81377 München
Germany

PD Dr. med. S. Tasci
Medizinische Klinik II
des Universitätsklinikums Bonn
Sigmund-Freud-Straße 25
53127 Bonn
Germany

Prof. Dr. med. K. Tatsch
Klinikum der Ludwig-Maximilians-Universität
München-Grosshadern
Klinik und Poliklinik für Nuklearmedizin
Marchioninistraße 15
81377 München
Germany

PD Dr. med. R. Tiling
Klinikum der Ludwig-Maximilians-Universität
München-Grosshadern
Klinik und Poliklinik für Nuklearmedizin
Marchioninistraße 15
81377 München
Germany

Prof. Dr. med. J.-C. Tonn
Klinikum der Ludwig-Maximilians-Universität
München-Grosshadern
Neurochirurgische Klinik und Poliklinik
Marchioninistraße 15
81377 München
Germany

Prof. Dr. R. Voltz
Klinik und Poliklinik für Palliativmedizin
Klinikum der Universität zu Köln
50924 Köln
Germany

PD Dr. med. M. Weckesser
Klinik und Poliklinik für Nuklearmedizin
Universitätsklinikum Münster
Albert-Schweitzer-Straße 33
48149 Münster
Germany

Dr. med. H. Wieder
Institut für Röntgendiagnostik
der Technischen Universität München
Klinikum rechts der Isar
Ismaninger Straße 22
81675 München
Germany

Prof. Dr. med. M. Wolff
Chirurgisches Zentrum
des Universitätsklinikums Bonn
Sigmund-Freud-Straße 25
53127 Bonn
Germany

PD Dr. rer. nat. S. Ziegler
Nuklearmedizinische Klinik und Poliklinik
der Technischen Universität München
Klinikum rechts der Isar
Ismaninger Straße 22
81675 München
Germany

1 PET and PET/CT: Basic Principles and Instrumentation

M.-J. Martínez, S. I. Ziegler, and Th. Beyer

Recent Results in Cancer Research, Vol. 170
© Springer-Verlag Berlin Heidelberg 2008

The increasing role of positron emission tomography (PET) in the diagnosis and staging of malignant disease and monitoring of therapy response can be attributed to significant improvements made in the performance of this imaging technology. Anticipated progress is frequently constrained by the physics of PET, and current designs of PET scanners aim at an ultimately high spatial resolution and sensitivity as well as improved signal-to-noise properties. Recent advances in the field of PET instrumentation include the introduction of novel scintillation crystal technology and detector electronics, as well as the widespread introduction of fast and efficient, iterative image reconstruction algorithms for fully three-dimensional (3D) PET data sets. These advances have led to a dramatic reduction in clinical imaging times while improving image quality. Finally, the combination of functional imaging and computed tomography (CT) within a combined PET/CT tomograph provides a tool to accurately localise functional abnormalities in an anatomical context. In addition, lengthy transmission scans can be eliminated in PET/CT examinations and the overall scan duration can be reduced by as much as 40%. A combined anatomical and functional clinical study can be completed in less than 30 min, thus allowing an increase in patient throughput. This chapter describes the basic principles of annihilation coincidence detection and the design and performance characteristics of PET detectors and scanners. Recent developments in PET scanner technology, from the introduction of new PET detectors to the combined PET/CT systems are discussed as well.

1.1 Positron Emission Tomography

1.1.1 Positron Emission and Coincidence Principle

The principles of imaging tissue function in vivo are summarised in Fig. 1.1. The PET process begins with the selection and production of a suitable molecular probe, a pharmaceutical labelled with a positron-emitting radionuclide, followed by the administration of the probe to the patient and finally the imaging of the distribution of the probe in the patient. Positron (β^+) emitters are neutron-deficient nuclei that gain stability through the transmutation of a proton (p) into a neutron (n). During this process, a positive electron, or positron (e^+), and an electron neutrino (v) are emitted:

$$p \rightarrow n + e^+ + v$$

The total available energy for the decay is shared between the positron and the neutrino. Thus, positrons show a continuous energy spectrum with a maximum value that depends on the specific radioisotope, typically in the range of a few kiloelectron volts to a few megaelectron volts. Once ejected, the positron loses

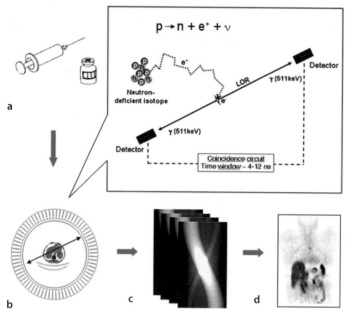

Fig. 1.1a–d. Principles of in vivo PET imaging: **a** A radiopharmaceutical is injected in the patient. **b** The positron annihilates with an electron of the surrounding tissue generating, thus two 511-keV photons which can be measured by the detection system. The co-linearity of both photons (electronic collimation) allows the annihilation events to be detected by two opposite detector units within a time window of typically 4–12 ns. **c** Measured coincidence data are stored in form of sinograms and **d** a coronal view of the reconstructed image mapping the utilisation of the radiotracer throughout the patient

kinetic energy to the surrounding material by ionisation and scattering processes. When the positron is almost at rest, usually within a few millimetres of the site of its origin, it interacts with an electron of the surrounding tissue. The positron and electron annihilate and two photons of 511 keV each are emitted back to back.

Annihilation events are registered by coincidence detectors consisting of two opposite detector units. Due to the co-linearity of the emitted gamma quanta (electronic collimation), the need for physical collimation that is known from SPECT imaging can be avoided. The two detector units will only detect events that occur within their sensitive volume. The line joining the pair of detectors is referred to as the line of response (LOR). Since the annihilation quanta are emitted simultaneously, the pair of detectors will identify an event as a coincidence event only if both photons are detected within a very short time interval set in the detection system and referred to as coincidence timing window.

Events coming from annihilation processes are referred to as true coincidence events. Unfortunately, not all acquired events contribute to the signal. Coincidence timing windows

in modern tomographs are set typically to 4–12 ns, depending on the detector material used (see Sect. 1.2.1). During this time, photons from unrelated positron-electron annihilations, referred to as random coincidence events (Fig. 1.2a), are detected as well. The random event rate in a pair of detectors is given by:

$$R_{randoms} = 2\tau \cdot S_1 \cdot S_2 \rightarrow$$

where τ is the width of coincidence timing window, and S_1 and S_2 are the single countrates in detector 1 and 2, respectively. Random countrates increase linearly with the width of the coincidence window and are proportional to the square of the singles rate incident on the detectors. Random events contribute to the noise in PET images and thus degrade image quality. Another contribution to background noise in PET images comes from scatter coincidence events. In a scatter event (Fig. 1.2b), one or both of the annihilation photons change their initial direction because of Compton interaction with surrounding tissues or even in the detectors, before being accepted as valid counts. The contribution of scatter radiation to the total countrate can be reduced by defining an energy window

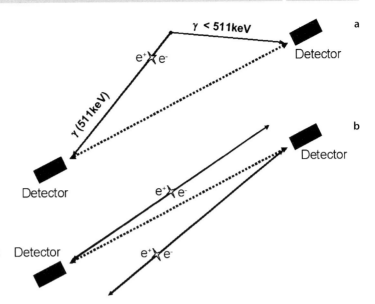

Fig. 1.2a,b. Additional contributions to PET data may come from **a** scatter of one or two photons which reach a detector pair in coincidence and **b** two annihilation photons from different decay processes which accidentally reach a detector pair (these events are called random coincidences)

with a lower threshold typically set at 350–400 keV. However, due to the limited energy resolution of a whole-body PET system, a large proportion of the scatter events falling within the standard energy window are considered as true coincidences. Scatter coincidences result in a misplacement of the annihilation events or, in other words, in assigning counts to an incorrect LOR. Scatter contributions increase with the patient size, being larger in 3D than in 2D acquisition mode (see Chap. 3).

There are a number of suitable radionuclides for medical applications of PET (Table 1.1). In oncology, however, the most important radiopharmaceutical is ^{18}F. ^{18}F is used to label substrates like glucose (^{18}F-FDG), which accumulates in locations with high glucose utilisation. Since tumours are hypermetabolic, ^{18}F-FDG becomes a sensitive biochemical indicator of malignancy. Given that ^{18}F can be routinely produced in a cyclotron and has a half-life of 109.8 min, making it suitable for remote transport, ^{18}F-FDG has become the workhorse in the diagnosis, staging of malignant disease and monitoring of response to therapy.

1.2 PET Detector and Tomograph Design

1.2.1 PET Detectors

Scintillator crystals are the most widely used detectors in PET. They become excited after the annihilation photons deposit their energy and de-excite by emitting visible scintillation light that can be detected by a photomultiplier. The main characteristics required for PET scintillator crystals are high mass density and atomic number, high light output, and fast response. High mass density and high atomic number, synonymous with high stopping power, are needed for high photo

Table 1.1. Half-life, maximum energy of beta particles and positron range of some isotopes commonly used in PET

Isotope	Half-life (min)	E_{max} (MeV)	Range in water (mm)	
			Max	Mean
^{11}C	20.4	0.96	4.1	1.1
^{13}N	9.96	1.19	5.1	1.5
^{15}O	2.03	1.73	7.3	2.5
^{18}F	109.8	0.63	2.4	0.6
^{68}Ga	68.3	1.89	8.2	2.9
^{82}Rb	1.25	3.40	14.1	5.9

absorption at 511 keV. A high light output, i.e. the number of useful photons created per incident amount of photon energy deposited in the crystal, leads to good energy resolution. This is particularly important for discriminating scattered radiation, as it reduces the statistical uncertainty on the energy measurement. A fast response, i.e. a fast rise time and a fast decay time with no afterglow, provides a narrower timing coincidence window and consequently a reduction in random coincidence countrate.

The first PET tomographs developed in the early 1970s used thallium-doped sodium-iodine crystals, NaI(Tl) [44], a scintillator that is widely employed in nuclear medicine gamma cameras to detect the 140-keV photons from the decay of ^{99m}Tc. This scintillator provides a very high light output, which leads to good energy resolution, but it presents a low stopping power for 511-keV photons. Therefore, to detect annihilation photons efficiently, thicker crystals than those used in gamma cameras are needed. In the late 1970s, bismuth germanate BGO was introduced [17]. Even though the light yield of BGO is 15% of NaI(Tl) and the decay time approximately 30% longer (Table 1.2), it became very successful owing to its higher atomic number and consequently higher detection efficiency. Since 1986, when the first multi-ring scanner, the Siemens ECAT 931 [50] was built, BGO became the PET scintillator material of choice.

However, the physical properties of BGO crystals limited the energy resolution and countrate performance of the multi-ring scanners and crystals with faster decay times and higher light output were sought. Therefore, in the 1990s, cerium-doped gadolinium oxyorthosilicate, GSO [52], and cerium-doped lutetium oxyorthosilicate, LSO [38], became available. LSO and GSO show higher light output, higher stopping power and faster response than BGO and therefore allow a significant improvement in countrate performance of the PET systems. The physical properties of these newer crystals are also compared in Table 1.2.

Scintillators in clinical PET are usually glued to photomultiplier tubes (PMTs). In the early PET systems, the detector unit consisted of a single scintillator crystal coupled to an individual PMT. The units were arranged in a single layer ring or in multiple rings around the patient. This design presented the drawback of limited spatial resolution, due to the large size of the PMTs, and an elevated system cost. In the mid 1980s, Casey and Nutt [15] decreased both complexity and cost in a single design; the block detector (Fig. 1.3). In this standard design, a large scintillator crystal, usually BGO or LSO, is coupled to four PMTs. The crystal is segmented by making partial cuts through the crystal with a fine saw to facilitate identification by PMTs of where a specific signal originated within the crystal. The cuts are filled with a reflective material that reduces and

Table 1.2. Physical properties of different scintillator crystals for PET

Property	NaI	BGO	LSO	GSO	LYSO[a]
Density (g/ml)	3.67	7.13	7.4	6.7	7.1
Effective Z	51	74	66	61	64
Attenuation length (cm)	2.88	1.05	1.16	1.43	1.1
Decay time (ns)	230	300	35–45	30–60	40
Photons/MeV	38,000	8,200	28,000	10,000	32,000
Light yield (% NaI)	100	15	75	25	75
Hygroscopic	Yes	No	No	No	No

[a] Values correspond to Lu:Y concentrations of 9:1. NaI, sodium iodide; GSO, gadolinium oxyorthosilicate; BGO, bismuth germanate; LSO, lutetium oxyorthosilicate; LYSO, lutetium-yttrium oxyorthosilicate

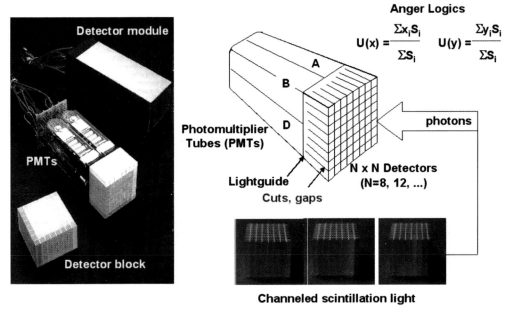

Fig. 1.3. The concept of the PET block design: a block of scintillator is partitioned into N × N small elements with saw cuts of different depths. The scintillator crystal is coupled to four photomultiplier tubes (*PMTs*). An incident annihilation photon deposits its energy in the scintillator crystal leading to the generation of scintillator light that can be detected by the PMTs. The sharing of the light between the PMTs depends on the depth of the cuts and allows the detector element to be identified by Anger Logics

controls optical cross-talks between array elements. To control the amount of light shared by the PMTs and thus locate a particular event, the length of the cuts varies within the crystal. Arrays of 8×8 or even 13×13 elements, each 4- to 6-mm wide and 20- to 30-mm thick, are normally used.

An alternative to the block detector design is the Anger-logic approach [2] in which a large area NaI(Tl) detector is read out by an array of PMTs. A light guide serves to spread the scintillator light to an appropriate number of PMTs. In this arrangement, the location of the photon interaction point within the crystal is given, as well, as the centroid of the signals in each of the PMTs. In order to detect coincidence events efficiently, the crystals must be thicker (25 mm). Consequently, the spatial resolution worsens as a result of increased Compton scattering within the NaI(Tl) crystal. Scanners with this detector geometry operate in 3D mode for increased sensitivity [33]. Recently, a pixelated detector design has been introduced [51]. In this design, individual small-area GSO detector elements (4×6 mm^2 surface and 20-mm depth) are coupled to a continuous light guide and placed on an array of PMTs. The advantage of this design is a more homogeneous light collection for all crystals, which allows for good energy resolution.

1.2.2 Scanner Design

Ring tomographs based on discrete crystals consist of some 10,000 detection elements arranged in several rings. The choice of the ring diameter implies a compromise between several factors such as scanner sensitivity (the smaller the diameter the larger the solid angle covered by the detectors and the higher the sensitivity), the fraction of scattered radiation, which is reduced with increased ring diameter, and the total cost. Typically, ring diameters range from 80 to 90 cm. The axial extent of ring tomographs varies from 15 to 18 cm. Annular lead shielding with an inner diameter equal to the patient port at the sides of the detector rings reduces the single-event rate originating from activity outside the FOV. As the number of random coincidences increases with the square of the single countrate, this shielding effectively reduces random background. Septa made of lead or tungsten between the detector slices were traditionally used in 2D acquisition mode to allow coincidences only within one transverse slice or direct neighbours. The septa reduce scatter contribution but they also reduce sensitivity. In order to increase sensitivity, scanners with retractable septa were designed [16], thus allowing emission scanning in both 2D and 3D mode (Fig. 1.4). In 3D acquisition, the acceptance angle is increased by removing the inter-pane septa, thus allowing coincidence events between different detector rings to be detected.

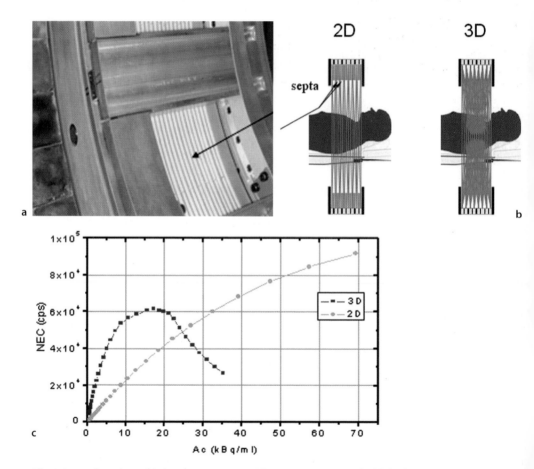

Fig. 1.4a–c. View of a multi-ring PET scanner **a** with inter-ring septa to shield the detector rings from out-of-plane scatter and random coincidences. **b** With the septa extended into the field-of-view (FOV), the number of active lines of response (LORs) is limited to those in-plane and small incident angles (*left*), whereas with the septa removed (*right*) the number of active LORs is greatly increased, thereby increasing sensitivity. **c** The noise equivalent countrate (*NEC*) as a function of activity concentration in the FOV for an LSO ACCEL scanner. The data show the significantly improved performance in 3D mode with the septa retracted, particularly at low-activity concentrations. NEC data courtesy of Siemens AG, Erlangen

1.3 Data Processing and Quantification in PET

1.3.1 Sinograms

Events acquired during a PET scan occur in a random order and are usually sorted into distinct angular directions before reconstruction. Figure 1.5 illustrates how data sorting is performed for the particular case of 2D acquisition. The data corresponding to a given transverse plane, referred to as direct coincidences, are stored in a 2D matrix, referred to as sinogram. Each matrix element represents the sum of all the events occurring in the same LOR, characterised by two coordinates: its angular orientation ö (vertical axis) and its distance from the centre of the gantry, s (horizontal axis). Each complete row in the sinogram therefore represents the parallel projection, at a given ö of the radioactivity distribution in the scanned object. When PET acquisition is performed in 3D mode, coincidences are also accepted in detector pairs which belong to different rings. In this case, PET raw data will contain both, direct and oblique sinograms, i.e. information of the LORs for direct and oblique coincidences. To increase the sensitivity of the system, many scanners combine the axial data into a single reconstructed image. The number of direct and oblique sinograms which are collapsed into one axial plane for image reconstruction defines the span of the system. Span should not be confused with the maximum number of ring detectors in 3D mode which are allowed to measure cross-coincidences. Another way of increasing the number of counts in a sinogram pixel is to combine angular samples. In scanners with small detectors, the number of sinogram rows can be reduced without greatly affecting the spatial resolution of the system. The reduction of angular samples is referred to as sinogram mashing. The mashing factor indicates how many times the angular samples have been reduced by half. For instance, a mashing factor of 1 means the number of rows is half the original one, a factor of 2 means the number of rows is reduced to 1/4 of the original, etc.

1.3.1.1 Static, Dynamic, Gated and List Mode Acquisition

In a static study, PET data are acquired over a period of time and the reconstructed image represents the time average of the radiotracer distribution. A static study is suitable when either physiologically induced time variations in the radiotracer distribution are very slow or when the countrate is so low that a long acquisition is required to obtain a satisfactory image quality.

Alternatively to static acquisition, dynamic and gated studies allow images to be visualised sequentially, like a movie. Dynamic studies display temporal changes in radiotracer distribution, and they are requested for kinetic parameter estimation.

In gated studies, PET acquisition is synchronised to an external signal, typically a cardiac or a respiratory signal, or both. The resulting gated images show the motion taking

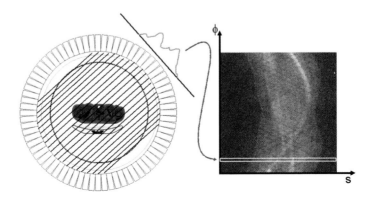

Fig. 1.5. Data sorting in the form of a sinogram for PET acquisition: sinogram rows are filled with the number of events that hit detector pairs along a set of LORs which have the same angular orientation (projections)

place during the cardiac or respiratory cycle of the patient. The most important application of gated studies is in the field of cardiology, and more recently the implementation in oncology studies to obtain respiration motion-free images and subsequently improve lesion detectability and quantification of lesions in the thorax region is under investigation [39].

List mode (LM) acquisition provides more detailed temporal information. PET data are stored at fixed time intervals, typically 10 ms, as a list of event type, detector pair number and time information. LM makes it possible to interleave the PET data with the status of an external signal, which allows the data to be reformatted into static, dynamic or gated sinograms upon completion of the acquisition.

1.3.2   Data Processing

In principle, the line integral along a given LOR should be proportional to the number of photons emitted along that line. In reality, a number of important corrections have to be applied to the sinogram data in order to obtain the true line integrals of the radiotracer concentration. The corrections involve detector sensitivity normalisation, dead-time, random, scatter and attenuation correction.

1.3.2.1 Normalisation

Lines-of-response in a PET data set have different sensitivities resulting from the variation in detector efficiency and further geometric effects. If not corrected for, these effects may lead to false quantification and artefacts in PET images. The process of correcting for these effects is referred to as normalisation. Variations in detector efficiency become particularly important in tomographs with full-ring geometry with up to 20,000 individual detector elements. One way to correct for differences in detector response is to expose each detector pair with the same radioactive source. Geometric effects are typically corrected using analytical methods [29]. From normalisation, individual correction factors can be derived for each detector pair

and further applied to the number of counts measured in that pair.

1.3.2.2 Detector Dead Time

Dead time is the time interval in which the detector ceases to respond because the system is processing a detected event. In block detectors, the dead time is mainly imposed by the integration amplifiers. To compensate for dead time, a multiplication factor can be applied to the measured counts. However, at high countrates this approach is no longer feasible. There are several ways to improve system dead time, and in general countrate performance, for instance using faster scintillator crystals, novel approaches to detector-PMT coupling or using faster electronics [45] for signal processing.

1.3.2.3 Randoms Correction

Random radiation arises not only from the radioactivity in the field of view (FOV) of the scanner, but also from the radioactivity outside the FOV, when one of the two photons from a given positron annihilation enters the scanner FOV and reaches the detectors. For whole-body imaging with 18F-FDG, the radiopharmaceutical distributes throughout the body, and radioactivity that localises in regions outside the FOV (e.g. the bladder) increases the overall random rate to a level that may exceed 50% of the total acquisition rate.

There are different methods to correct for accidental coincidences. One of the most widely used is the delayed coincidence window method in which a delayed timing window, usually with the same time width as the coincidence timing window, is defined. This window only samples random events which can be subtracted from the prompts during acquisition (online subtraction). Online subtraction is often used in commercial scanners, since it requires little disk space. Alternatively, random rates can be estimated from single event rates (Eq. 2) and be subtracted from the measured prompts [19]. The main drawback when using this approach is the difficulty of estimating the dead time and τ accurately.

1.3.2.4 Scatter Correction

Since scatter events result in misplacement of true events, scatter correction becomes an important issue for PET quantification. There are many techniques that can be used for scatter correction and that fall mainly into three categories: (a) techniques based on measurement with multiple energy windows [47], (b) techniques based on pre- or postreconstruction filtering and/or subtraction operations [5] and (c) techniques based on estimation of scatter distribution [42, 55].The suitability of any of these approaches depends on several aspects such as the acquisition mode (2D or 3D), scanner design or scanned body part.

1.3.2.5 Attenuation Correction

Attenuation correction is the most important correction in PET and it accounts for the removed annihilation events from a LOR due to Compton interaction. For whole-body imaging of large patients, the attenuation correction factors along LORs through the abdomen and shoulders can be significantly high, and cause an amplification of the intrinsic noise in the PET emission data. The importance of correcting for attenuation is shown in Figure 1.6, which shows the uncorrected image (Fig. 1.6a) and the attenuation-corrected image (Fig. 1.6b). Increased uptake in the skin and lungs, as well as nonuniform recovery of uptake in the liver and spleen, are well-known features of nonattenuation corrected ^{18}F-FDG-PET images.

Due to the co-linearity of the two emitted quanta, the total attenuation for a specific LOR does not depend on where the annihilation process occurs. Thus, a transmission measurement can be used for the calculation of the attenuation correction factors as given in Figure 1.7. The transmission measurement is normally done using a coincidence-based attenuation scan [14]. Typically, this scan is performed with three [68]Ge rod sources which rotate around the patient. Transmission scans range from 3 to 10 min and must cover the same axial range as the emission scan. One way to reduce the duration of the transmission scan is to segment the low-statistics transmission im-

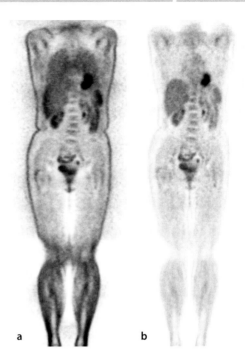

Fig. 1.6a,b. Coronal view through a whole-body FDG PET image of a patient: **a** the image has been reconstructed without attenuation correction and **b** the image is attenuation-corrected. Lungs, skin and periphery of lever show an artificially increased radiotracer uptake in the uncorrected image (**a**) as compared to the corrected image (**b**)

age into a small number of tissue types with a priori known attenuation coefficients [56].

1.3.2.6 Absolute Quantification

Once all the corrections have been applied to the sinogram, the resulting voxel intensity is directly proportional to the true amount of radioactivity in that voxel. To obtain the absolute activity value, a cross-calibration, typically with a cylinder containing a uniform solution of known activity concentration, is performed. The calibration factor (CF) is defined as:

$$CF = \frac{counts\ per\ pixel}{radionuclide\ concentration\ in\ cylinder\left(kBq\,/\,cm^{3}\right)}$$

To attain the activity concentration of a given voxel, its contents should be divided by the CF. The effectiveness of cross-calibration mandates an accurate scatter correction of the measured data, especially when acquiring in 3D mode when a significant contribution of scatter events to the measured data is expected.

1.3.3 Reconstruction

Since the PET raw data are essentially parallel projections of the tracer distribution, techniques based on reconstruction from projections are used to recover the 3D tracer

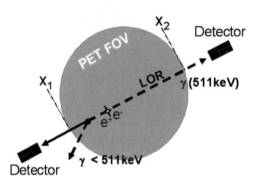

$$I = I_0 \int_{x_1}^{x_2} e^{-\mu(x, E_{PET})dx}$$

a

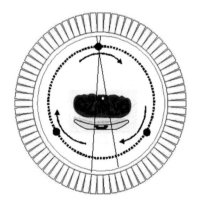

$$ACF = \frac{I_0}{I} = \frac{Blank\ scan}{Transmission}$$

b

distribution. Reconstruction algorithms are optimised for 2D data, and 3D reconstruction algorithms, which require much greater computational time, do not yet play an important role in clinical routine. PET data acquired in 3D acquisition mode are usually reduced into a set of 2D data before image reconstruction by means of faster rebinning methods such as Fourier rebinning (FORE) [22].

Until a few years ago, the most common reconstruction method in PET has been submitted to 2D filtered back-projection (FBP), an analytical approach based on the inverse 2D radon transform [28] of the projected data. Projection data are back-projected homogeneously along the corresponding LOR. Before the forward projection, the data are mathematically processed by means of a special function called a filter, which cancels out the positive counts in areas of zero activity. The choice of the filter is determined by the type of study and statistical quality of the data. In general, filtering with a function that eliminates high spatial frequencies will decrease the noise in the image but it affects the spatial resolution. Thus, it is desirable to do as little filtering as possible in order to preserve resolution and with it quantitative accuracy in the image.

Recently, iterative methods based on the maximum-likelihood estimation of the tracer distribution have been implemented and nowadays are commonly used in clinical routine. Briefly, iterative methods start with an assumed image, compute projections from the image, compare the original projection data and update the image based upon the differ-

Fig. 1.7a,b. The physics of PET attenuation and procedure for correction of the attenuation effect: **a** an annihilation photon scatters in the patient and the event is removed from a LOR. The attenuated activity (I) is given by the nonattenuated activity (I_0) multiplied by an attenuation factor computed as shown as the integral along the corresponding LOR within the patient. **b** Up to three 68Ge rotating sources can be used to measure the attenuation correction factors. The (I_0/I) ratio is estimated from a blank scan acquired without a patient and a transmission scan acquired with the patient positioned in the scanner

ence between the calculated and the actual projections. Iterative algorithms accurately model the radiation physics and take into account normalisation and detector effects, leading to more realistic images with highly improved noise properties. However, given their slow convergence, the implementation in clinical routine has only been possible with the introduction of faster algorithms such as ordered subset expectation maximisation

(OSEM) [30] or the row action maximum likelihood (RAMLA) [11]. Further progress has been made by incorporating attenuation information into the reconstruction model in the form of weighting factors. Figure 1.8 shows an FDG whole-body scan acquired in 3D mode and reconstructed using (Fig. 1.8a) attenuation-weighted OSEM (AWOSEM) [18] and (Fig. 1.8b) FBP. The overall image quality is superior with AWOSEM.

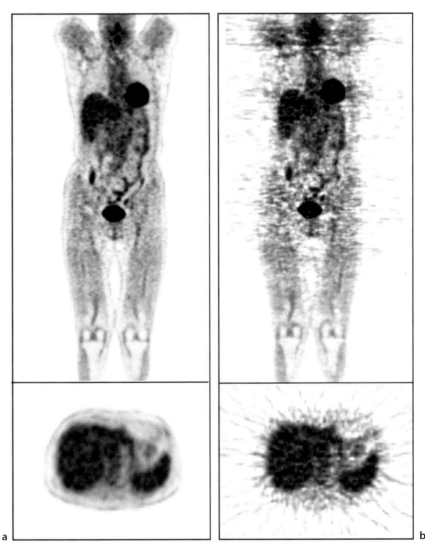

a   b

Fig. 1.8a,b. Coronal (*top*) and transverse (*bottom*) views of a ^{18}F-FDG whole-body scan acquired in 3D mode and reconstructed using **a** Fourier rebinning (FORE) and ordered subset expectation maximisation (OSEM) and **b** 2D filtered back-projection

1.3.4 Scanner Performance

1.3.4.1 Spatial Resolution: Limiting Factors

The spatial resolution of a scanner represents its ability to distinguish small structures after image reconstruction. In scanners with discrete detector elements, the spatial resolution is primarily determined by the size of the individual crystals However, other factors may further degrade the spatial resolution of a scanner such as the effective positron range and the depth of interaction (DOI) effect.

The effective positron range is defined as the average distance from the emitting nucleus to the end of the positron range, measured perpendicular to a line defined by the direction of the annihilation quanta (Fig. 1.9a). In whole-body scanners, the effect of noncolinearity in the emitted quanta and blurring from the positron range results in a degradation that extends from a few tenths of a millimetre up to a few millimetres. The DOI effect, on the other hand, is related to the depth of the detector crystals, which is approximately 2–3 cm. Due to their energy, annihilation photons can travel several

millimetres before interacting with the crystal. The photon may even travel through one crystal to the adjacent one. As a result the LOR is misplaced. This effect is more pronounced for a source located away from the centre of the FOV, due to the angulation between detectors (Fig. 1.9b). For a BGO whole-body scanner, measurements show that because of DOI, the spatial resolution degrades from 4.5 mm near the centre of the scanner to 8.9 mm for a radial distance of 20 cm [1].

The limited spatial resolution becomes apparent in the images as a blurring effect. More importantly, quantification in small structures may also be affected, since the activity appears to be distributed over a larger area. In the same way, the activity value within a voxel will always contain some contribution from adjacent voxels. This effect is referred to as partial volume effect (PVE) and will result in an over- or underestimation of activity concentrations depending on the regional distribution of the radiotracer. The errors introduced by PVE are less when the size of the structure of interest is large compared to the spatial resolution of the system, typically twice the spatial resolution.

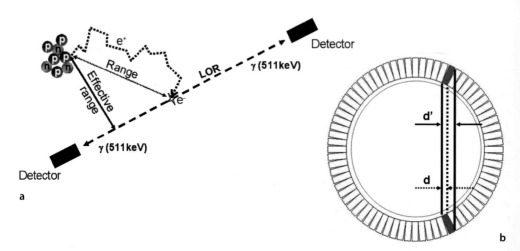

Fig. 1.9a,b. Factors affecting the spatial resolution on PET scanners. **a** Blurring due to positron range effects, the perpendicular distance from the decaying nucleus to the line defined by the two 511-keV annihilation photons is referred to as the effective positron range. **b** The apparent width of a detector element, d', increases with increasing radial offset in a ring PET scanner. Because the depths at which the gamma rays interact within the scintillator crystal are unknown, the annihilation event for a pair of photons recorded in coincidence could have occurred anywhere between the two solid lines. The magnitude of the effect depends on the source location, the diameter of the scanner, and the length and width of the crystal elements

1.3.4.2 Noise-Equivalent Countrate

Random, scatter, and count rate performance depend on the scanned object and PET scanner geometry. A parameter which describes the influence of those factors on the overall ability of the scanner to measure the true events count-rate is referred to as noise equivalent countrate (NEC) and it is defined as:

$$NEC = \frac{T^2}{T + S + KR}$$

where T is the true events countrate, S the scatter countrate, R the random countrate and K is a factor that depends on the method used for random subtraction: 2 for on-line random subtraction (see Sect. 1.3.2.3) and 1 for noise-less random subtraction. Figure 4c shows an example of a NEC curve as a function of activity concentration in a 20-cm diameter, 70-cm-long phantom [NEMA NU 2001 protocol; 20]. The significant improvement in the 3D NEC, and hence signal to noise, at lower activity concentrations is clear from the curves. Even though it is not trivial to extrapolate from performance curves to clinical situations, countrate performance curves provide a tool for scanner performance comparison.

1.3.4.3 Routine Quality Assurance

Since most of the clinical PET scanners contain approximately 20,000 scintillation crystals coupled to hundreds of photomultipliers, a defect in one or more detector units may cause serious image artefacts. To prevent image artefacts from defective detector modules and to check system stability, daily scanner quality control procedures are necessary. In most PET scanners, constancy checks are performed by comparing a reference blank scan obtained during the last setup with a daily acquired blank scan using rotating rod sources. The difference between both scans is characterised by the average variance, a parameter that is a sensitive indicator of all types of detector problems. When the average variance value is elevated, sinograms of the actual blank scan should be checked carefully. If no rotat-

ing rods are present, as is the case for most of the PET scanners in the PET/CT tomographs, the daily quality control is performed with a cylindrical phantom filled with a known activity concentration.

1.4 Combined PET/CT Imaging

1.4.1 Motivation: Challenge of Stand-Alone PET

The major drawback of standard PET is that the images are of substantially lower resolution than, for example, those of CT and MRI. The lack of anatomical detail in PET results in poor localisation of lesions and poor demarcation of lesion borders. Moreover, lesions are often complex, with some portions being more active metabolically than others. To complement molecular and anatomical information such as that obtained by PET and CT, respectively, and thus facilitate a more accurate diagnosis [54], both retrospective software-based approaches and, later, hardware-based approaches to combined dual-modality imaging have been introduced. While fully or semi-automated software algorithms register almost any complementary images of the thorax, for example, in a few minutes [48], they fail to align independently acquired image volumes extending over larger axial ranges (e.g., whole-body imaging).

Hardware-based approaches to anato-metabolic imaging [54] in humans have existed for combined PET/CT since 1998 [53]. Combined PET/CT tomographs can acquire molecular and anatomical information in a single examination without moving the patient [6], thus minimizing any intrinsic spatial misalignment. The almost simultaneous acquisition of such complementary information has been shown to lead to superior diagnostic information compared to separated PET and CT imaging [33]. Total examination times with PET/CT are significantly reduced in comparison to standard PET imaging times since the available CT transmission information is used for attenuation correction of the complementary PET emission data [34]. In addition, scanner and operational costs could potentially be reduced, since standard PET transmission sources become obsolete in PET/CT imaging [46]. Taking together the benefits of intrinsically aligned PET and CT data, shorter scan times and logistical advantages in patient management with PET/CT, combined PET/CT imaging has become a state-of-the-art tool for patient management in clinical oncology.

1.4.2 PET/CT Tomograph Designs

A first approach to hardware fusion as an alternative to the more traditional software fusion methods was discussed by Hasegawa and colleagues [27] who presented a dual-modality imager capable of acquiring both CT and SPECT data in a single imaging session. This work was transferred to the field of complementary CT and PET imaging by Townsend and Beyer [53]

who completed the design, construction and clinical operation of the first combined, dual-modality PET/CT tomograph in 1998.

An important issue of combining PET and CT from the technological point of view is to correlate the position of the patient in both systems, independently of the patient's weight and the region of the body scanned. Given that in commercial PET/CT designs both scanning modalities are axially displaced, the design of a novel patient support system that does not promote a relative vertical deflection between the CT and the PET as it extends into the gantry becomes critical. Nowadays, two ways of combining both scanners are found in the commercially available PET/CT tomographs (Fig. 1.10). The first one is the integrated scanner design, in which both scanners are located within a common gantry. The second approach is having two gantries that are separated by a small axial gap (Fig. 1.10a).

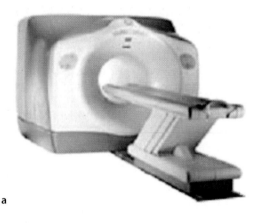

a

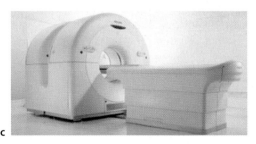

c

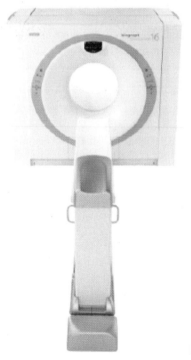

b

Fig. 1.10a–c. Some of the commercially available dual-modality PET/CT scanners: **a** GEMINI by Philips Medical Systems, **b** Biograph Sensation 16 by Siemens Medical Solutions and **c** Discovery LS by General Electric

1.4.2.1 CT Components of PET/CT

Most clinical CT systems in PET/CT tomographs present a partial-ring detector fan- or cone-beam geometry rotating together with an x-ray tube. This configuration is known as third-generation geometry, also referred to as spiral geometry because of the effective path the x-ray beam describes around the patient during a CT acquisition performed with continuous bed motion. Initially, combined imaging of the heart was not the primary objective of PET/CT imaging, as illustrated by the incorporation of only mid-range CT components in the first generations of combined tomographs [31]. The main application of PET/CT in oncology was to supplement the limited anatomical background information of PET with the intrinsically associated anatomy as imaged by

CT. While, the first PET/CT scanners employed 1- to 2- and 4-slice CT systems; more recent PET/CT designs, however, employ CT systems with up to 64 detector rows [37] and thus offer the potential of defining and evaluating acquisition protocol standards for imaging the heart.

1.4.2.2 PET Components of PET/CT

In all commercial PET/CT designs, PET components typically correspond to commercially available stand-alone PET systems with a few modifications. PET detector materials used in commercial PET/CT systems include BGO, LSO and GSO (Table 1.3), four vendors offer exclusively 3D PET designs without septa installed, while one vendor promotes 3D as an option to standard 2D PET imaging with removable

Table 1.3. Characteristics of selected commercial PET/CT systems

PET/CT System PET component	Biograph 16 (high resolution) Accel	Gemini GXL Allegro	Discovery ST Advance NXi
Scintillator	LSO	GSO	BGO
Detector dimensions (mm)	4×4x25	4×6×30	6.3×6.3×30
Axial field of view (cm)	16.2	18	15.7
Sensitivity (cps/kBq)	4.5	8.3	9.3 (3D)
Peak NECR (kcps)	93	70	63 (3D)
Transverse resolution (mm)	4.5	5.1	6.2 (3D)
Axial resolution	5.6	5.5	7.0 (3D)
2D mode availability	No	No	Yes
Attenuation correction mode	CT	CT&^{137}Cs	CT
CT component	**Somatom Sensation 16**	**Brilliance CT-16**	**Lightspeed CVT**
Detector type	UFC	CdWO$_4$	Ceramic
Slices	16	16	16
Fastest rotation time (s)	0.42	0.5	0.5
Transverse field of view (cm)	50	50	50
Minimum slice width (mm)	0.75	0.75	--
CT patient port (cm)	70	70	70

Data were obtained from the vendors of PET/CT systems: Siemens (Biograph 16), Philips (Gemini GXL), and GE Healthcare (Discovery ST). Performance data are obtained according to NEMA NU-2001

septa in the combined gantry. Scatter and random countrates in 3D PET/CT acquisition are higher because of the larger bore diameter of the common gantry. However, recent developments involving faster electronics and improved signal processing [45] take full advantage of the properties of the LSO and GSO fast scintillator crystals leading to a considerable improvement in the sensitivity and countrate performance.

1.4.3 PET/CT Acquisition

1.4.3.1 Standard 18F-FDG-PET/CT Imaging Protocol for Oncology

For oncology purposes, a standard 18F-FDG-PET/CT acquisition protocol consists of three steps: (1) patient preparation and positioning, (2) the transmission scan, and (3) the emission scan. After patient preparation and positioning, a localisation scan (Fig. 1.11) is done. This localisation scan, referred to as either a topogram or scout scan, is acquired with the x-ray tube/detector assembly locked at a given position, usually frontal, and the patient pallet moving continuously into the gantry. The topogram is used to define the axial examination range of the combined study. Thus, the axial extent of the complementary CT and PET acquisition are matched to ensure fully quantitative attenuation and scatter correction of the emission data, and to avoid any over- or underscanning of the patient in case of limited or extensive disease, respectively. Next, the patient is moved to the start position of the CT scan, which typically is acquired in spiral mode. Contrary to standard PET protocols, contamination of the transmission data from the injected emission activity is virtually nonexistent due to the larger source strength of the x-ray source [7]. Thus, post-injection CT transmission becomes standard in PET/CT. Following the completion of the CT scan, the patient is shifted to the FOV of the PET, towards the rear of the combined gantry, where emission scanning is performed in the caudocranial direction, starting at the pelvis region to limit artefacts from the tracer metabolite excretion into the urinary system. Emission data can be acquired in 2D or 3D, depending on the PET system configuration. Depending on the axial co-scan range and the PET acquisition time for an individual bed position, the combined scanning can be completed in 30 min or less. Based on the standard acquisition scheme that involves a transmission and an emission scan, all PET images are reconstructed after (CT-based) attenuation correction. The reconstruction method of choice is based on iterative reconstruction techniques that involve an attenuation-weighted ordered subset approach or a RAMLA approach.

1.4.3.2 CT-Based Attenuation Correction

The transformation of the CT transmission information to attenuation coefficients and, subsequently, to attenuation maps is based on work by LaCroix et al. [36]. First the CT images are transformed into attenuation images at some estimated effective CT energy. Then the attenuation image at the relevant emission energy is multiplied by the ratio of attenuation coefficients of water at that effective CT energy (40–70 keV) and the emission energy, respectively. While this simple scaling approach works well for soft tissues, serious overestimation of the attenuation coefficients of cortical bone is observed [36]. To account for the larger energy difference between CT and PET, the original scaling approach was modified [34]. Instead of a linear scaling with a single scale factor, a bi-linear scaling was developed [34, 25] to account for the nonlinear energy dependencies of the photoelectric and Compton effect, which dominate at lower (i.e. CT) and higher (i.e. PET) energies, respectively (Fig. 1.12). Today all CT-based attenuation correction algorithms in commercial PET/CT systems are based exclusively on bi-linear scaling methods [13, 34].

1.4.4 PET/CT Image Artefacts: Origins, Appearance and Corrections

In general, artefacts may arise from technical or methodological pitfalls and affect the accuracy of diagnostic imaging. These artefacts can be interpreted as structures in the images

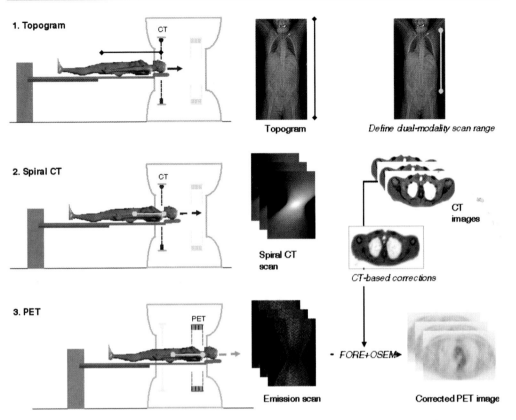

Fig. 1.11. A typical PET/CT examination protocol. Following the administration of the PET radiopharmaceutical and uptake, the patient is positioned on the scanner bed, and a topogram scan (overview) is acquired to determine the range of the PET/CT examination as indicated in *yellow*. Subsequently, a CT scan is acquired in spiral mode. Note that IV and/or oral CT contrast agents can be administered, when indicated, prior to the spiral CT scan. After the completion of the CT exam, the patient is moved to the PET field of view, and the emission scanning commences. CT images can be used for CT-based quantitative corrections of the PET emission data. At the end of the exam, co-registered PET and CT images are available to the user and can be viewed in fused mode or separately

Fig. 1.12. Plot of a typical bi-linear algorithm used for the computation of PET attenuation correction factors (ACFs) from CT images. PET ACFs (y-axis) are calculated from x-ray linear attenuation factors in HU (x-axis). The linear trends correspond to a mixture of air and water (soft tissue) and of water and bone (bone tissue)

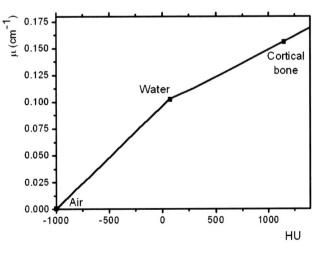

that are not typically present but that are produced by an external agent or action. Artefacts from CT may propagate into the PET images whenever the CT is used for attenuation of the PET data. Though these artefacts can generally be recognised on the CT and therefore on the fused PET/CT images, they are harder to detect on the attenuation-corrected PET alone. Such artefacts can arise directly or be complementary to other effects, leading to a wide range of possible artefacts on the CT images and on the corresponding attenuation-corrected PET images. It is, therefore, highly recommended to review not only the corrected PET and fused PET/CT images, but also the uncorrected PET images to identify any methodology-based image distortions.

Metal implants or other high-density materials such as ceramic fillings, a pacemaker, or chemotherapy infusion have been shown to yield artefacts on the CT images [24, 21], which may translate into artefacts in the corresponding corrected emission data [12, 32]. In the presence of higher-density implants, the bi-linear algorithm will overestimate the attenuation of the implants and thus lead to an overestimated tracer concentration in the vicinity of these implants (Fig. 1.13). Intravenous (IV) contrast and/or oral contrast, on the other hand, use substances with high atomic numbers such as iodine to increase the attenuation of the vessels, or the bowel, and intestines and are administered to the patient to enhance the visualisation of structures such as the vas-

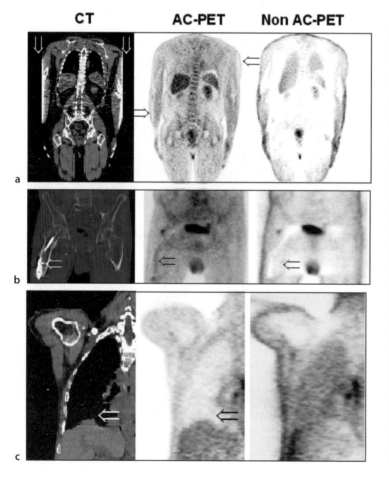

CT   AC-PET   Non AC-PET

Fig. 1.13a-c. Whole-body FDG-PET/CT studies in which CT artefacts propagate into PET imaging when using CT-based attenuation correction. **a** Artefacts in arm regions in CT images (*left*) due to the truncation of the CT field of view lead to falsely reduced activities at the periphery of the patient. No abnormal tracer distribution appears in the uncorrected image (*right*). **b** Artefacts on CT images (*left*) due to metal implants lead to an artefactual increase in the corrected activity in close vicinity of the teeth, as visible in the attenuation corrected image (*centre*). However, no abnormal tracer distribution appears in the uncorrected image (*right*). **c** The presence of high-density CT contrast media in a given organ leads to increased activities in the corresponding organ (*centre*) while no abnormal tracer distribution appears in the uncorrected image (*right*)

cular system or the digestive tract in clinical CT and PET/CT scans. In the presence of CT contrast agents, the routine CT-based attenuation correction algorithm will incorrectly segment and scale the enhanced structures above the threshold of soft tissue and bone resulting in a bias in the attenuation factors (Fig. 1.14a) that could potentially generate artefacts in the corrected PET images when the contrast-enhanced CT scan is used to generate the attenuation coefficients [3, 23] (Fig. 1.14b, c). Contrast administration and acquisition protocol parameters of PET/CT exams may, however, be modified so as to provide useful diagnostic information at no cost of image artefacts [4, 9].

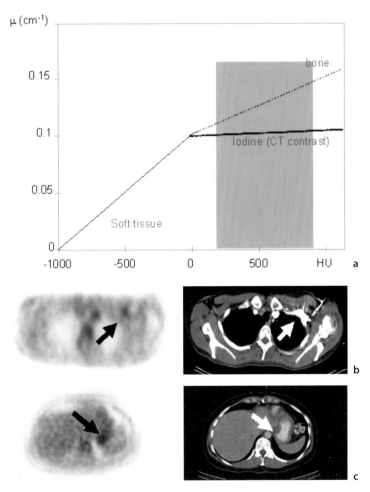

Fig. 1.14a–c. Example of a table to translate CT attenuation values (HU) into attenuation values at 511 keV (**a**). The bi-linear approach accounts for soft tissues and bone. The theoretical transformation for iodinated contrast agents is also shown. The range of CT attenuation values for IV contrast (*light blue*) and positive oral contrast (*blue*) is also indicated. It is clear from this table that contrast-enhanced pixel values are overestimated from the bi-linear scaling approach. In practice, this may lead to a artificially increased uptake patterns on attenuation-corrected PET when the contrast-enhanced CT scan is used. **b** Mono-phase IV contrast (300 mg/ml iodine), **c** positive oral contrast

Mismatch artefacts may arise from the discrepancy of the respiration protocols during standard CT and PET examinations when CT is used for PET attenuation correction [6, 26, 43]. For optimum CT image quality, patients are required to hold their breath during a clinical CT, while patients breathe quietly during a PET scan. List mode or PET gated studies [40] have proven to reduce respiration-induced smearing effects of structures or lesions affected by the respiration movement and therefore to provide a more accurate value of activity uptake (Fig. 1.13). However, in the absence of widely available respiratory gating mechanisms for PET, alternatives have to be found to match the morphology of the patient, as captured by CT, with the PET tracer distribution that is imaged over several breathing cycles. Limited breath-hold protocols are feasible routinely and have been shown to reduce respiration-induced artefacts in single- or dual-row PET/CT systems [8]. Muscle relaxation may lead as well to spatial misalignment of the CT and PET images. When a typical whole-body PET/CT exam (Fig. 1.10) is performed, head and neck regions have the largest time difference between PET and CT scans and the likelihood of muscle relaxation is within that time is rather high. Furthermore, inadequate patient physical restraints may lead to particularly large misalignment effects and can invalidate the fusion of the resulting PET/CT images. Despite careful patient instruction and preparation prior to the PET/CT exam, more serious motion artefacts may, nevertheless, occur. Patients may attempt to shift their body into a different position during the PET/CT exam if they feel discomfort or if the scan procedure is too lengthy. This motion is in addition to any motion from muscle relaxation, and sometimes may cause extensive, rather than local, mis-registration of functional and anatomical information.

Whenever whole-body PET/CT imaging protocols are based on standard PET-only imaging protocols, patients are positioned with their arms alongside the body. If the CT is acquired with the arms down, beam hardening and scatter effects are more pronounced and cause well-known streak artefacts that de-grade the CT image quality, making the identification and localisation of smaller lesions a challenge. Additionally, in almost all available PET/CT systems today the measured transverse FOV of the CT is 50 cm, whereas that of the PET is approximately 60 cm. This difference in the FOV values between CT and PET may lead to truncation artefacts when large patients are imaged or when they are being positioned away from the in-plane centre of the PET/CT gantry. The use of CT truncated images for attenuation correction of PET images may lead to an incorrect radiotracer distribution [10], as shown in Figure 1.13. Detruncation algorithms that recover truncated projections can be implemented on commercially available CT systems [41].

1.5   Future Trends

1.5.1   Future Trends in PET Instrumentation

PET detectors and instrumentation have developed into sophisticated clinical tools, but work is underway to develop higher-sensitivity, higher-resolution tomographs. Continuous research and development in the area of new scintillation materials has given way to other promising alternatives such as lutetium aluminium perovskite (LuAP) and lutetium pyrosilicate (LPS). Both potential candidates present characteristics that allow an improved system time resolution and therefore potential improvement of scanner performance. Another promising material for 3D acquisition is lanthanum bromide doped with cerium (LaBr (Ce)), which, since its melting point is similar to NaI(Tl) (800–900°C), would be produced more cost effectively than LSO or GSO. Additionally, with these scintillators time-of-flight scanners – which use the time difference between the two coincidence photons to better locate the annihilation position of the emitted positron – become feasible.

In addition, new detector designs, which have already been employed in small animal PET tomographs, may find their way to clinical systems. One example is the phoswich detector which uses two layers of different scintillator materials, typically LSO and GSO, which have different decay times. By monitoring the decay time of the signal pulse, the event can be located. The advantage of this design is that the depth at which the interaction of the annihilation photon occurs within the scintillator crystal, which is unknown, is defined better since each individual crystal layer has half the depth of that in the standard block. However, this results in an increased cost from the coupled scintillator crystals manufacture.

1.5.2 Future Trends in PET/CT

State-of-the-art PET/CT tomographs combine the latest imaging technologies in spiral, multi-slice CT and 3D PET employing novel scintillator materials.

With the new PET scanners and its improved spatial resolution, sensitivity and scanner performance, and the introduction of 64-slice CT machines, the PET/CT field of application, currently focused on diagnosis, staging of malignancy and the monitoring of therapy response in oncology, will expand to cardiology. It will also increase scanner speed and therefore patient throughput. If PET and CT gating acquisition protocols are finally implemented, the use of PET/CT for radiotherapy planning will improve. Since both scanners in PET/CT devices are fully 3D volume imaging scanners, advances in both cone-beam reconstruction algorithms for CT imaging and 3D iterative algorithms for PET, as well as superior scatter correction methods will greatly improve image quality. Additionally, new imaging protocols that help to minimise the presence of artefacts in CT images still need to be developed. New detruncation algorithms with enhanced CT image recovery which are currently under development [49] will contribute to this.

Ongoing research is aimed at closely integrating the hardware components of combined PET/CT systems and providing novel acquisition and image review tools for new diagnostic

and therapeutic medical applications in oncology and beyond.

1.5.3 Implication for Clinical Applications

Combined PET/CT is a noninvasive imaging modality for acquiring and reviewing both the anatomy and the molecular pathways of a patient within a single examination. PET/CT outperforms PET in clinical diagnosis and therapy monitoring, and therefore acts as a catalyst to state-of-the-art nuclear medicine imaging.

Since PET/CT tomographs represent hardware combinations of existing PET and CT technology, all instrumentation aspects of combined PET/CT imaging are understood and can be addressed with respect to specific imaging situations. This includes an understanding of the PET scanner performance in the presence of increased randoms rates from the enlarged gantry opening as well as the pitfalls in CT-based attenuation correction. By drawing from the experiences in stand-alone PET and CT imaging, which have been in coexistence and in steady support of physicists and mathematicians, PET/CT can be made the standard in diagnostic oncology imaging and lead the way to assessing the clinical efficacy of multi-modality imaging, including PET/MR. Nevertheless, the greatest challenge arises from local, institutional issues that have prevented health authorities outside the US from accepting PET/CT (or PET) as a valuable, cost-effective imaging modality.

Obviously, the clinical adoption and integration of new imaging technologies such as PET/CT is more efficient if imaging experts, namely nuclear medicine physicians and radiologists, cooperate during the preparation, installation and operational phase of the combined system. Most importantly, aside from how the PET/CT is being operated and used, the ultimate objective should be to provide the patient with the best diagnosis possible and to ensure that the results of the combined examination, whenever indicated, are being utilised to provide the best knowledge possible for therapy planning and follow-up.

References

1. Adam LE, Zaers J, Ostertag H, Trojan H, Bellemann ME, Brix G (1997) Performance evaluation of the whole-body PET scanner ECAT EXACT HR+ following the IEC standard. IEEE Trans Nucl Sci 44:1171–2179
2. Anger HO (1958) Scintillation camera. Rev Sci Instr 29:21–23
3. Antoch G, Freudenberg LS, Egelhof T, Stattaus J, Jentzen W, Debatin JF, Bockisch A (2002) Focal tracer uptake: a potential artifact in contrast-enhanced dual-modality PET/CT scans. J Nucl Med 43:1331–1342
4. Antoch G, Jentzen W, Freudenberg LS, Stattaus J, Mueller SP, Debatin JF, Bockisch A (2003) Effect of oral contrast agents on computed tomography-based positron emission tomography attenuation correction in dual-modality positron emission tomography/computed tomography imaging. Invest Radiol 38:781–789
5. Bailey DL, Meikle SR (1994) A convolution-subtraction scatter correction method for 3D PET. Phys Med Biol 39:411–424
6. Beyer T, Townsend DW, Brun T, Kinahan PE, Charron M, Roddy R, Jerin J, Young J, Byars L, Nutt R (2000a) A combined PET/CT scanner for clinical oncology. J Nucl Med 41:1361–1379
7. Beyer T, Townsend DW, Nutt R, Charron M, Kinahan PE, Meltzer C (2000b) Combined PET/CT imaging using a single, dual-modality tomograph: a promising approach to clinical oncology of the future. In: Wieler H, Coleman R (eds) PET in clinical oncology. Steinkopff Verlag, Darmstadt, pp 101–223
8. Beyer T, Antoch G, Blodgett T, Freudenberg LF, Akhurst T, Mueller S (2003) Dual-modality PET/CT imaging: the effect of respiratory motion on combined image quality in clinical oncology. Eur J Nucl Med Mol Imaging 30:581–596
9. Beyer T, Antoch G, Bockisch A, Stattaus J (2005) Optimized intravenous contrast administration for diagnostic whole-body 18F-FDG PET/CT. J Nucl Med 46:421–435
10. Beyer T, Bockisch A, Kuhl H, Martinez MJ (2006) Whole-Body 18F-FDG PET/CT in the presence of truncation artifacts. J Nucl Med 47:91–99
11. Browne J, de Pierro AB (1996) A row-action alternative to the EM algorithm for maximizing likelihood in emission tomography. IEEE Trans Med Imag, 15:681–699
12. Bujenovic S, Mannting F, Chakrabarti R, Ladnier D (2003) Artifactual 2-deoxy-2-[(18)F]fluoro-D-glucose localization surrounding metallic objects in a PET/CT scanner using CT-based attenuation correction. Mol Imaging Biol 5:21–22
13. Burger C, Goerres G, Schoenes S, Buck A, Lonn AH, Von Schulthess GK (2002) PET attenuation coefficients from CT images: experimental evaluation of the transformation of CT into PET 511-keV attenuation coefficients. Eur J Nucl Med Mol Imaging 29:921–927
14. Carson RE, Daube-Witherspoon ME, Green MV (1988) A method for postinjection PET transmission measurements with a rotating source. J Nucl Med 29:1551–1567
15. Casey ME, Nutt R (1986) Multicrystal two dimensional BGO detector system for positron emission tomography. IEEE Trans Nucl Sci 33:461–463
16. Cherry SR, Dahlbom M, Hoffman EJ (1992) High sensitivity, total body PET scanning using 3D data acquisition and reconstruction. IEEE Trans Nucl Sci 39:1081–1092
17. Cho ZH, Farukhi MR (1977) Bismuth germanate as a potential scintillation detector in positron cameras. Nucl Med 18:841–844
18. Comtat C, Kinahan PE, Fessler JA, Beyer T, Townsend DW, Defrise M, Michel C (2002) Clinically feasible reconstruction of 3D whole-body PET/CT data using blurred anatomical labels. Phys Med Biol 47:1–20
19. Cooke BE, Evans AC, Fanthome EO, Alarie Ras AM (1984) Performance figure and images from the Therascan 3128 positron emission tomograph. IEEE Trans Nucl Sci 31:641–644
20. Daube-Witherspoon ME, Karp JS, Casey ME, DiFilippo FP, Hines H, Muehllehner G, Simcic V, Stearns CW, Adam LE, Kohlmyer S, Sossi V (2002) PET performance measurements using the NEMA NU 1 2001 standard. J Nucl Med 43:1391–1409
21. De Man B, Nuyts J, Dupont P, Marchal G, Suetens P (1999) Metal streak artifacts in X-ray computed tomography: a simulation study. IEEE Trans Nucl Sci 46:691–696
22. Defrise M, Kinahan PE, Townsend DW, Michel C, Sibomana M, Newport DF (1997) Exact and approximate rebinning algorithms for 3-D PET data. IEEE Trans Med Imaging 16:141–158
23. Dizendorf E, Hany TF, Buck A, von Schulthess GK, Burger C (2003) Cause and magnitude of the error induced by oral CT contrast agent in CT-based attenuation correction of PET emission studies. J Nucl Med 44:731–738
24. Duerinckx AJ, Macovski A (1978) Polychromatic streak artifacts in computed tomography images. Comput Assist Tomogr 2:481–487
25. Fleming JS (1989) A technique for using CT images in attenuation correction and quantification in SPECT. Nucl Med Commun 10:81–87
26. Goerres GW, Kamel E, Heidelberg TN, Schwitter MR, Burger C, von Schulthess GK (2002) PET-CT image co-registration in the thorax: influence of respiration. Eur J Nucl Med Mol Imaging 29:351–360
27. Hasegawa BH, Lang, TH, Brown EL et al (1993) Object specific attenuation correction of SPECT with correlated dual-energy x-ray CT. IEEE Trans Nucl Sci 40:1241–1252
28. Herman GT (1980) Image reconstruction from projections: the fundamental of. computerized tomography. Academic Press, New York
29. Hoffman EJ, Guerrero TM, Germano G, Digby WM, Dahlbom M (1989) PET system calibrations and

corrections for quantitative and spatially accurate images. Nucl Sci IEEE Trans 36:1101–1112

30. Hudson HM, Larkin RS (1994) Accelerated image reconstruction using ordered subsets of projection data. IEEE Trans Med Imaging 13:601–609

31. Kalender WA, Vock P, Polacin A, Soucek M (1990) Spiral-CT: a new technique for volumetric scans. I. Basic principles and methodology. Rontgenpraxis 43:321–330

32. Kamel EM, Burger C, Buck A, von Schulthess GK, Goerres GW (2003) Impact of metallic dental implants on CT-based attenuation correction in a combined PET/CT scanner. Eur Radiol 13:721–728

33. Karp JS, Muehllehner G, Mankoff DA, Ordonez CE, Ollinger JM, Daube-Witherspoon ME, Haigh AT, Beerbohm DJ (1990) Continuous-slice PENN-PET: a positron tomograph with volume imaging capability. J Nucl Med 31:611–627

34. Kinahan PE, Townsend DW, Beyer T, Sashin D (1998) Attenuation correction for a combined 3D PET/CT scanner. Med Phys 25:2041–2053

35. Kluetz PG, Meltzer CC, Villemagne VL, Kinahan PE, Chander S, Martinelli MA, Townsend DW (2000) Combined PET/CT imaging in oncology. impact on patient management. Clin Positron Imaging 3:221–230

36. LaCroix KJ, Tsui BMW, Hasegawa BH, Brown JK (1994) Investigation of the use of x-ray CT images for attenuation compensation in SPECT. IEEE Trans Nucl Sci 41:2791–2799

37. Leschka S, Alkhadhi H, Plass A, Desbiolles L, Grunenfelder J, Marincek B, Wildermuth S (2005) Accuracy of MSCT coronary angiography with 64-slice technology: first experience. Eur Heart J 26:1481–1487

38. Melcher CL, Schweitzer JS (1992) Cerium-doped lutetium oxyorthosilicate: a fast, efficient new scintillator. IEEE Trans Nucl Sci 39:501–505

39. Nehmeh SA, Erdi YE, Ling CC, Rosenzweig KE, Schoder H, Larson SM, Macapinlac HA, Squire OD, Humm JL (2002) Effect of respiratory gating on quantifying PET images of lung cancer. J Nucl Med 43:871–881

40. Nehmeh SA, Erdi YE, Rosenzweig KE, Schoder H, Larson SM, Squire OD, Humm JL (2003) Reduction of respiratory motion artifacts in PET imaging of lung cancer by respiratory correlated dynamic PET: methodology and comparison with respiratory gated PET. J Nucl Med 44:1641–1648

41. Ohnesorge B, Flohr T, Schwarz K, Heiken JP, Bae KT (2000) Efficient correction for CT image artifacts caused by objects extending outside the scan field of view. Med Phys 27:31–36

42. Ollinger JM (1996) Model-based scatter correction for fully 3D PET. Phys Med Biol 41:151–176

43. Osman MM, Cohade C, Nakamoto Y, Wahl RL (2003) Respiratory motion artifacts on PET emission images obtained using CT attenuation correction on PET-CT. Eur J Nucl Med Mol Imaging 30:601–606

44. Phelps M, Hoffman E, Mullani N, Ter-Pogossian M (1975) Application of annihilation coincidence detection to transaxial reconstruction tomography. J Nucl Med 16:211–224

45. Puterbaugh KC, Breeding JE, Musrock MS, Seaver C, Casey ME, Young JW (2003) Performance comparison of a current LSO PET scanner versus the same scanner with upgraded electronics. IEEE Nucl Sci Symp 1931–1935.

46. Schulthess GKV (2000) Cost considerations regarding an integrated CT-PET system. Eur Radiol 10: S377–S380

47. Shao L, Freifelder R, Karp JS (1994) Triple energy window scatter correction technique in PET. IEEE Trans Med Imaging 13:641–648

48. Slomka PJ, Dey D, Przetak C, Aladl UE, Baum RP (2003) Automated 3-dimensional registration of stand-alone (18)F-FDG whole-body PET with CT. J Nucl Med 44:1151–1167

49. Sourbelle K, Kachelriess M, Kalender WA (2005) Reconstruction from truncated projections in CT using adaptive detruncation. Eur Radiol 15:1001–1014

50. Spinks TJ, Guzzardi R, Bellina CR (1988) Performance characteristics of a whole-body positron tomograph. J Nucl Med 29:1831–1841

51. Surti S, Karp JS, Freifelder R, Liu F (2000) Optimizing the performance of a PET detector using discrete GSO crystals on a continuous lightguide. IEEE Trans Nucl Sci 47:1031–1036

52. Takagi K, Fukazawa T (1983) Cerium-activated Gd[sub 2]SiO[sub 5] single crystal scintillator. Appl Phys Lett 42:41–45

53. Townsend DW, Beyer T (2002) A combined PET/CT scanner: the path to true image fusion. Br J Radiol 75:S21–S20

54. Wahl RL, Quint LE, Cieslak RD, Aisen AM, Koeppe RA, Meyer CR (1993) "Anatometabolic" tumor imaging: fusion of FDG PET with CT or MRI to localize foci of increased activity. J Nucl Med 34:1191–1197

55. Watson CC (2000) New, faster, image-based scatter correction for 3D PET. IEEE Trans Nucl Sci 47:1581–1594

56. Xu M, Cutler PD, Luk WK (1996) Adaptive, segmented attenuation correction for whole-body PET imaging. IEEE Trans Nucl Sci 43:331–336

2 Radiopharmacy

R. Michael

Recent Results in Cancer Research, Vol. 170
© Springer-Verlag Berlin Heidelberg 2008

The field of radiochemistry/radiopharmacy deals with the production, testing and application of radioactive drugs. Radiopharmacy has been gaining increasing significance with the further development of PET technology and advances in nuclear medicine and radiation oncology therapy. The recent development of PET scan technology, particularly in combination with computed tomography (PET/CT), has largely established the use of PET as a diagnostic method in oncology. This development increasingly demands the synthesis of radiopharmaceuticals as a further basis for the development of the PET method.

According to the definition given by the German Drug Law (AMG), radiopharmaceuticals are diagnostically or therapeutically applied drugs that consist of or contain radioactive substances (Table 2.1). In the simplest case, unbound radionuclides are used as drugs, e.g., $[^{18}F]$fluoride. The radioactive nuclides are usually bound to organic molecules with pharmacokinetics enabling a high uptake in the target organ. Radioactive nuclides are selected according to their physical properties. Nuclides with suitable physical data for external radiation measurement are used in diagnostics (gamma or positron radiation), while beta emitters with a low range and high efficiency are applied for therapy.

Conventional nuclear medical diagnostics are performed with iodine isotopes or otherwise largely with metals such as technetium or indium, which can only bind to organic molecules by complex bonds. Impairment of the biological properties can hardly be avoided in this connection. The radionuclides used in PET differ not only in their basically distinct physical properties such as radioactive decay and half-life (Table 2.2), but also in their more extensive synthesis potentialities. In contrast to the usual analog labeling of radioactive compounds in SPECT, the radionuclides F-18 and C-11 mainly used in oncological PET diagnostics can label endogenous compounds or drugs without substantially changing their structure or pharmacological properties. Particularly C-11 enables authentic labeling of endogenous substances.

Table 2.1. Definition of radiopharmaceuticals used for diagnosis and therapy according to the German Drug Law (AMG)

§ 2 AMG (German Drug Law)

Pharmaceuticals are substances intended to reveal or influence the texture, condition, or function of the body or of an emotional state.

§ 4 AMG (German Drug Law)

Radiopharmaceuticals are drugs that consist of or contain radioactive substances and spontaneously emit ionising radiation and are intended to be used based on those characteristics.

Table 2.2. Physical properties of the most important radionuclides in nuclear medical diagnostics

Nuclide	Decay mode	γ-Energy	Half-life	Application
Tc-99m	γ	140	6 h	SPECT
In-111	γ	250	72 h	
I-123	γ	160	13 h	
F-18	β⁺	511	110 min	PET
C-11	β⁺	511	20 min	
N-13	β⁺	511	10 min	
O-15	β⁺	511	2 min	

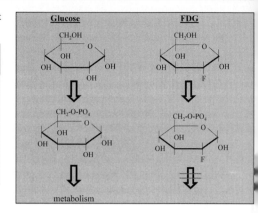

Fig. 2.1. F-18-FDG as an example of blocked metabolism

An extremely small amount of substance in the subphysiological range is characteristic for the PET radiopharmaceuticals used only for diagnostic purposes and also designated as PET tracers. Since the injected substance amounts range from nanomoles to picomoles, physiological concentrations are not impaired or influenced. Pharmacological impairments or side effects are not to be expected with the low substance amounts.

In vivo tracer distribution can be monitored by external radioactivity measurement. The diagnostic applicability of a radionuclide is dependent not only on its physical properties but also on its biochemical tracer properties. A high selective tracer uptake in target vs adjacent tissue is required. Transport to the tumor tissue and trapping in the cells must relate to the physical half-life to achieve an adequately high radioactive signal. Another tracer prerequisite is sufficient retention time for detection in the cell. The metabolic behavior of the tracer is decisive here. The substance should pass through only one or a few defined metabolic steps in the target organ. Biologically effective substances will undergo multiple chemical changes to block their metabolism.

A typical example for this concept of blocked metabolism is F-18 FDG, a glucose molecule with an F-18 atom instead of a hydroxyl group at position 2. The substance is largely taken up by cells with increased glucose consumption and, like glucose, undergoes hexokinase-catalyzed phosphorylation. Further metabolism is blocked, however, and the substance remains in the cells for an adequately long period of time (Fig. 2.1).

Besides meeting biochemical demands, a PET pharmaceutical must also fulfill special radiochemical requirements. Since PET nuclides are characterized by a short physical half-life, they must be produced at the place where they are used. A complete PET center consists of a cyclotron, radiochemical and radiopharmaceutical laboratories, and a PET scanner (Fig. 2.2). This combination requires particularly intensive cooperation between physicians and scientists. F-18 compounds are a certain exception, since they can be readily transported into the close proximity of the cyclotron. However, transport over a distance of 200 km is economically questionable and hardly justifiable for radiation protection reasons.

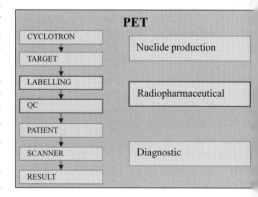

Fig. 2.2. Complete PET center: flow chart

The short half-life of the PET nuclides necessitates fast synthesis methods. Equilibrium reactions common in organic chemistry cannot be performed because the nuclide would largely decay in the time required (Fig. 2.3). Multistep synthesis or intermediate purification is problematic for the same reason.

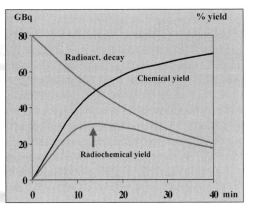

Fig. 2.3. Interaction between radioactive decay and duration of synthesis using C-11 synthesis as an example

Another problem is the low concentration of nuclides produced in the cyclotron in nca (no-carrier-added) form. For example, 3.7 GBq C-11 has a mass of 10^{-10} g. Known organic synthesis pathways often cannot be successfully used in this concentration range, and completely new synthesis pathways must be developed.

Because of the high initial activity (more than 100 GBq F-18), high radiation energy and requisite speed, it is virtually impossible to perform manual synthesis. In recent years, a number of companies have developed computer-guided synthesis modules for PET tracer production that enable fully automatic performance of all synthesis steps (Fig. 2.4). The modules are usually placed in airtight "hot cells" shielded with 75 mm of lead.

Apart from complying with radiation protection standards, it is necessary to meet the GMP (good manufacturing practice) criteria for drug production must be met, particularly those expressed in the guidelines for manufacturing sterile pharmaceutical products. It is

only possible to fulfill both these requirements with technologically complex facilities and an adequate number of well-qualified employees.

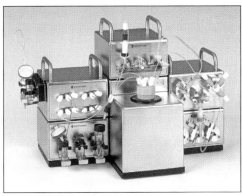

Fig. 2.4. Synthesis modules for PET tracer production. Source: Eckert & Ziegler AG Berlin

The substance most commonly used worldwide in oncological PET diagnostics is 2-[^{18}F]fluoro-2-desoxy-D-glucose (FDG). FDG is the only PET radiopharmaceutical that is an approved drug and can thus be readily used for diagnostic purposes. Because of its great importance, FDG will be briefly described in terms of its manufacture and quality control as a representative example of PET radiopharmaceuticals in general.

The first radiochemical FDG synthesis was published in 1978 [12], an electrophilic synthesis with the initial reactant [^{18}F]F$_2$. The now internationally prevailing nucleophilic FDG synthesis was developed in 1986 [8].

The passage from F-18 production in the cyclotron to FDG injection involves multiple steps (Fig. 2.5). The target material for producing F-18 in the cyclotron is water enriched to more than 97% with the stable oxygen atom O-18. The no-carrier-added F-18 fluoride generated by proton irradiation is transported to the synthesis module by a thin plastic tube. Using an ion exchanger, the F-18 fluoride is separated from the target water and purified. When placed in absolutely water-free acetonitrile in the presence of a phase-transfer

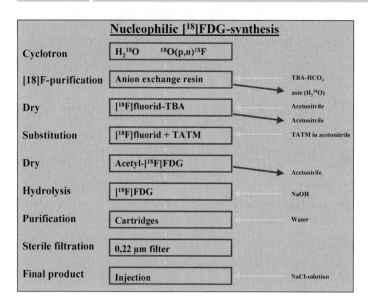

Fig. 2.5. F-18-FDG synthesis

catalysator, the F-18 fluoride reacts with the mannose triflate precursor (TATM) protected with acetyl groups. After nucleophilic substitution at 90°C, the solvent is evaporated. The protecting groups are split from the intermediate tetra-acetyl FDG by hydrolysis with NaOH [6]. Purification is achieved by passing the reaction product through a combination of cartridges. A physiological injection solution is produced by sterile filtration after adding a defined amount of NaCl solution (Fig. 2.6).

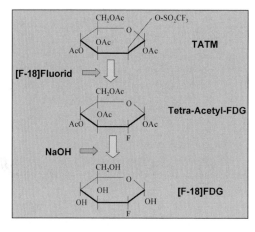

Fig. 2.6 Nucleophilic F-18-FDG synthesis

Before being administered to patients, each production batch must be submitted to an identity check and a contamination check. Procedures and threshold values for possible contaminations are stipulated in the European Pharmacopoiea monographs Fludeoxyglucosi (^{18}F) Solutio Iniectabilis and Radioactive Drugs.

The first step of quality control takes place directly after synthesis while the FDG is being transported to the PET scanner. Fast analytic methods are used to check the identity of the substance and determine several essential quality parameters: radiochemical purity, solvent residues, and pH. The substance is released after these tests. Its application as an injection solution is only justified after its written release.

Checking further quality characteristics (Table 2.3) – particularly radionuclide purity, chemical purity, sterility, and freedom from pyrogens – takes longer than the decay time of F-18 permits and can thus only be done after the drug has been administered. This procedure of parametric release requires precise validation of the production process and continuous in-process control.

With this procedure, about 60 GBq of F-18 FDG can be produced, regardless of the cyclo-

Table 2.3. F-18-FDG quality characteristics

Quality criteria	Method	Limit	Quality criteria	Method	Limit
Solution	Visually	Clear	Color	Visually	Colorless or slightly yellow
pH	Potentiometer	4.5–7.0	Isotonicity	Osmometer	270–330 mosm/kg
Identification					
FDG	HPLC	RT = RT$_{Ref.}$	F-18	Spectroscopy	511 keV
Purity					
Radionuclidic purity	Spectroscopy	> 99%	Radionuclidic purity	Half-life	105–115 min
Organic solvents	GC	Acetonitrile <0.38 mg/ml	Chemical purity	HPLC	Impurity < 0.4 mg/ml
Radiochemical purity	TLC	FDG > 97%	Radiochemical purity	HPLC	FDG > 97%
Apyrogenicity	Limulus test	< 17.5 IU/ml	Sterility	Direct membrane method	Sterile

tron type, synthesis module, or exposure time. It must be taken into account, however, that more than half the radioactivity decays through transport and waiting times. With an average distance between the cyclotron and PET scanner, FDG synthesis requires about 5 h from the start of irradiation to the application of the injection solution (Fig. 2.7). This also means that FDG production often involves night work.

Given the many technologically complicated processes, occasional defective syntheses cannot be completely excluded, especially since manual intervention during the process is virtually impossible for radiation protection reasons. Synthesis can only be repeated after decay and purification of the synthesis module, which is very time-consuming because of the length of exposure required. Resultant stress for examiners and patients is unfortunately unavoidable.

FDG-PET does have several important limitations and not all oncological questions can be answered with FDG [18]. Thus there is still an ongoing search for new tracers that are specific for certain tumor types. Moreover, old developments have been revitalized by new technologies combining PET and CT (PET/CT). Several

tracers that may become important in the future will be specified here. It must be stressed that, despite promising approaches, there are no completed studies that would enable drug approval for any tracer other than FDG.

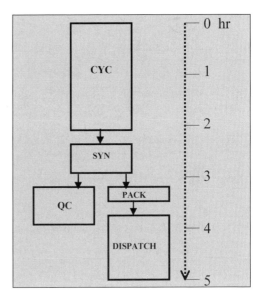

Fig. 2.7. FDG synthesis: time from start of irradiation to shipping

A large number of radioactive drugs have been described for application in PET diagnostics, but most of them have not achieved clinical significance. One of the oldest PET tracers is F-18 fluoride for scintigraphy of skeletal metastases [4]. However, it was diagnostically used in only a few centers. With the development of PET/CT, F-18 fluoride has gained considerable importance in the diagnostics of bone metastases [5]. Particularly in the lower extremities, F-18 fluoride is markedly superior to the Tc-99m compounds commonly used for nuclear medical diagnostics in the skeletal system [2].

Choline is a building block of membrane lipid synthesis; the molecule has known selectivity in the metabolism of prostate cancer. Prostate cancer cells have a very fast metabolism. C-11 choline, which was first synthesized by Hara et al. [9], already accumulates in prostate cancer after 5 min. F-18-labeled choline derivatives were soon developed because of their longer half-life. Imaging is now most commonly done with F-18 fluoroethylcholine [10], which is similar to C-11 choline in its cellular uptake and phosphorylation.

An alternative for diagnosing prostate cancer is C-11 acetate [14, 23, 19] which was originally developed for myocardial diagnostics. Acetate largely enters lipid metabolism in tumor cells and accumulates in the cells like choline. In working with C-11 compounds, it must be considered, however, that the cyclotron and radiochemistry facility must be near the PET scanner and that only two patients can be examined with one production batch. A radiochemical production in a short synthesis time has recently been described [21].

Proliferation measurements have a high application potential in oncological PET diagnostics . Detection of DNA synthesis with thymidine enables a sensitive follow-up. However, the fact that thymidine is metabolized very rapidly renders it unsuitable for imaging. The breakdown is blocked by substitution with fluorine. The development of F-18 FLT (3'-deoxy-3' [F-18] fluorothymidine) [15] has provided a substance that could play an important role in tumor treatment follow-up [20].

The use of radiolabeled amino acids has long been discussed, particularly for brain tumor diagnostics [13]. Apart from C-11 methionine, particularly F-18 FET ([18F]fluoroethyl tyrosine) has gained wide acceptance as a diagnostic agent [22, 1]. FET PET is useful particularly in planning therapy in glioblastoma is [17]. A practicable automated synthesis method has only recently been developed [7].

Hypoxic tumor components are associated with an impaired oxygen supply. They are considerably more therapy-resistant than other tissues. F-18 FMISO (fluoromisonidazole) can serve as an example of a marker for hypoxic tumor tissue. The accumulation of FMISO probably correlates with a reduced oxygen concentration in tumor tissue. The demonstration of hypoxic tissue enables more specific therapy. However, hypoxia markers are still in the initial stage of clinical testing. An automated synthesis has been described [16].

A nuclide untypical for PET examinations is the positron emitter Ga-67 with a half-life of 2.8 days. Ga-67 is not produced in the cyclotron but in a Ge68/Ga-68 generator and is therefore also available for PET scanners that are not situated near a cyclotron. Ga-68 is clinically used for labeling DOTA-conjugated peptides [11], which are specifically bound to receptors of neuroendocrine tumors. Ga-68-DOTA-conjugated peptides can be labeled in high yield [3]. Production at the PET scanner and not in a laboratory equipped for work with positron emitters requires special radiation protection measures and highly developed automation.

References

1. Been LB, Suurmeijer AJ, Cobben DC, Jager PL, Hoekstra HJ, Elsinga PH (2004) [18F]FLT-PET in oncology: current status and opportunities. Eur J Nucl Med Mol Imaging 31:1659–1672
2. Blake GM, Park-Hohlohan SJ, Fogelman I (2002) Quantitative studies of bone in postmenopausal woman using 18F-Fluoride and 99mTc-Methylene Diphosphonate. J Nucl Med 43:338–345
3. Breeman WA, de Jong M, de Blois E, Bernard BF, Konijnenberg M, Krenning EP (2005) Radiolabelling DOTA-peptide with 68Ga. Eur J Nucl Med 32:478–485
4. Charkes ND, Makler PT, Philips C (1978) Studies of skeletal tracer kinetics. I. Digital-computer solution

of a five compartment model of [18F]fluoride kinetics in humans. J Nucl Med 19:1301–1309

5. Evan-Sapir E, Metser U, Flusser G, Zuriel L, Kollender Y, Lerman H, Lievshitz G, Ron I, Mishani E (2004) Assessment of malignant skeletal disease: initial experience with 18F-fluoride PET/CT and comparison between 18F-fluoride PET and 18F-fluoride PET/CT. J Nucl Med 45:272–278

6. Füchtner F, Steinbach J, Mäding P, Johannsen B (1995) Basic hydrolysis of 2-[18F]Fluoro-1,3,4,6-tetra-O-acetyl-D-glucose in the preparation of 2-[18F]Fluoro-2-deoxy-D-glucose. Appl Radiat Isot 47:61–66

7. Hamacher K, Coenen HH (2002) Efficient routine production of the 18F-labelled amino acid O-(2[18Ffluoroethyl)-L-tyrosine. Appl Radiat Isot 57:853–856

8. Hamacher K, Coenen HH, Stöcklin G (1986) Efficient stereospecific synthesis of NCA 2[18F]fluoro-2-deoxy-D-glucose using aminopolyether supported nucleophilic substitution. J Nucl Med 27:235–238

9. Hara T, Kosake N, Kondo S, Kondo T (1998) PET imaging of prostata cancer using carbon-11-cholin. J Nucl Med 39:990–995

10. Hara T, Kosaka N, Kishi H (2002) Development of 18F-fluorethylcholinfor cancer imaging with PET: synthesis, biochemistry, and prostata cancer imaging. J Nucl Med 43:187–199

11. Hofmann M, Maecke H, Borner R, Weckesser E, Schoffski P, Oei L, Schumacher J, Henze M, Heppeler A, Meyer J, Knapp H (2001) Biokinetics and imaging with the somatostatin receptor PET radioligand (68Ga)-DOTA-TOC: preliminary data. Eur J Nucl Med 28:1751–1757

12. Ido T, Wan CN, Cassela V, Fowler JS, Wolf AP (1978) Labeled 2-deoxy-D-glucose analogs. 18F-labeled 2-deoxy-2-fluoro-D-glucose, 2-deoxy-2-fluoro-D-mannose and 14C-2-deoxy-2-fluoro-D-glucose. J Label Compds Radiopharm 14:175–183

13. Jager PL, Vaalburg W, Pruim J, de Vries EGE, Langen KJ, Piers DA (2001) Radiolabeled amino acids: basic aspects and clinical applications in oncology. J Nucl Med 42:432–445

14. Kotzerke J, Volkmer BG, Glatting G, van den Hoff J, Gschwend JE, Messer P, Reske SN, Neumaier B (2003) Intraindividual comparison of [11C]acetate and [11C]choline PET for detection of metastases of prostata cancer. Nuklearmedizin 42:25–30

15. Machulla HJ, Blocher A, Kuntzsch M, Piert M, Wei R, Grierson JR (2000) simplified labeling approach for synthesizing 3'-Deoxy-3'-[18F]fluorothymidine ([18F]FLT. J Radioanalyt Nucl Chem 243:843–846

16. Oh SJ, Chi DY, Mosdzianowski C, Kim JY, Gil HS, Kang SH, Ryu JS, Moon DH (2005) Fully automated synthesis of [18F]fluoromisonidazole using a conventional [18F]FDG module. Nucl Med Biol 32:899–905

17. Plotkin M, Gneveckow U, Meier-Hauff K, Amthauer H, Feussner A, Denecke T, Gutberlet M, Jordan A, Felix R, Wust P (2006) 18F-FET PET for planning of thermotherapy using magnetic nanoparticles in recurrent glioblastoma. Int J Hypertherm 22:319–325

18. Reske SN, Kotzerke L (2001) FDG-PET for clinical use. Eur J Nucl Med 28:1707–1723

19. Sandblom G, Sorensen J, Lundin N, Haggman M, Malmstrom PU (2006) Positron emission tomography with C11-acetate for tumor detection and localization in patients with prostata-specific antigen relapse after radical prostatectomy. Urology 67:996–1000

20. Shields AF, Grierson JR, Dohmen BM, Machulla HJ, Stayanoff JC, Lawhorn-Crews JM, Obradovich JE, Muzik O, Manger TJ (1998) Imaging proliferation in vivo with [F-18]FLT and positron emission tomography (PET). Nat Med 4:1334–1336

21. Soloviev D, Tamburella C (2006) Captive solvent [11C]acetate synthesis in GMP conditions. Appl Rad Isot 64:995–1000

22. Weber WA, Wester HJ, Groscu AL, Herz M, Dzewas B, Feldmann HJ, Molls M, Stöcklin G, Schwaiger M (2000) O-(2-[18F]Fluoroethyl)-L-tyrosine and L-[methyl-11C]methionine uptake in brain tumours: initial results of a comparative study. Eur J Nucl Med 27:542–549

23. Yoshimoto M, Waki A, Obata A, Furukawa T, Yonekura Y, Fujibayashi Y (2004) Radiolabeled cholin as a proliferation marker: comparison with radiolabeled acetate. Nucl Med Biol 31:859–865

3 Brain Tumors

G. Pöpperl, K. Tatsch, F.-W. Kreth, and J.-C. Tonn

Recent Results in Cancer Research, Vol. 170

Primary brain tumors may develop from different cell types including glial cells, neurons, neuroglial precursor cells, the meninges, cells of the hypophysis, or lymphocytes. The incidence of primary brain tumors varies between subtypes which are classified by the World Health Organization (WHO) based on their cellular origin, the clinical course and histological appearance of the neoplasms, immunophenotypic features, and the molecular/cytogenic profile. The most frequent and difficult to treat primary brain tumors are gliomas, which are divided into two main categories: astrocytic and oligodendroglial tumors. Glial tumors are graded pathologically on the basis of the most malignant area identified regarding the presence or absence of nuclear atypia, mitosis, microvascular proliferation, and necrosis. Accurate pathological grading is essential because it defines treatment and prognosis. The histological features of the tumor and the patient's age and performance status are major prognostic factors and have more influence than any specific therapy on patient's outcome [48, 3]. Malignant high-grade astrocytomas, anaplastic astrocytoma, and glioblastoma multiforme are the most common glial tumors, with an annual incidence of three to four per 100,000 population. At least 80% of malignant gliomas, especially in the elderly, are glioblastomas. Life expectancy of patients with high-grade gliomas is still highly unfavorable. Standard therapeutic regimens, which include surgery, radiation therapy, and systemic chemotherapy have resulted in median survival times only ranging from 1 year for glioblastoma to approximately 3 years for anaplastic astrocytoma [7, 12]. Over the past few decades, therefore, therapy for gliomas has become more aggressive with neurosurgeons, neuro-oncologists, and radio-oncologists struggling to achieve longer disease-free intervals and prolong survival. For this purpose various alternative treatments including high-dose radiation beam therapy, radiosurgery, radioactive seed implantation, and other locoregional approaches such as radioimmunotherapy, interstitial photodynamic laser thermotherapy, or convection enhanced delivery of chemotherapeutic drugs have become promising adjuncts. Multimodal treatment tailored to the specific patient's pathology becomes more and more clinical reality in many centers. However, it goes along with an increasing spectrum of therapy-induced, reactive changes, which challenge diagnostic methods.

Cranial computed tomography (CT) and magnetic resonance imaging (MRI) with and without contrast media are widely used for diagnosis of brain tumors. Besides information on the size and localization of the tumor, especially MRI provides information on infiltration of surrounding structures and can assess secondary phenomena such as mass effect, edema, and signs of increased intracranial pressure or hemorrhage. CT is used for detection of intratumoral calcifications, which may confirm the diagnosis of oligodendrogliomas. Although CT and MRI are without doubt unsurpassed diagnostic modalities for the detection of cerebral lesions, these methods also have limitations. For example, they may not clearly differentiate neoplastic from some benign diseases when establishing the primary diagnosis or in delineating tumor borders. Furthermore, especially the broad variety of treatment effects concurrent with space-occupying edema and contrast enhancement do not always allow to reliably separate tumor recurrence from therapy-induced changes.

Clinical use of positron emission tomography (PET), which provides biochemical and molecular information, is expanding and its value has been primarily investigated in patients with gliomas as the most frequent and difficult to treat primary brain tumors. In contrast to morphological imaging modalities, PET depicts the metabolic state of gliomas and may help to overcome the above-mentioned diagnostic limitations by adding functional information. Over the last two decades, an increasing number of strategies highlighting various metabolic pathways have been followed to evaluate PET imaging for primary diagnosis, classification, characterization, preoperative evaluation, and especially for posttherapeutic assessment of gliomas. The main functions studied so far are glucose metabolism using 2-[^{18}F]fluoro-2-deoxy-D-glucose (FDG) and amino acid transport and partly incorporation using amino acids such as [methyl-^{11}C]-l-methionine (MET) or O-(2-[^{18}F]fluoroethyl)-l-tyrosine (FET).

This chapter focuses predominantly on the use of these well-established tracers. It summarizes the data in the literature on the current understanding of these techniques and addresses their major applications. Finally, it also briefly touches other metabolic pathways such as proliferation, membrane or lipid biosynthesis, tumor hypoxia or angiogenesis.

3.1   Primary and Differential Diagnosis of Gliomas

In patients who become clinically suspicious of brain tumor, MRI and CT are the first-line imaging modalities for detecting even small lesions and usually establish the differential diagnosis between normal brain tissue and malignant or nonmalignant lesions. However, in some cases differential diagnosis between a malignant and benign origin may be difficult. In those cases PET can help to further characterize (not to detect!) the lesion.

Differential diagnoses of low-grade gliomas showing only little or no contrast enhancement on MRI mainly consist of gliosis, demyelinating lesions, vascular abnormalities such as cavernomas or venous angiomas, or posttraumatic scar. Since all of these tumoral and nontumoral lesions present with FDG uptake lower or close to that of normal white matter, FDG seems to be a less valuable tracer to differentiate them. Contrast-enhancing lesions with mass effect and perifocal edema may represent high-grade gliomas. The most important differential diagnoses are florid inflammatory lesions such as brain abscesses, ischemic or hemorrhagic infarcts, or other malignancies such as metastases or cerebral lymphomas. The main limitation of FDG is the high glucose consumption of normal grey matter. FDG uptake even in high-grade tumors, therefore, is often similar to that in normal grey matter and for that reason often indistinguishable from normal brain tissue or benign lesions. Detection of small lesions is especially problematic in this respect. Another drawback of FDG in the assessment of unclear brain lesions is its lack of specificity for malignancy. Elevated glucose metabolism may also be seen in florid inflammatory lesions, in recent ischemic infarcts, in some benign tumors (e.g., meningiomas, benign pituitary adenomas) or during epileptic seizures. The few studies that have addressed the ability of FDG-PET to differentiate between neoplastic and non-neoplastic lesions conclude that this tracer has drawbacks in the primary evaluation of unclear brain lesions. Therefore, in discriminating nontumoral and tumoral lesions in patients with suspected glioma, amino acid tracers seem superior to FDG-PET. In a series of

196 consecutive patients, Herholz et al. [25] demonstrated increased amino acid uptake in nearly all patients with gliomas, even in those with low-grade types. Increased uptake provided a 79% correct differentiation between glioma and nontumoral lesions based on a simple threshold value (1.47) for MET uptake in the most active lesion area relative to the contralateral side. In this study, nontumoral lesions mainly comprised chronic or subacute ischemic or inflammatory demyelinating lesions that had been examined because a tumor could not be definitely excluded by initial CT or MRI studies. The remaining nontumoral lesions consisted of reactive gliosis, dysplasia heterotopia, hematoma, cyst of the pineal body, cavernoma, or post-traumatic scar in individual cases. Based on these findings, a negative amino acid PET scan excludes the presence of glioma with high probability [25]. According to data in the literature, gliosis [4] and demyelinating lesions [2] present only with minor or no tracer accumulation, as little as cavernous angiomas [17] showing pathologic uptake. In contrast, low-grade gliomas present with elevated uptake in most cases [25, 32, 42, 57]. Two representative examples for the differentiation of a low-grade glioma from a nonmalignant lesion using FET PET are shown in Figure 3.1.

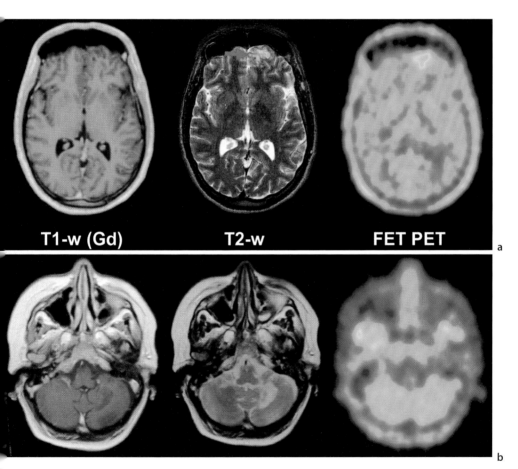

Fig. 3.1a,b. Differential diagnosis of two unclear brain lesions suspicious for low-grade gliomas, both showing signal hyperintensities on T2-weighted MRI but no contrast enhancement on T1-weighted images. Stereotactic biopsy was performed in both cases revealing (**a**) a protoplasmatic astrocytoma WHO II in the left frontal lobe showing focal tumoral uptake on FET PET and (**b**) demyelinating lesion (no tumor) showing no pathological FET uptake

Notably, data in acute cerebral infarcts or active inflammation are somewhat contradictory and require further clarification. Increased uptake of MET was described in the latter [27, 28, 69], whereas in vitro and animal studies have suggested that uptake of other amino acid tracers such as FET was not increased in activated white blood cells of experimental soft tissue infection [31] or only slightly and to a similar extent increased in experimental lesions with and without inflammatory cells. This observation indicates that this slight FET uptake was due to a disruption of the blood-brain barrier rather than due to trapping by macrophages [64]. For the subgroup of vascular abnormalities, dynamic analysis of amino acid tracer uptake may help to further characterize suspect lesions by comparing their kinetic properties with blood pool activity. As shown by Weckesser et al. in a case of giant aneurysm, the diagnosis of vascular abnormality could be confirmed by dynamic evaluation [74]. Overall, quantitative and dynamic evaluation of amino acid PET may contribute to the characterization and differentiation of gliomas from nontumoral lesions.

3.2   Tumor Delineation

Exact delineation of gliomas has essential impact on further treatment strategies. On the one hand, surgical resection should be as complete as possible but at the same time largely sparing of functionally intact normal brain tissue; on the other hand, precise determination of tumor borders is in particular mandatory in cases of nonresectable tumors to define the optimal volume for radiation therapy. Concerning tumor delineation from surrounding normal brain tissue, radiolabeled amino acid tracers seem superior to FDG. Especially brain tumors, which appear hypo- or isometabolic compared to cortical uptake and which are located in or near the grey matter, can only be partially identified, with FDG hampering a clear definition of tumor boundaries [75]. As reported by Spence et al. [66], delineation of gliomas using FDG-PET could perhaps be improved by delayed interval imaging since comparisons between tumor and grey matter showed preferential retentions in the tumors relative to grey matter at delayed time points. However, the question remains of whether this is a practicable approach in clinical routine and whether it is worthwhile, a necessary question since many studies have shown encouraging results of improved tumor delineation using amino acid tracers [25, 32]. Already in 1989 Mosskin et al. [39] used stereotactic serial biopsies to document that the real tumor size was better reflected by MET PET compared to morphologic imaging with CT or MRI. Recent studies confirm that MET detects solid parts of brain tumors as well as the infiltration area with high sensitivity and specificity and therefore will guide improved management of patients with brain tumors [36]. Similar results have been published for FET [47], suggesting that the combined use of MRI and FET PET significantly improves the accuracy in distinguishing glioma tissue from peritumoral brain tissue, especially in brain lesions without disruption of the blood–brain barrier and widespread signal hyperintensities in T2-weighted MRI. While the area showing contrast enhancement on MRI in most cases underestimates the real tumor size, taking into account the entire lesion showing signal hyperintensities in T2-weighted MRI overestimates the tumor size. A representative example is shown in Figure 3.2.

Especially in pretreated patients following surgery [22] and/or radiation therapy [21] MET PET markedly improves delineation of residual/recurrent tumor tissue and posttherapeutic changes and herewith helps to define optimal volume for percutaneous [22] or stereotactic radiation therapy [21]. Following combined treatment planning concept using functional (MET PET) and morphological (MRI/CT) imaging modalities, survival times were significantly longer compared to treatment planning based on morphological data alone [21].

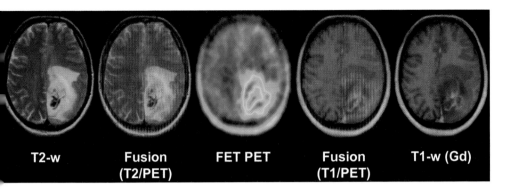

Fig. 3.2. MRI and FET PET images and the respective fused images of a patient with glioblastoma. While signal hyperintensities on T2-weighted MRI overestimate the real tumor size by also delineating perifocal but nontumoral changes, the contrast-enhancing area seems to underestimate the tumor size, as suggested by FET PET

3.3 Biopsy Planning

Brain tumors may consist of different parts and are histologically often heterogeneous with respect to tumor grading. Stereotactic biopsy aims to obtain representative specimen out of the tumor sites with the highest tumor grade and malignancy. However, CT- or MRI-guided stereotactic biopsy does not always provide reliable diagnoses and estimation of tumor grading. Therefore, various techniques have been developed to integrate PET images routinely into the planning of stereotactic brain biopsy, in order to take advantage of the metabolic information provided by PET. First experience with PET-guided biopsies was gained with FDG, which is proposed to locate areas with the highest cell density and turnover. Different groups showed an improvement in the diagnostic yield in stereotactic biopsy by getting samples from the areas with the highest FDG uptake [23, 24]. Levivier et al. [37] found a statistically significant difference in the distribution of histological diagnoses between CT- and PET-guided trajectories, suggesting that FDG-PET may help in selecting targets for biopsy sampling that are the most representative ones for tumor diagnosis and grading. However, experience with FDG-PET has also shown some limitations: targeting may be difficult in lesions with hypo- or isometabolic glucose metabolism, such as in low-grade tumors. Furthermore, problems can arise in defining the borderline between tumoral and cortical FDG uptake, when the hypermetabolic lesion is located near or within the grey matter.

Therefore, amino acid tracers have also been tested as additive or even alternative tracers and have been reported as very helpful in determining the optimal biopsy site [20, 50]. In this context, Pirotte et al. [49] concluded that MET is a good alternative to FDG for target selection, especially in patients showing no or equivalent FDG uptake to that of grey matter. The same group also demonstrated in different patient populations (including children) that PET-guided stereotactic biopsy provided accurate histological diagnoses in most individuals, allowed reducing the number of trajectories in lesions located in high-risk or functional areas, and was also helpful in better understanding and management of complex cases [50, 51]. More recent studies extended the experience to FET [18, 47] and also demonstrated that the combined use of MRI and FET PET in patients with gliomas significantly improves the identification of cellular glioma tissue and, thus, has considerable impact on target selection for biopsies. A very difficult clinical setting in this context is to target a representative area for biopsy in brain lesions presenting with abnormalities in T2-weighted MRI but without relevant contrast enhancement. Data from Pauleit et al. [47] clearly demonstrated that tumor tissue was only found in approximately 50% of

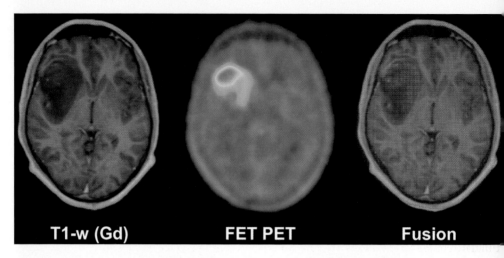

Fig. 3.3. Images of a patient with histopathologically proven mixed glioma (WHO III, oligoastrocytoma Fusion of MRI and FET PET guides the stereotactic biopsy by showing high metabolic activity only in the rostral part of the tumor. While biopsy from this area led to the diagnosis of an oligoastrocytoma, a secon biopsy taken from the dorsal part was only categorized as diffuse astrocytoma (WHO II)

biopsies taken from areas with increased signal on T2-weighted images and that the integration of FET PET significantly improved the accuracy of MRI for the distinction of cellular glioma tissue from peritumoral brain tissue. A representative example for the advantages of PET-guided biopsy is shown in Figure 3.3.

3.4 Grading and Malignant Progression

According to the WHO system, tumor grading is based on histological criteria such as presence or absence of nuclear atypia, mitosis, microvascular proliferation and necrosis [34]. Accurate pathological grading is essential because it determines treatment and prognosis. The histological features of glioma are one of the major prognostic factors and (unfortunately as yet) have more influence on the outcome than any specific therapy [48, 63].

Since it has previously been shown that FDG uptake correlates well with the histological grading of gliomas [1, 15], this method has been considered as a highly valuable diagnostic tool. Cut-off levels for the tumor-to-white-

matter (1.5) and the tumor-to-cortex uptake ratio (0.6) have proven to accurately differ entiate between low- and high-grade tumor [46]. Furthermore, FDG-PET may help in th challenging assessment of low-grade glioma. Since these tumors may remain apparentl dormant for many years or may dedifferenti ate and progress at unpredictable time point: opinions on the best time point for treatmer vary widely. Patients with biopsy-proven low grade gliomas and tumoral FDG uptake highe than the white matter have a higher risk fc malignant transformation compared to thos with no areas of FDG uptake higher than whit matter [10]. If those patients could be identi fied by FDG-PET, needless treatment of low grade tumors could be avoided.

The role of radiolabeled amino acids or ar alogs for tumor grading is more controversi: [14, 18, 42, 47, 61]. Even though amino acid up take has been shown to correlate with cell pro liferative activity [42, 61], microvessel densit [35], and seems to represent a prognostic factc [11], the use of standard ratio methods con paring the tumoral amino acid uptake with th uptake within the normal cortical brain in th late uptake phase (from 20 min after injectio onward), which are the most widely reporte echniques in the literature, has indeed shown slight but not statistically significant increase rom low- to high-grade tumors, however, with substantial overlap between the tumor classifications. Therefore, for neither primary [18, 2, 47] nor recurrent tumors [52], the clinically most important differentiation between ow and high grade, especially between WHO grades II and III, was tumor grading reliably chieved using this approach. Figure 3.4 illustrates the different uptake patterns of FDG nd the amino acid tracer FET in low and high grade gliomas.

Recently, however, debate on tumor grading with amino acid tracers has been newly timulated based on the results of a PET study, n which FET uptake kinetics have been described to differ significantly between newly diagnosed low- and high-grade tumors [74]. Based on their results, the authors hypothesized that differentiation between low- and igh-grade glioma might be possible by taking heir different kinetic behaviors into account.

In a recent FET PET study, the kinetic data f 45 multimodally pretreated patients actu-

ally confirmed a highly statistically significant difference between low- and high-grade recurrent tumors only in the early uptake phase. In contrast to the standard ratio method, which was not able to distinguish between low- and high-grade tumors on a statistically significant level, detailed analysis of the time course of FET uptake provided a high sensitivity and specificity of 92%, respectively, for differentiating low- from high-grade recurrent gliomas. While steadily increasing uptake until the end of the acquisition period pointed to reactive posttherapeutic changes or low-grade tumors, decreasing values following an early peak indicated recurrent glioblastoma or dedifferentiation of initially low-grade tumors [55].

3.5 Prognosis

Patronas et al. pioneered the use of FDG-PET results as prognostic factor in gliomas, showing that FDG uptake correlated well with survival [46]. The results of other authors using FDG-

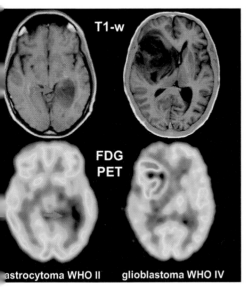
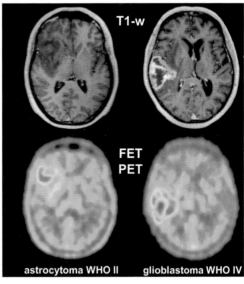

Fig. 3.4a,b. T1-weighted MRI images and (a) FDG PET in comparison to (b) FET PET of a patient with low-nd high-grade glioma, respectively. While FDG PET shows an uptake close to that of white matter in the low-rade astrocytoma (WHO II) (*red arrow*), the glioblastoma presents with higher uptake compared to normal ortex. In contrast, FET PET shows increased uptake in low- and high-grade glioma and therefore seems to e less valuable for tumor grading (using the most widely applied tumor/normal cortex ratio method)

PET as prognostic indicator agreed with those findings [10, 60]. A recent report even claimed that FDG-PET is better than pathological grading for determination of prognosis in gliomas [45]. In patients with biopsy-proven low-grade gliomas, FDG uptake that was higher than the uptake in normal white matter represents a significantly higher risk of malignant transformation compared to patients whose tumors show no areas of uptake greater than in white matter [9].

Although the prognosis depends on the histological tumor grade [12, 43] and the correlation between the tumor grade and the degree of amino acid tracer uptake in the late uptake phase seems to be poor, a recent study of Kim et al. [33] showed that MET PET was a significant prognostic factor independent of tumor grading and that MET was even superior to FDG. MET uptake correlated well with cellular proliferation markers (Ki-67, PCNA) [33, 61] and therefore may be a useful biological prognostic marker in glioma patients. Other authors also agree that baseline MET uptake is an important prognostic indicator for patients with low-grade [57], high-grade [11], and also with pretreated recurrent tumors [72] and that high uptake is statistically associated with a poor survival time.

3.6   Diagnosis of Recurrence

During long-term follow-up, an early and reliable differentiation of therapy-induced reactive changes (such as radiation necrosis) from tumor recurrence is necessary to determine the most appropriate further treatment. While radiation necrosis may be treated by steroids or in extensive cases by debulking surgery, recurrent tumor requires continuation of therapy, changing ineffective treatment, or palliative care only. Structural imaging methods are of limited value in this setting [40, 70], since recurrent tumor and posttherapeutic lesions may both appear as a mass lesion coming along with edema and contrast enhancement due to a breakdown of the blood-brain barrier.

For years, FDG-PET was considered as the gold standard for the differential diagnosis between recurrent glioma and radiation necrosis. A preliminary study by Patronas et al. [46] even suggested that FDG was both 100% sensitive and specific in its ability to differentiate recurrent tumor from necrosis. Several subsequent studies later on supported a high sensitivity and specificity of FDG-PET in this context [16, 41, 71]. However, more recent studies have questioned the efficacy and usefulness of FDG-PET for this purpose and reported specificities as low as 40% [44, 59] especially in tumors that are WHO grade II or III or in small tumor volumes. Another general drawback is that glucose metabolism is also increased in inflammatory tissue, generating the main source of false-positive FDG-PET findings in oncology [67]. This disadvantage of FDG comes up especially in patients after high-dose radiation beam therapy, radiosurgery, or other locoregional approaches delivering high local radiation doses such as radioactive seed implantation or radioimmunotherapy. In those cases a persistent FDG accumulation surrounding the treated area caused by a marked increase in macrophage infiltrates can be observed independent of the presence of recurrent tumor [38]. Furthermore, evaluation of FDG-PET may be hampered in patients receiving steroid treatment by a generalized reduction in cerebral glucose metabolism [19].

Ogawa et al. [41] were one of the first groups reporting on amino acid PET for detection and differential diagnosis of tumor recurrence and found that the use of MET in addition to FDG improved the accuracy to differentiate recurrent brain tumor with FDG hypometabolism from radiation injury. In a recent study van Laere and co-workers [72] compared the single and combined use of FDG and MET for evaluation of brain tumor recurrence and progression. The combined use of both tracers resulted in the highest accuracy (83%), sensitivity (95%) and specificity (60%) in detecting recurrence. While sensitivity decreased for MET alone (75%), specificity increased (70%). They concluded that both tracers provide independent and synergistic prognostic information and that MET can be considered a he agent of choice for the diagnosis of recurrence. Similarly, Thiel et al. supported the impact of MET PET for differential diagnosis of recurrent tumor and reactive posttherapeutic lesions [68]. FET PET was also able to distinguish reliably between tumor recurrence and therapy-induced benign changes in multimodally pretreated glioma patients using a simple threshold value for the tumor to background ratio [52] and demonstrated higher sensitivity and specificity for the diagnosis of recurrence (sensitivity, 100%; specificity 92%) than conventional MRI (sensitivity 93%; specificity 50%) [56]. Figure 3.5 shows two examples or recurrence and radiation injury compared with the respective MRI images.

3.7 Monitoring Therapy

Immediately after therapy, a critical question regarding further therapeutic strategies is whether treatment has been effective or not. Chemotherapy could be discontinued by early detection of its inefficacy thus avoiding many side effects. Similarly, during radiation therapy dose escalation is only advisable if viable tumor tissue is still present after standard therapy.

Some studies have shown that high FDG uptake preceding therapy is a strong indicator of more aggressive tumors and shorter survival [1, 10, 45]; however, only a few studies investigated the FDG uptake at various time points after therapy (and these studies primarily focused on radiation therapy). The results of an immediate (within 2 weeks) postradiation scan alone were not related to survival [65]. Serial evaluation of metabolic activity with PET has provided more accurate prognostic information than a single evaluation [62]. Generally, assessing therapy response with pre- to immediate posttreatment comparisons seemed to better reflect therapeutic efficacy since some authors concordantly have shown that an in-

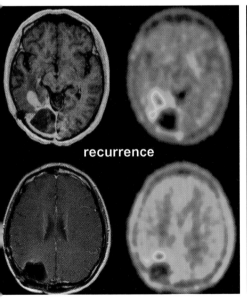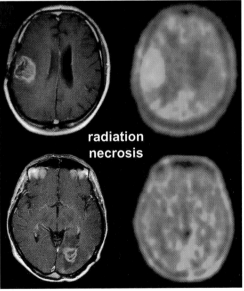

b

Fig. 3.5a,b. T1-weighted MRI and FET PET images of two cases with (**a**) recurrent high-grade tumors (histopathologically proven glioblastoma in the upper row and WHO III anaplastic astrocytoma in the lower row), showing increased nodular FET uptake. MRI images show concordant contrast enhancement in one case (upper row) but normal findings without suspicious contrast enhancement in the other case (lower row). **b** Radiation necrosis both showing no or only a little FET uptake but intense contrast enhancement on MRI, which was rated as tumor recurrence in both cases. Stereotactic biopsy, however, revealed no vital tumor cells but rather necrotic tissue

crease in FDG uptake was correlated with longer survival, whereas a decrease in metabolism was associated with poorer outcome after radio- [65] or chemotherapy [8].

Data on monitoring therapy with amino acid tracers is also limited, but promising. MET PET used for monitoring the effects of radiation therapy [58], systemic chemotherapy [26, 58], or brachytherapy with ^{125}I-seeds [73] has been shown to address therapeutic efficacy during and after these modalities. FET PET is also a valuable tool in monitoring therapeutic effects, which has been proven for locoregional approaches such as intralesional radioimmunotherapy [54] or convection-enhanced delivery of paclitaxel [53]. In long-term follow-up, stable or decreasing homogeneous FET uptake even in contrast-enhancing lesions was suggestive of reactive changes, whereas increasing ratios in more nodular-type lesions always appeared to be indicative of recurrence. Therefore,

FET PET seems more reliable than MRI for this purpose since the latter is often hampered by reactive alterations of the blood-brain barrier and the expanding edema that follows such aggressive local approaches and may mimic inefficacy or recurrence. Most importantly, amino acid PET successfully differentiates between recurrent tumor and radiation necrosis and, in contrast to FDG, shows a high tumor-to-nontumor contrast even in small recurrent tumors. A representative example of a patient monitored with serial FET and FDG-PET scans following locoregional radioimmunotherapy is shown in Figure 3.6, clearly illustrating the advantages of amino acid imaging in depicting the recurrent tumor and also in assessing the metabolic response of the recurrent tumor on chemotherapy.

Possibly another promising indicator regarding the clinically most important question of early treatment response might be the

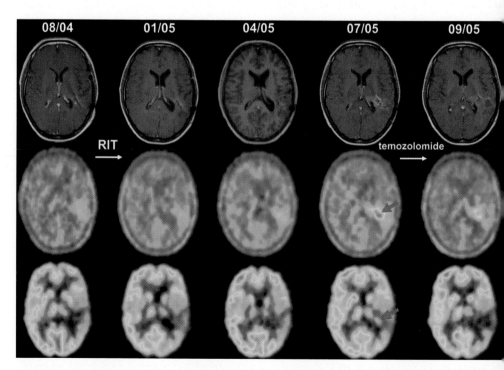

Fig. 3.6. Representative MRI and PET images of a patient following surgery and radiation therapy for glioblastoma monitored with serial FET and FDG PET scans following locoregional radioimmunotherapy. The images clearly illustrate the advantages of amino acid imaging compared to FDG PET and MRI in depicting the recurrent tumor (*red arrow*) and also in assessing the metabolic response of the recurrent tumor on chemotherapy with temozolomide

measurement of tumor proliferation using [18F]fluorothymidine (FLT). To date, however, data on early imaging of drug-induced changes in cell proliferation of brain tumors is still lacking.

3.8 Perspectives

Multimodal imaging integrating morphologic (MRI, CT) and metabolic information should advance our current understanding of complex glioma pathology. Since in recent years various new tumor-specific therapeutic regimens acting on a molecular level have come to the forefront, it is imperative that we further investigate and develop methods reflecting molecular pathology and therapeutic processes as they progress over time.

At present, the routinely used PET tracers add not only useful but indispensable information concerning the differential diagnosis of brain tumors, tumor delineation and grading, estimation of prognosis, biopsy planning, as well as therapy monitoring and assessment of posttherapeutic follow-up. While FDG currently is still considered as the first-choice tracer for tumor grading or estimation of malignant transformation of initially low-grade tumors, there is rapidly increasing evidence that radiolabeled amino acids may have superior properties in delineation of tumor borders, biopsy planning, evaluation of treatment effects, and in the differentiation of recurrent tumor and reactive posttherapeutic changes after conventional treatment. In recent years, especially [18F]-labeled amino acid tracers have gained importance based on the possibility of their widespread use even in hospitals lacking an onsite cyclotron. In the future, however, most of the applications mentioned above should take into account analysis of tracer kinetics. This could further strengthen the role of this technique.

Furthermore, current experience with PET imaging following standard treatment has to be expanded to the new fields of therapeutic options, especially locoregional therapeutic approaches or approaches acting on the molecular level. In this context, new aspects of brain tumor imaging will arise from the possibility of noninvasive imaging gene expression. Location, magnitude, and extent of expression of an exogenous gene introduced by gene therapy into patients with gliomas can be monitored by PET using [124I]FIAU – a specific marker substrate for gene expression of HSV-1-thymidine kinase [29]. Imaging gene expression will make it possible to determine the dimension of transduced cell function and vector-mediated gene expression, which can then be correlated with therapeutic effects thus, enabling assessment of gene therapy protocols for clinical application [30].

Imaging tumor hypoxia using misonidazole derivates is another aspect that deserves further investigation. Preliminary clinical data suggest that late [18F]FMISO PET images provide a spatial description of hypoxia in brain tumors that is independent of blood-brain barrier disruption and tumor perfusion [5]. Since hypoxic tissue is relatively resistant to radiation therapy, perfusion-hypoxia patterns may lead to a better prediction of treatment response in glioma patients. Preliminary clinical results addressing proliferation of brain tumor using FLT also show great promise. FLT uptake correlated well with the proliferation index Ki-67 and revealed predictive power with respect to tumor progression and patient survival [6]. Membrane biosynthesis as assessed by PET and radiolabeled choline derivates may also yield diagnostic information. DeGrado et al. introduced [18F]fluorocholine (FCH) for brain tumor imaging [13]. Contrary to amino acid tracers such as MET or FET, however, FCH is also accumulated in inflammatory cells [76], and therefore its specificity for tumor detection especially in pretreated patients might be limited. Future studies are needed to determine its advantages and limitations in vivo. More recently, [18F]Galacto-RGD (arginine-glycine-aspartic acid) has been developed for PET imaging of alpha(v)beta(3) integrin expression, a receptor involved in tumor angiogenesis, which may also play a role in imaging high-grade gliomas. This tracer offers a new strategy for noninvasive monitoring of molecular processes and may provide helpful information for planning and controlling therapy targeting the alpha(v)beta(3) integrin [3].

In conclusion, FDG and amino acid tracers are mature tracers for routine application in the diagnostic work-up of gliomas while for all other tracers mentioned, extended clinical studies have yet to assess their full benefits. However, the latter tracers offer new perspectives and should encourage us to continue and extend PET research in this exciting field.

References

1. Alavi JB, Alavi A, Chawluk J, Kushner M, Powe J, Hickey W, Reivich M (1988) Positron emission tomography in patients with glioma. A predictor of prognosis. Cancer 62:1074–1078
2. Becherer A, Karanikas G, Szabo M, Zettinig G, Asenbaum S, Marosi C, Henk C, Wunderbaldinger P, Czech T, Wadsak W, Kletter K (2003) Brain tumour imaging with PET: a comparison between [^{18}F]fluorodopa and [^{11}C]methionine. Eur J Nucl Med Mol Imaging 30:1561–1567
3. Beer AJ, Haubner R, Goebel M, Luderschmidt S, Spilker ME, Wester HJ, Weber WA, Schwaiger M (2005) Biodistribution and Pharmacokinetics of the {alpha}v{beta}3-Selective Tracer ^{18}F-galacto-RGD in cancer patients. J Nucl Med 46:1333–1341
4. Braun V, Dempf S, Weller R, Reske SN, Schachenmayr W, Richter HP (2002) Cranial neuronavigation with direct integration of (^{11})C methionine positron emission tomography (PET) data – results of a pilot study in 32 surgical cases. Acta Neurochir (Wien) 144:777–782; discussion 782
5. Bruehlmeier M, Roelcke U, Schubiger PA, Ametamey SM (2004) Assessment of hypoxia and perfusion in human brain tumors using PET with ^{18}F-fluoromisonidazole and ^{15}O-H$_2$O. J Nucl Med 45:1851–1859
6. Chen W, Cloughesy T, Kamdar N, Satyamurthy N, Bergsneider M, Liau L, Mischel P, Czernin J, Phelps ME, Silverman DH (2005) Imaging proliferation in brain tumors with ^{18}F-FLT PET: comparison with ^{18}F-FDG. J Nucl Med 46:945–952
7. Davis FG, Freels S, Grutsch J, Barlas S, Brem S (1998) Survival rates in patients with primary malignant brain tumors stratified by patient age and tumor histological type: an analysis based on surveillance, epidemiology, and end results (SEER) data, 1973–1991. J Neurosurg 88:1–10
8. De Witte O, Hildebrand J, Luxen A, Goldman S (1994) Acute effect of carmustine on glucose metabolism in brain and glioblastoma. Cancer 74:2836–2842
9. De Witte O, Levivier M, Violon P, Salmon I, Damhaut P, Wikler D Jr, Hildebrand J, Brotchi J, Goldman S (1996) Prognostic value positron emission tomography with [^{18}F]fluoro-2-deoxy-D-glucose in the low grade glioma. Neurosurgery 39:470–476; discussion 476–477
10. De Witte O, Lefranc F, Levivier M, Salmon I, Brotchi J, Goldman S (2000) FDG-PET as a prognostic factor in high-grade astrocytoma. J Neurooncol 49:157–163
11. De Witte O, Goldberg I, Wikler D, Rorive S, Damhaut P, Monclus M, Salmon I, Brotchi J, Goldman S (2001) Positron emission tomography with injection of methionine as a prognostic factor in glioma. J Neurosurg 95:746–750
12. DeAngelis LM (2001) Brain tumors. N Engl J Med 344:114–123
13. DeGrado TR, Baldwin SW, Wang S, Orr MD, Liao RP, Friedman HS, Reiman R, Price DT, Coleman RE (2001) Synthesis and evaluation of (^{18})F-labeled choline analogs as oncologic PET tracers. J Nucl Med 42:1805–1814
14. Derlon JM, Bourdet C, Bustany P, Chatel M, Theron J, Darcel F, Syrota A (1989) [^{11}C]L-methionine uptake in gliomas. Neurosurgery 25:720–728
15. Di Chiro G (1987) Positron emission tomography using [^{18}F] fluorodeoxyglucose in brain tumors. A powerful diagnostic and prognostic tool. Invest Radiol 22:360–371
16. Di Chiro G, Oldfield E, Wright DC, De Michele D, Katz DA, Patronas NJ, Doppman JL, Larson SM, Ito M, Kufta CV (1988) Cerebral necrosis after radiotherapy and/or intraarterial chemotherapy for brain tumors: PET and neuropathologic studies. AJR Am J Roentgenol 150:189–197
17. Ericson K, von Holst H, Mosskin M, Bergstrom M, Lindqvist M, Noren G, Eriksson L (1986) Positron emission tomography of cavernous haemangiomas of the brain. Acta Radiol Diagn (Stockh) 27:379–383
18. Floeth FW, Pauleit D, Wittsack HJ, Langen KJ, Reifenberger G, Hamacher K, Messing-Junger M, Zilles K, Weber F, Stummer W, Steiger HJ, Woebker G, Muller HW, Coenen H, Sabel M (2005) Multimodal metabolic imaging of cerebral gliomas: positron emission tomography with [^{18}F]fluoroethyl-L-tyrosine and magnetic resonance spectroscopy. J Neurosurg 102:318–327
19. Fulham MJ, Brunetti A, Aloj L, Raman R, Dwyer AJ, Di Chiro G (1995) Decreased cerebral glucose metabolism in patients with brain tumors: an effect of corticosteroids. J Neurosurg 83:657–664
20. Goldman S, Levivier M, Pirotte B, Brucher JM, Wikler D, Damhaut P, Dethy S, Brotchi J, Hildebrand J (1997) Regional methionine and glucose uptake in high-grade gliomas: a comparative study on PET-guided stereotactic biopsy. J Nucl Med 38:1459–1462
21. Grosu AL, Weber WA, Franz M, Stark S, Piert M, Thamm R, Gumprecht H, Schwaiger M, Molls M, Nieder C (2005a) Reirradiation of recurrent high grade gliomas using amino acid PET (SPECT)/CT/MRI image fusion to determine gross tumor volume

for stereotactic fractionated radiotherapy. Int J Radiat Oncol Biol Phys 63:511–519

22. Grosu AL, Weber WA, Riedel E, Jeremic B, Nieder C, Franz M, Gumprecht H, Jaeger R, Schwaiger M, Molls M (2005b) L-(methyl-^{11}C) methionine positron emission tomography for target delineation in resected high-grade gliomas before radiotherapy. Int J Radiat Oncol Biol Phys 63:64–74

23. Hanson MW, Glantz MJ, Hoffman JM, Friedman AH, Burger PC, Schold SC, Coleman RE (1991) FDG-PET in the selection of brain lesions for biopsy. J Comput Assist Tomogr 15:796–801

24. Herholz K, Pietrzyk U, Voges J, Schroder R, Halber M, Treuer H, Sturm V, Heiss WD (1993) Correlation of glucose consumption and tumor cell density in astrocytomas. A stereotactic PET study. J Neurosurg 79:853–858

25. Herholz K, Holzer T, Bauer B, Schroder R, Voges J, Ernestus RI, Mendoza G, Weber-Luxenburger G, Lottgen J, Thiel A, Wienhard K, Heiss WD (1998) ^{11}C-methionine PET for differential diagnosis of low-grade gliomas. Neurology 50:1316–1322

26. Herholz K, Kracht LW, Heiss WD (2003) Monitoring the effect of chemotherapy in a mixed glioma by C-11-methionine PET. J Neuroimaging 13:269–271

27. Ishii K, Ogawa T, Hatazawa J, Kanno I, Inugami A, Fujita H, Shimosegawa E, Murakami M, Okudera T, Uemura K (1993) High L-methyl-^{11}C]methionine uptake in brain abscess: a PET study. J Comput Assist Tomogr 17:660–661

28. Jacobs A (1995) Amino acid uptake in ischemically compromised brain tissue. Stroke 26:1859–1866

29. Jacobs A, Voges J, Reszka R, Lercher M, Gossmann A, Kracht L, Kaestle C, Wagner R, Wienhard K, Heiss WD (2001) Positron-emission tomography of vector-mediated gene expression in gene therapy for gliomas. Lancet 358:727–729

30. Jacobs AH, Voges J, Kracht LW, Dittmar C, Winkeler A, Thomas A, Wienhard K, Herholz K, Heiss WD (2003) Imaging in gene therapy of patients with glioma. J Neurooncol 65:291–305

31. Kaim AH, Weber B, Kurrer MO, Westera G, Schweitzer A, Gottschalk J, von Schulthess GK, Buck A (2002) ([18])F-FDG and ([18])F-FET uptake in experimental soft tissue infection. Eur J Nucl Med Mol Imaging 29:648–654

32. Kaschten B, Stevenaert A, Sadzot B, Deprez M, Degueldre C, Del Fiore G, Luxen A, Reznik M (1998) Preoperative evaluation of 54 gliomas by PET with fluorine-18-fluorodeoxyglucose and/or carbon-11-methionine. J Nucl Med 39:778–785

33. Kim S, Chung JK, Im SH, Jeong JM, Lee DS, Kim DG, Jung HW, Lee MC (2005) ^{11}C-methionine PET as a prognostic marker in patients with glioma: comparison with ^{18}F-FDG PET. Eur J Nucl Med Mol Imaging 32:52–59

34. Kleihues P, Cavenee WK (2000) Tumors of the nervous system. Pathology and genetics. IARC Press, Lyon, France

35. Kracht LW, Friese M, Herholz K, Schroeder R, Bauer B, Jacobs A, Heiss WD (2003) Methyl-^{11}C]-l-methionine uptake as measured by positron emission tomography correlates to microvessel density in patients with glioma. Eur J Nucl Med Mol Imaging 30:868–873

36. Kracht LW, Miletic H, Busch S, Jacobs AH, Voges J, Hoevels M, Klein JC, Herholz K, Heiss WD (2004) Delineation of brain tumor extent with ^{11}C]L-methionine positron emission tomography: local comparison with stereotactic histopathology. Clin Cancer Res 10:7163–7170

37. Levivier M, Goldman S, Pirotte B, Brucher JM, Baleriaux D, Luxen A, Hildebrand J, Brotchi J (1995) Diagnostic yield of stereotactic brain biopsy guided by positron emission tomography with ^{18}F]fluorodeoxyglucose. J Neurosurg 82:445–452

38. Marriott CJ, Thorstad W, Akabani G, Brown MT, McLendon RE, Hanson MW, Coleman RE (1998) Locally increased uptake of fluorine-18-fluorodeoxyglucose after intracavitary administration of iodine-131-labeled antibody for primary brain tumors. J Nucl Med 39:1376–1380

39. Mosskin M, Ericson K, Hindmarsh T, von Holst H, Collins VP, Bergstrom M, Eriksson L, Johnstrom P (1989) Positron emission tomography compared with magnetic resonance imaging and computed tomography in supratentorial gliomas using multiple stereotactic biopsies as reference. Acta Radiol 30:225–232

40. Nelson SJ (1999) Imaging of brain tumors after therapy. Neuroimaging Clin N Am 9:801–819

41. Ogawa T, Kanno I, Shishido F, Inugami A, Higano S, Fujita H, Murakami M, Uemura K, Yasui N, Mineura K et al (1991) Clinical value of PET with ^{18}F-fluorodeoxyglucose and L-methyl-11C-methionine for diagnosis of recurrent brain tumor and radiation injury. Acta Radiol 32:197–202

42. Ogawa T, Shishido F, Kanno I, Inugami A, Fujita H, Murakami M, Shimosegawa E, Ito H, Hatazawa J, Okudera T et al (1993) Cerebral glioma: evaluation with methionine PET. Radiology 186:45–53

43. Ohgaki H, Kleihues P (2005) Population-based studies on incidence, survival rates, and genetic alterations in astrocytic and oligodendroglial gliomas. J Neuropathol Exp Neurol 64:479–489

44. Olivero WC, Dulebohn SC, Lister JR (1995) The use of PET in evaluating patients with primary brain tumours: is it useful? J Neurol Neurosurg Psychiatry 58:250–252

45. Padma MV, Said S, Jacobs M, Hwang DR, Dunigan K, Satter M, Christian B, Ruppert J, Bernstein T, Kraus G, Mantil JC (2003) Prediction of pathology and survival by FDG PET in gliomas. J Neurooncol 64:227–237

46. Patronas NJ, Di Chiro G, Brooks RA, DeLaPaz RL, Kornblith PL, Smith BH, Rizzoli HV, Kessler RM, Manning RG, Channing M, Wolf AP, O'Connor CM (1982) Work in progress: [18]F] fluorodeoxyglucose and positron emission tomography in the evaluation of radiation necrosis of the brain. Radiology 144:885–889

47. Pauleit D, Floeth F, Hamacher K, Riemenschneider MJ, Reifenberger G, Muller HW, Zilles K, Coenen HH, Langen KJ (2005) O-(2-[18F]fluoroethyl)-l-tyrosine PET combined with MRI improves the diagnostic assessment of cerebral gliomas. Brain 128:678–687

48. Perry A, Jenkins RB, O'Fallon JR, Schaefer PL, Kimmel DW, Mahoney MR, Scheithauer BW, Smith SM, Hill EM, Sebo TJ, Levitt R, Krook J, Tschetter LK, Morton RF, Buckner JC (1999) Clinicopathologic study of 85 similarly treated patients with anaplastic astrocytic tumors. An analysis of DNA content (ploidy), cellular proliferation, and p53 expression. Cancer 86:672–683

49. Pirotte B, Goldman S, David P, Wikler D, Damhaut P, Vandesteene A, Salmon L, Brotchi J, Levivier M (1997) Stereotactic brain biopsy guided by positron emission tomography (PET) with [F-18]fluorodeoxy-glucose and [C-11]methionine. Acta Neurochir Suppl (Wien) 68:133–138

50. Pirotte B, Goldman S, Salzberg S, Wikler D, David P, Vandesteene A, Van Bogaert P, Salmon I, Brotchi J, Levivier M (2003) Combined positron emission tomography and magnetic resonance imaging for the planning of stereotactic brain biopsies in children: experience in 9 cases. Pediatr Neurosurg 38:146–155

51. Pirotte B, Goldman S, Massager N, David P, Wikler D, Lipszyc M, Salmon I, Brotchi J, Levivier M (2004) Combined use of 18F-fluorodeoxyglucose and 11C-methionine in 45 positron emission tomography-guided stereotactic brain biopsies. J Neurosurg 101:476–483

52. Popperl G, Gotz C, Rachinger W, Gildehaus FJ, Tonn JC, Tatsch K (2004) Value of O-(2-[18F]fluoroethyl)- l-tyrosine PET for the diagnosis of recurrent glioma. Eur J Nucl Med Mol Imaging 31:1464–1470

53. Popperl G, Goldbrunner R, Gildehaus FJ, Kreth FW, Tanner P, Holtmannspotter M, Tonn JC, Tatsch K (2005) O-(2-[18F]fluoroethyl)-l-tyrosine PET for monitoring the effects of convection-enhanced delivery of paclitaxel in patients with recurrent glioblastoma. Eur J Nucl Med Mol Imaging 32:1018–1025

54. Popperl G, Goetz C, Rachinger W, Schnell O, Gildehaus FJ, Tonn JC, Tatsch K (2006a) Serial O-(2-[18F]fluoroethyl)-l-tyrosine PET for monitoring the effects of intracavitary radioimmunotherapy in patients with malignant glioma. Eur J Nucl Med Mol Imaging 33:792–800

55. Popperl G, Kreth FW, Herms J, Koch W, Mehrkens JH, Gildehaus FJ, Kretzschmar HA, Tonn JC, Tatsch K (2006b) Analysis of 18F-FET PET for grading of recurrent gliomas: is evaluation of uptake kinetics superior to standard methods? J Nucl Med 47:393–403

56. Rachinger W, Goetz C, Popperl G, Gildehaus FJ, Kreth FW, Holtmannspotter M, Herms J, Koch W, Tatsch K, Tonn JC (2005) Positron emission tomography with O-(2-[18F]fluoroethyl)-l-tyrosine versus magnetic resonance imaging in the diagnosis of recurrent gliomas. Neurosurgery 57:505–511; discussion 511

57. Ribom D, Eriksson A, Hartman M, Engler H, Nilsson A, Langstrom B, Bolander H, Bergstrom M, Smits A (2001) Positron emission tomography (11C-methionine and survival in patients with low-grade gliomas. Cancer 92:1541–1549

58. Ribom D, Schoenmaekers M, Engler H, Smits A (2005) Evaluation of 11C-methionine PET as a surrogate endpoint after treatment of grade 2 gliomas. J Neurooncol 71:325–332

59. Ricci PE, Karis JP, Heiserman JE, Fram EK, Bice AN, Drayer BP (1998) Differentiating recurrent tumor from radiation necrosis: time for re-evaluation of positron emission tomography? AJNR Am J Neuroradiol 19:407–413

60. Rozental JM, Levine RL, Nickles RJ (1991) Changes in glucose uptake by malignant gliomas: preliminary study of prognostic significance. J Neurooncol 10:75–83

61. Sato N, Suzuki M, Kuwata N, Kuroda K, Wada T, Beppu T, Sera K, Sasaki T, Ogawa A (1999) Evaluation of the malignancy of glioma using 11C-methionine positron emission tomography and proliferating cell nuclear antigen staining. Neurosurg Rev 22:210–214

62. Schifter T, Hoffman JM, Hanson MW, Boyko OB, Beam C, Paine S, Schold SC, Burger PC, Coleman RE (1993) Serial FDG-PET studies in the prediction of survival in patients with primary brain tumors. J Comput Assist Tomogr 17:509–561

63. Scott JN, Rewcastle NB, Brasher PM, Fulton D, MacKinnon JA, Hamilton M, Cairncross JG, Forsyth P (1999) Which glioblastoma multiforme patient will become a long-term survivor? A population-based study. Ann Neurol 46:183–188

64. Spaeth N, Wyss MT, Weber B, Scheidegger S, Lutz A, Verwey J, Radovanovic I, Pahnke J, Wild D, Westera G, Weishaupt D, Hermann DM, Kaser-Hotz B, Aguzzi A, Buck A (2004) Uptake of 18F-fluorocholine, 18F-fluoroethyl-L-tyrosine, and 18F-FDG in acute cerebral radiation injury in the rat: implications for separation of radiation necrosis from tumor recurrence. J Nucl Med 45:1931–1938

65. Spence AM, Muzi M, Graham MM, O'Sullivan F, Link JM, Lewellen TK, Lewellen B, Freeman SD, Mankoff DA, Eary JF, Krohn KA (2002) 2-[(18)F]Fluoro-2-deoxyglucose and glucose uptake in malignant gliomas before and after radiotherapy: correlation with outcome. Clin Cancer Res 8:971–979

66. Spence AM, Muzi M, Mankoff DA, O'Sullivan SF, Link JM, Lewellen TK, Lewellen B, Pham P, Minoshima S, Swanson K, Krohn KA (2004) 18F-FDG PET of gliomas at delayed intervals: improved distinction between tumor and normal gray matter. J Nucl Med 45:1653–1659

67. Strauss LG (1996) Fluorine-18 deoxyglucose and false-positive results: a major problem in the diagnostics of oncological patients. Eur J Nucl Med 23:1409–1415

68. Thiel A, Pietrzyk U, Sturm V, Herholz K, Hovels M, Schroder R (2000) Enhanced accuracy in differential diagnosis of radiation necrosis by positron emission tomography-magnetic resonance imaging coregis-

tration: technical case report. Neurosurgery 46:232–234

69. Tsuyuguchi N, Sunada I, Ohata K, Takami T, Nishio A, Hara M, Kawabe J, Okamura T, Ochi H (2003) Evaluation of treatment effects in brain abscess with positron emission tomography: comparison of fluorine-18-fluorodeoxyglucose and carbon-11-methionine. Ann Nucl Med 17:47–51

70. Valk PE, Dillon WP (1991) Radiation injury of the brain. AJNR Am J Neuroradiol 12:45–62

71. Valk PE, Budinger TF, Levin VA, Silver P, Gutin PH, Doyle WK (1988) PET of malignant cerebral tumors after interstitial brachytherapy. Demonstration of metabolic activity and correlation with clinical outcome. J Neurosurg 69:830–838

72. Van Laere K, Ceyssens S, Van Calenbergh F, de Groot T, Menten J, Flamen P, Bormans G, Mortelmans L (2005) Direct comparison of ^{18}F-FDG and ^{11}C-methionine PET in suspected recurrence of glioma: sensitivity, inter-observer variability and prognostic value. Eur J Nucl Med Mol Imaging 32:39–51

73. Voges J, Herholz K, Holzer T, Wurker M, Bauer B, Pietrzyk U, Treuer H, Schroder R, Sturm V, Heiss WD (1997) ^{11}C-methionine and ^{18}F-2-fluorodeoxyglucose positron emission tomography: a tool for diagnosis of cerebral glioma and monitoring after brachytherapy with 125I seeds. Stereotact Funct Neurosurg 69:129–135

74. Weckesser M, Langen KJ, Rickert CH, Kloska S, Straeter R, Hamacher K, Kurlemann G, Wassmann H, Coenen HH, Schober O (2005) O-(2-[(^{18})F] fluorethyl)-l: -tyrosine PET in the clinical evaluation of primary brain tumours. Eur J Nucl Med Mol Imaging 32:422–429

75. Wong TZ, van der Westhuizen GJ, Coleman RE (2002) Positron emission tomography imaging of brain tumors. Neuroimaging Clin N Am 12:615–626

76. Wyss MT, Weber B, Honer M, Spath N, Ametamey SM, Westera G, Bode B, Kaim AH, Buck A (2004) ^{18}F-choline in experimental soft tissue infection assessed with autoradiography and high-resolution PET. Eur J Nucl Med Mol Imaging 31:312–316

4   PET/CT Imaging in Head and Neck Tumors

R. Rödel

Recent Results in Cancer Research, Vol. 170
© Springer-Verlag Berlin Heidelberg 2008

4.1   Introduction

Head and neck cancer is the 10th most common cancer in the world [49], accounting for 2%–5% of all malignant cancers [4, 13, 44]. The incidence worldwide is greater than 35,000 cases per year with approximately 20 in 100,000 males, who are affected twice as often as females. The incidence is increasing, particularly in younger patients and in women [39]. More than 20% of patients diagnosed with head and neck cancer will develop a second or third primary tumor, due to susceptibility of the mucosa to carcinomatous change [11].

The 5-year survival rates for head and neck cancer depend on stage and site of tumor (40%–95% for stage I and II and 0%–50% for stage III and IV); for all stages combined the range is between 35% and 50%, probably in part due to late presentation [33]. The annual mortality rate for head and neck cancer is of the same magnitude as that of malignant melanoma or cervical cancer [12].

Most tumor lesions (80%–90%) are histopathologically squamous cell carcinomas, which are graded depending on the degree of cornification; others are adenocarcinoma, lymphoma, sarcoma and metastases from remote organs [11, 38]. The highly enhanced glucose utilisation of malignant squamous cell carcinoma compared to normal tissue can be demonstrated by positron emission tomography (PET) using fluoro-2-deoxy-D-glucose (FDG-PET) [36]. PET has proved to be a useful tool to differentiate between malignant and benign lesions as well as to stage lymph nodes, which is indispensable for adequate tumor treatment (for a review see [28]).

Although it is highly sensitive, PET may provide imprecise anatomic localisation of radiotracer uptake, especially in the complicated anatomical situation of the head and neck. Additional anatomical information can be provided by computer tomography (CT), which may demonstrate PET-negative tumors. When using separate PET and CT scanners at different times, information from fused imaging is limited because identical bedding in the different scanners is not always achieved and anatomical changes (i.e. embossment) may occur between investigation dates. Computerised co-registration of CT and PET (PET/CT), which is done nearly simultaneously in a single integrated scanner, can eliminate these shortcomings and unifies functional and anatomical information by imaging fusion techniques.

The 511-keV annihilation radiation in PET is partly absorbed in the patient's body, so that attenuation correction is essential from a technical point of view. In doing so, attenuation correction coefficients for human tissue densities are derived from CT data, where x-rays have shown an energy range between 40 and 140 keV. The use of intravenous contrast agents is expected to affect the CT-based attenuation correction for PET, since the high attenuation of contrast agents at x-ray energies does not apply to annihilation energy. This could lead to an overestimation of FDG accumulation in PET. In addition, the attenuation of intravenous contrast agent changes quickly after injection so that the sequential emission scans (PET) will have different distributions compared to transmission scans (CT) [29].

The aim of this retrospective study was to evaluate the feasibility and the benefit of clinical findings by comparing the results of the individual procedures (PET and CT) with the additional diagnostic information of the fused PET/CT images. In addition, attention is turned to the influence of intravenous contrast agents on the quality and accuracy of attenuation-corrected PET and hence PET/CT.

4.2 Methods

The patient population consisted of 85 patients (mean age, 58.7 ± 13.5 years; 61 males, 23 females) who had undergone clinical examinations in otorhinolaryngology and were suspected of having head and neck cancer. The patients received whole-body scans on a dual modality PET/CT system (Siemens biograph) 90 min after intravenous injection of 370 MBq [F-18]FDG. To reduce the effect of respiratory motion of the lungs, the PET scans were done with preferably flat respiration. CT was performed with 40 mAs, 130 kV, in 5-mm slices and a pitch of 1.5. Fifty-one patients were scanned with no or with only oral administration of contrast agents, 34 patients were scanned after intravenous administration of iodinated contrast agent (Ultravist 300, 120 ml at whole-body scan and 60 ml at head and neck scan) with an automatic injector. CT data were used for attenuation correction of PET emission images. Both PET and CT images were reconstructed in 5-mm slices in the coronal, sagittal and transversal planes. An uptake value higher than 3.0 was defined as abnormal accumulation of FDG outside normal anatomic structures and under the influence of asymmetry.

The images were reviewed independently by two experienced blinded investigators on a workstation (Siemens E.SOFT V) linked to the PET/CT scanner. The results of PET and CT imaging were compared concerning the diagnostic impact of the CT scan to FDG-PET images and the additional value of fused imaging. The reference standard was histological appearance of lesions and clinical follow-up in cases where biopsy results were not available.

4.3 Results

4.3.1 Conspicuous Findings

The total number of lesions detected with PET or CT with abnormal FDG uptake in PET or a conspicuous sign in CT was 260. These findings were classified as malignant in 155 lesions on CT images and 226 lesions on FDG-PET images, as suspicious for malignancy in 47 lesions on CT and 12 on FDG-PET and as benign in 47 lesions on CT and 27 on FDG-PET. The number of concordant findings was 172 (66.2%) and the number of discordant findings was 88 (33.8%). Discrepancies occurred mainly in the mediastinum, the primary tumor site and in the lungs (Table 4.1). A representative example is shown in Figure 4.1. After image fusion, only 15 lesions (5.8% of all and 17.0% of discrepant findings) in nine patients could not be classified as either malignant or benign.

Table 4.1. Localisation and number of discrepant findings in PET and CT

Localisation	No. of discrepant findings
Mediastinum	22
Lymph nodes, cervical, axillary	19
Primary tumor	18
Lung	16
Soft tissue, bones	8
Others	5

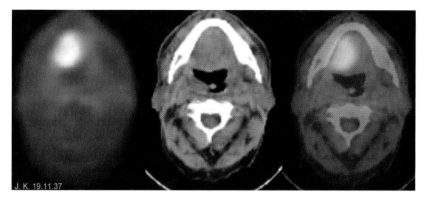

Fig. 4.1. Focal accumulation of FDG (*left*) with no suspicious finding in CT (*middle*). Fusion of PET and CT images (*right*) give evidence for malignant tumor in the base of the oral cavity. Histology revealed squamous cell carcinoma

4.3.2 Histopathology

Histology revealed predominately squamous cell carcinoma in 49 patients (57.7%), undifferentiated carcinoma in seven patients (8.2%), metastases of bronchial cell carcinoma in five patients (5.9%) and others in 16 patients (18.8%) (Table 4.2). In seven patients (8.2%), there was no evidence of malignancy (inflammation, sarcoidosis, or hyperplasia) from the histopathological examination.

Table 4.2. Histological findings in 85 patients with head and neck tumors

Histology	No. of patients	Percentage
Squamous cell carcinoma	48	57.7
Adenocarcinoma	3	3.5
Bronchial carcinoma	5	5.9
Undifferentiated carcinoma	7	8.2
Benign lesion	7	8.2
Others	14	16.5

4.3.3 Detection of Primary Tumors

Primary lesions were present in 46 patients; among these there were 13 recurrent diseases. Histology revealed squamous cell carcinoma in 30 patients (16 with moderate differentia-

tion, eight with medium grade differentiation and six with cornification grading missing). Others (n=8) were mainly adenocarcinoma, undifferentiated carcinoma and adenocystic carcinoma. Eight lesions were of benign origin according to histological findings (inflammation, cyst, or sarcoidosis). In PET, 36 out of 38 (sensitivity, 94.7%; specificity, 37.5%) malignant tumors were detected, the two missing lesions were moderate differentiated squamous cell carcinoma. CT detected 21 malignant lesions (sensitivity, 61.8%; specificity, 50.0%); on histology, the missing lesions showed squamous cell carcinoma, undifferentiated carcinoma, adenocarcinoma and adenocystic carcinoma. With PET/CT image fusion, the detection rate was 37 out of 38 (97.4%) for malignant tumors. Sensitivity was calculated to be 94.7% and specificity 42.9%. However, due to the small number of samples, the 95% confidence interval for specificity in PET, CT and PET/CT was not in the acceptable range so that reliable statistical significance cannot be presented as yet. With or without administration of intravenous contrast agent, there were only marginal changes in the detection rates.

4.3.4 Detection of Recurrent Tumors

Among all primary tumors, there were 13 lesions which could be classified as recurrent tumors. Histological examination revealed squamous cell carcinoma in 12 cases (nine with moderate differentiation, one with medium grade differentiation and two with cornification grading missing). One recurrent tumor was a malignant fibrous histiocytoma. PET produced correct diagnosis in all 13 lesions, whereas in CT only seven lesions (53.9%) were suggested to be malignant and the other six cases to be inconspicuous. With fusion of PET and CT images, the detection rate was still 100%, whereas CT improved the anatomical localisation in all cases. The administration of intravenous contrast agent had no influence on the detection rate with PET or image fusion. Because of the low detection rate with CT imaging alone, no reliable statement can be made concerning the influence of intravenous contrast agent administration.

4.3.5 Detection of Unknown Primary

Thirty-five patients were presented with metastatic cancer of unknown primary origin (CUP). From biopsy results, there were 19 patients with squamous cell carcinoma (ten with moderate differentiation, seven with medium grade differentiation, two with missing cornification grading), five with undifferentiated carcinoma and 11 with other histological findings (melanoma, bronchial cell carcinoma, transitional cell tumor, or adenocarcinoma). With PET, a primary tumor could be detected in 15 patients (42.8%). A representative example is shown in Figure 4.2. Among these there were nine cases with squamous cell carcinoma (eight with moderate differentiation, one with

medium grade differentiation). CT was able to identify the primary tumor in seven patients (20%), lesions which were also seen in PET. Histological examination of the metastases for undetected primary origin revealed in ten cases squamous cell carcinoma (two with moderate differentiation, six medium grade differentiation and two without missing cornification grading), in five cases undifferentiated carcinoma and in five cases others (melanoma, bronchial cell carcinoma, thyroid cancer, or muciferous carcinoma). With no or only oral contrast administration in 22 patients, the detection rate was higher for PET (45.5%) and CT (22.7%) compared to 13 patients who received intravenous contrast agent (PET 38.5% and CT 15.4%).

4.3.6 Benefit in Diagnosis for All Lesions by Fusion of CT and PET

Taking into account all 260 lesions after fusion of PET and CT images, 58 lesions found in CT and 27 lesions found in PET had to be reclassified. The results of reclassifying are presented for the two acquisition modes separately: no/oral contrast agent vs intravenous contrast agent. With no or only oral administration of contrast agent, mainly the equivocal findings in CT (18%) had to be reclassified in malignant lesions, but they were reduced to 8% with administration of intravenous contrast agent (Table 4.3). The equivocal findings in PET (5%) had to be reclassified as benign findings when no or only oral administration of contrast agent was administrated, but in return there

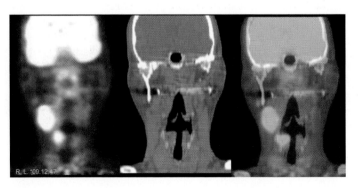

Fig. 4.2. Patient with CUP. Two hot spots without anatomical relation in PET (*left*) and no finding in CT (*middle*). Fusion of PET and CT (*right*) shows location of lymph node level III on right side of the larynx. Histological finding after PET/CT and endoscopy proved diagnosis of laryngeal cancer

Table 4.3. Reclassification of findings in PET and CT due to diagnosis by image fusion (PET/CT) by histological findings compared to cases with no or only oral contrast agent administration vs. intravenous contrast agent administration

Change of finding	No/oral contrast		IV contrast	
	No. of findings	%	No. of findings	%
CT equivocal → CT malignant	27	18	8	8
CT equivocal → CT benign	4	3	5	5
CT malignant → CT benign	2	1	4	4
CT no evidence → CT malignant	2	1	6	6
Total	**35**	**23**	**23**	**23**
PET equivocal → PET malignant	0	0	0	0
PET equivocal → PET benign	7	5	5	5
PET malignant → PET benign	3	2	8	8
PET no evidence → PET malignant	3	2	1	1
Total	**13**	**9**	**14**	**14**

was an increasing percentage of changes from malignant to benign tumors (Table 4.3).

The administration of iodinated contrast agent had no influence on the sensitivity in PET (95%), but led to a reduction of specificity from 65% to 50% (Fig. 4.3), although the accuracy was reduced only marginally from 90% to 88%. For CT, the administration of iodinated contrast agent yielded improved sensitivity (from 80% to 93%), specificity (from 76% to 80%) and accuracy (from 79% to 90%). For fused PET/CT images, the administration of iodinated contrast agent had no influence on sensitivity (96%), specificity was improved (from 78% to 82%) and the accuracy was nearly unchanged (from 92% to 93%) (Fig. 4.3).

4.4 Discussion

The accuracy and usefulness of FDG-PET in patients with head and neck tumors presented in the literature can be confirmed by our results, with recent published data demonstrating sensitivities between 81% and 98% for primary tumors and between 83% and 100% for recurrent tumors with FDG-PET [5, 8–10, 23–25, 31, 32, 34, 37, 40, 42, 46, 48]. In our patient population, the sensitivity of 94.7% for primary tumors and 100% for recurrent tumors lies in the upper range. On the other hand, lesions with inflammatory processes adversely affected the low specificity of FDG-PET in our patient population. For CT, the sensitivity for detecting primary (61.8%) and recurrent tumors (53.9%) was lower than for PET, in accordance with other recent studies, with specificity between 52% and 88% for primary tumors and 52% and 86% for recurrent tumors [5, 8–10, 23, 31, 32, 34, 42]. With image fusion, the sensitivity was enhanced to 97.4% and the rate of false positive findings in PET was reduced, resulting in an increased specificity for combined PET/CT of 42.9%. This can be compared to the only published study by Zimmer et al. [50] where a sensitivity of 95% and specificity of 60% was reported for recurrent head and neck cancer with image-fused PET/CT.

Our rate (42.8%) for detecting a primary tumor in patients with CUP on FDG-PET lies in the upper range (9%–50%), which has been reported in other recent studies [1, 5, 6, 8, 17–19, 21, 27, 35, 37, 45], but there are also two out-

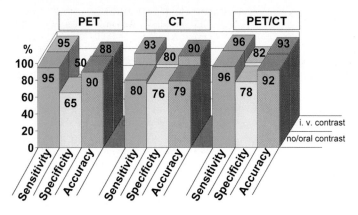

Fig. 4.3. Final results of sensitivity, specificity and accuracy for 245 lesions in 85 patients with head and neck tumors in the acquisition mode with no or only oral contrast agent and administration of intravenous contrast agent

standing results with detection rates of 75% reported by Kresnik et al. [22] in 15 CUP patients and by Pöpperl et al. [34] in four CUP patients with FDG-PET. In our patient population with CT alone, the detection rate was lower and CT did not contribute to the sensitivity in combined PET/CT as found in other studies [8, 14, 22, 34, 37, 41]. In contrast to these results, there are some studies with combined PET/CT which show an improvement in the detection rate between 57% and 75% [14, 30, 34]. Our results show, however, that CT is helpful in anatomic localisation of PET findings, as mentioned in other studies [30, 41]. Given the small number of samples, it seems that the administration of intravenous contrast agent exerts a negative influence on detection of primary tumors in patients with CUP, but a higher number of patients with enhanced CT scans will be needed to establish greater precision.

By fusing PET and CT images, the interpretation of all findings is improved compared to PET or CT alone. The benefit is a reduction in the number of discordant findings from 33.8% to 5.8% of all lesions. This compares well with results from Schöder et al. who found that PET/CT had an effect on patient care in 18% of 68 patients [41]. Statistical significance is presented for all lesions with an improvement in sensitivity, specificity and accuracy with combined PET/CT compared to PET or CT alone (Fig. 4.3). Similar results have been found by other authors who used combined PET/CT (Table 4.4) [2, 3, 16, 41, 43]. The benefit from fused images is highest compared to CT, particularly without intravenous administration of iodinated contrast agent. With administration of intravenous contrast agent, the accuracy of CT imaging increases, but this reduces the significance of PET, which can be explained

Table 4.4. Overall findings for head and neck tumors. Comparison of performance with FDG-PET, CT and combined PET/CT in recent studies which used combined PET/CT (references in square brackets)

	PET	CT	PET/CT
Sensitivity (%)	87 [3]	74–91 [3, 43]	96–100 [2, 8, 16, 41]
Specificity (%)	91 [3]	75–98.5 [3, 43]	77–98.5 [2, 3, 16, 43]
Accuracy (%)	90 [3, 41]	74 [3]	88–96 [3, 16, 41]

by overcorrection of attenuation due to CT/x-rays [7, 29]. On the other hand, intravenous contrast agents may substantially enhance the CT image quality and the significance of image interpretation in the head and neck [20]. With the exception of demonstrating mediastinal nodes, enhanced CT is estimated not to be statistically significant in the outcome of standard uptake values [15, 47]. For head and neck tumors, it can be concluded from our results that there is no significant improvement in sensitivity and accuracy when using enhanced CT for combined PET/CT.

4.5 Conclusion

With combined PET/CT as a simultaneous investigation with FDG, PET and CT, we are able to provide reliable diagnoses in head and neck cancer in approximately 94% of all lesions and roughly 90% of all affected patients. Approximately 97% of all primary malignant tumors and all recurrent tumors can be detected. PET/CT has a great impact, especially on the follow-up of affected patients, since morphological evaluation after surgery or radiation therapy may be highly complicated. Combined PET/CT with image fusion is highly recommended in evaluating patients with head and neck cancer. For combined PET/CT, the significance of enhanced CT with intravenous administration of an iodinated agent is only marginal compared to native CT scans or administration of only oral contrast agent.

References

1. Alberini JL, Belhocine T, Hustinx R, Daenen F, Rigo P (2003) Whole-body positron emission tomography using fluorodeoxyglucose in patients with metastases of unknown primary tumors (CUP syndrome). Nucl Med Commun 24:1081–1086
2. Babin E, Hamon M, Benateau H, Desmonts C, Comoz F, Goullet de Rugy M, Bequignon A, Chesnay E (2004) Interest of PET/CT scan fusion to assess mandible involvement in oral cavity and oropharyngeal carcinomas. Ann Otolaryngol Chir Cervicofac 121:235–240
3. Branstetter BF 4th, Blodgett TM, Zimmer LA, Snyderman CH, Johnson JT, Raman S, Meltzer CC (2005) Head and neck malignancy: is PET/CT more accurate than PET or CT alone? Radiology 235:580–586
4. Canto MT, Devesa SS (2002): Oral cavity and pharynx cancer incidence rates in the United States, 1975–1998. Oral Oncol 38:610–617
5. Bender H, Straehler-Pohl HJ (1999) In Wieler HJ (ed) PET in der klinischen Onkologie. Steinkopff, Darmstadt, pp 133–147
6. Bohuslavizki KH, Klutmann S, Kroger S, Sonnemann U, Buchert R, Werner JA, Mester J, Clausen M (2000) FDG PET detection of unknown primary tumors. J Nucl Med 41:816–822
7. Bokisch A, Beyer T, Antoch G, Freudenberg LS, Kuhl H, Debattin JF, Muller SP (2004) Positron emission tomography/computed tomography – imaging protocols, artifacts, and pitfalls. Mol Imaging Biol 6:188–199
8. Bruschini P, Giorgetti A, Bruschini L, Nacci A, Volterrani D, Cosottini M, Ursino F, Mariani G, Fattori B (2003) Positron emission tomography (PET) in the staging of head and neck cancer: comparison between PET and CT. Acta Otorhinolarnygol Ital 223:446–453
9. Dresel S, Schwenzer K, Brinkbaumer K, Schmid R, Szeimies U, Popperl G, Hahn K (2001) [[F-18]FDG imaging of head and neck tumors: comparison of hybrid PET, dedicated PET and CT. Nuklearmedizin 40:172–178
10. Dresel S, Grammerstorff J, Schwenzer K, Brinkbaumer K, Schmid R, Pfluger T, Hahn K (2003) [18F]FDG imaging of head and neck tumors: comparison of hybrid PET and morphological methods. Eur J Nucl Med Mol Imaging 30:995–1003
11. Eakin R (2001) Head and neck cancer. In: Spence RAJ, Johnston PG (eds) Oncology. Oxford University Press, Oxford, pp 191–208
12. Edwards D (1997) Face to Face. King's Fund, London
13. Forastiere A, Koch W, Trotti A, Sidransky D (2001) Head and neck cancer. N Engl J Med 346:1890–1900
14. Freudenberg LS, Fischer M, Antoch G, Jentzen W, Gutzeit A, Rosenbaum SJ, Bockisch A, Egelhof T (2005) Dual modality of 18F-fluorodeoxyglucose-positron emission tomography/computed tomography in patients with cervical carcinoma of unknown primary Med Princ Pract 14:155–160
15. Goerres GW, von Schulthess GK, Steinert HC (2004) Why most PET of lung and head and neck cancer will be PET CT. J Nucl Med 45[Suppl 1]:66s–71s
16. Goshen E, Davidson T, Yahalom R, Talmi YP, Zwas ST (2006) PET/CT in the evaluation of patients with squamous cell cancer of the head and neck. Int J Oral Maxillofac Surg 35:332–336
17. Haas I, Hoffmann TK, Engers R, Ganzer U (2002) Diagnostic strategies in cervical carcinoma of an unknown primary (CUP). Eur Arch Otorhinolaryngol 259:325–333

18. Johansen J, Eigtved A, Buchwald C, Theilgaard SA, Hansen HS (2002) Implication of ^{18}F-fluoro-2-deoxy-D-glucose positron emission tomography on management of carcinoma of unknown primary in the head and neck: a Danish cohort study. Laryngoscope 112:2009–2014

19. Jungehulsing M, Scheidhauer K, Damm M, Pietrzyk U, Eckel H, Schicha H, Stennert E (2000) 2[F]-fluoro-2-deoxy-D-glucose positron emission tomography is a sensitive tool for the detection of occult primary cancer (carcinoma of unknown primary syndrome) with head and neck lymph node manifestation. Otolaryngol Head Neck Surg 123:294–301

20. Keberle M, Tschammler A, Berning K, Hahn D (2001) Spiral CT of the neck: when do neck malignancies delineate best during contrast enhancement? Eur Radiol 11:1986–1990

21. Kole AC, Nieweg OE, Pruim J, Hoekstra HJ, Koops HS, Roodenburg JL, Vaalburg W, Vermey A (1998) Detection of unknown occult primary tumors using positron emission tomography. Cancer 82:1160–1166

22. Kresnik E, Mikosch P, Gallowitsch HJ, Kogler D, Wiesser S, Heinisch M, Unterweger O, raunik W, Kumnig G, Gomez I, Grunbacher G, Lind P (2001) Evaluation of head and neck cancer with ^{18}F-FDG PET: a comparison with conventional methods. Eur J Nucl Med 28:816–821

23. Kunkel M, Forster GJ, Reichert TE, Jeong JH, Benz P, Bartenstein P, Wagner W, Whiteside TL (2003) Detection of recurrent oral squamous cell carcinoma by [^{18}F]-2-fluorodeoxyglucose-positron emission tomography: implications for prognosis and patient management. Cancer 98:2257–2265

24. Lapela M, Eigtved A, Jyrkkio S, Grenman R, Kurki T, Lindholm P, Nuutinen J, Sutinen E, Solin O, Bjornskov I, Bretlau P, Friberg L, Holm S, Jensen M, Sand Hansen H, Minn H (2000) Experience in qualitative and quantitative FDG PET in follow-up of patients with suspected recurrence from head and neck cancer. Eur J Cancer 36:858–867

25. Li P, Zhuang H, Mozley PD, Denittis A, Yeh D, Machtay M, Smith R, Alavi A (2001) Evaluation of recurrent squamous cell carcinoma of the head and neck with FDG positron emission tomography. Clin Nucl Med 26:131–135

26. Lowe VJ, Boyd JH, Dunphy FR, Kim H, Dunleavy T, Collins BT, Martin D, Stack BC Jr, Hollenbeak C, Fletcher JW (2000) Surveillance for recurrent head and neck cancer using positron emission tomography. J Clin Oncol 18:651–658

27. Mantaga, P, Baum RP, Hertel A, Adams S, Niessen A, Sengupta S, Hor G (2003) PET with 2-[F-18]-fluoro-2-deoxy-D-glucose (FDG) in patients with cancer of unknown primary (CUP): influence on patients' diagnostic and therapeutic management. Cancer Biother Radiopharm 18:47–58

28. Menda Y, Grha, MM (2005) Update on F-18- Fluorodeoxyglucose/positron emission tomography and positron emission tomographay/computed tomography imaging of squamous head and neck cancers. Semin Nucl Med 35:214–219

29. Nakamoto Y, Chin BB, Kraitchman DL, Lawler LP, Marshall LT, Wahl RL (2003) Effects of nonionic intravenous contrast agents at PET/CT imaging: phantom and canine studies. Radiology 227:817–824.

30. Nanni C, Rubello D, Castellucci P, Farsad M, Franchi R, Toso S, Barile C, Rampin L, Nibale O, Fanti S (2005) Role of 18F-FDG PET-CT imaging for the detection of an unknown primary tumor: preliminary results in 21 patients. Eur J Nucl Med Mol Imaging 32:589–592

31. Ng SH, Yen TC, Liao CT, Chang JT, Chan SC, Ko SF, Wang HM, Wong HF (2005) ^{18}F-FDG PET and CT/MRI in oral cavity squamous cell carcinoma: a prospective study of 124 patients with histologic correlation. J Nucl Med 46:1136–143

32. Nowak B, Di Martino E, Janicke S, Cremerius U, Adam G, Zimny M, Reinartz P, Bull U (1999) Diagnostic evaluation of malignant head and neck cancer by F-18-FDG PET compared to CT/MRI. Nuklearmedizin 38:312–318

33. Otto, S. Oncology Nursing . 4th ed. London: Mosby; 2001

34. Pöpperl G, Lang S, Dagdelen O, Jager L, Tiling R, Hahn K, Tatsch K (2002) Correlation of FDG-PET and MRI/CT with histopathology in primary diagnosis, lymph node staging and diagnosis of recurrence of head and neck cancer. Fortschr Röntgenstr 174:714–720

35. Regelink G, Brouwer J, de Bree R, Pruim J, van der Laan BF, Vaalburg W, Hoekstra OS, Comans EF, Vissink A, Leemans CR, Roodenburg JL (2002) Detection of unknown primary tumors and distant metastases in patients with cervical metastases: value of FDG-PET versus conventional modalities. Eur J Nucl Med Mol Imaging 29:1024–1030

36 Reske SN, Kotzerke J (2001) FDG-PET for clinical use. Eur J Med 28:1707–1723

37. Reske SN, Dankerl A, Glatting G, Mottaghy FM, Blumstein NM (2004) Stellenwert der PET bei Kopf-Hals-Tumoren. Laryngorhinootologie 83:391–406

38 Schantz SP, Harrison LB, Forastiere AA (1996) Tumors of the nasal cavity and paranasal sinuses, nasopharynx, oral cavity and oropharynx. In: De Vita VT, Hellmann S, Rosenberg SA (eds): Cancer, principles and practice of oncology. Lippincott-Raven, NewYork, pp 741–801

39. Schantz SP, Yu G (2002) Head and neck cancer incidence trends in Young Americans, 1973–1997, with a special analysis for tongue cancer. Arch Otolaryngol Head Neck Surg 128:268–274

40. Schmidt M, Schmalenbach M, Jungehulsing M, Theissen P, Dietlein M, Schroder U, Eschner W, Stennert E, Schicha H (2004) ^{18}F-FDG PET for detecting recurrent head and neck cancer, local lymph node involvement and distant metastases. Comparison of qualitative visual and semiquantitative analysis. Nuklearmedizin 43:91–101

41. Schöder H, Yeung HW, Gonen M, Kraus D, Larson SM (2004) Head and neck cancer: clinical usefulness

and accuracy of PET/CT image fusion. Radiology 231:65–72

42. Schöder H, Yeung HW (2004) Positron emission imaging of head and neck cancer, including thyroid carcinoma. Semin Nucl Med 34:180–97

43. Schwartz DL, Ford E, Rajendran J, Yueh B, Coltrera MD, Virgin J, Anzai Y, Haynor D, Lewellyn B, Mattes D, Meyer J, Phillips M, Leblanc M, Kinahan P, Krohn K, Eary J, Laramore GE (2005) FDG-PET/CT imaging for preradiotherapy staging of head-and-neck squamous cell carcinoma. Int J Radiat Oncol Biol Phys 61:129–136

44. Spence RAJ, Johnston PG (2001) Oncology. Oxford University Press, Oxford

45. Stoeckli SJ, Mosna-Firlejczyk K, Goerres GW (2003) Lymph node metastasis of squamous cell carcinoma from an unknown primary: impact of positron emission tomography. Eur J Nucl Med Mol Imaging 30:411–416

46. Wong RJ, Lin DT, Schoder H, Patel SG, Gonen M, Wolden S, Pfister DG, Shah JP, Larson SM, Kraus DH (2002) Diagnostic and prognostic value of [^{18}F]fluorodeoxyglucose positron emission tomography for recurrent head and neck squamous cell carcinoma. J Clin Oncol 20:4199–4208

47. Yau YY, Chan WS, Tam YM, Vernon P, Wong S, Coel M, Chu SK (2005) Application of intravenous contrast in PET/CT: does it really introduce significant attenuation correction error? J Nucl Med 46:283–291

48. Yen TC, Chang YC, Chan SC, Chang JT, Hsu CH, Lin KJ, Lin WJ, Fu YK, Ng SH (2005) Are dual-phase ^{18}F-FDG PET scans necessary in nasopharyngeal carcinoma to assess the primary tumor and loco-regional nodes? Eur J Nucl Med Mol Imaging 32:541–548

49. Yeole BB, Sankaranarayanan R, Sunny L, Swaminathan R, Parkin DM (2000) Survival from head and neck cancer in Mumbai (Bombay), India. Am Cancer Soc 89:437–444

50. Zimmer LA, Snyderman C, Fukui MB, Blodgett T, McCook B, Townsend DW, Meltzer CC (2005) The use of combined PET/CT for localizing recurrent head and neck cancer: the Pittsburgh experience. Ear Nose Throat J 84:108–110

5 PET and PET/CT in Thyroid Cancer

H. Palmedo and M. Wolff

Recent Results in Cancer Research, Vol. 170
© Springer-Verlag Berlin Heidelberg 2008

5.1 Background

Thyroid cancer can be divided into three main groups: tumors with follicle cell differentiation (differentiated thyroid cancer), tumors with C-cell differentiation (medullary thyroid cancer), and anaplastic carcinomas. The insular carcinoma takes an intermediate place between differentiated and anaplastic cancer. Within the category of differentiated cancers, a distinction is made between papillary and follicular tumors. Papillary tumors are found most frequently and several subtypes are defined referring to tumor capsule invasion, the extent of invasion, the presence of sclerosis and oncocytic or oxyphil cells. The last subtype is also called Hürthle-cell carcinoma and is of critical importance because iodine uptake is often low or completely missing. C-cell cancer can develop spontaneously or be genetically determined as familial medullary cancer or in a multiple endocrine neoplasia (MEN-2a/MEN-2b).

Differentiated thyroid cancer (DTC) occurs in three to five per 100,000 inhabitants and represents about 1% of all malignant tumors [33]. Incidence increases with age, as shown in autopsy studies, with rates of occult thyroid cancer in up to 35% of cases. This might be explained by the biological behavior of DTC known to be a very slowly growing tumor entity. An absolute increase of DTC is observed after ionizing radiation of the thyroid during childhood. Whether an increased iodine sup-

ply leads to a higher rate of DTC is not clear. However, there is a relative shift in histological findings from follicular to more frequent papillary cancers after better iodine supply.

Important prognostic factors are age, tumor stage, and histopathological grading. The TNM classification according to the recommendations of the International Union Against Cancer/Union Internationale Contre le Cancer (UICC) [32] is given in Table 5.1. Histopathological grading is based on the evaluation of nuclear atypia, the extent of necrosis, and vascular invasion [1]. Follicular carcinomas generally exhibit more frequent distant metastases in the lungs and bones than papillary cancers. These tend to spread in the cervical and mediastinal regional lymph nodes, a stage that most authors, in contrast to other tumors, consider not to be associated with a poorer prognosis for the group of differentiated tumors. In most cases, prognosis is favorable [10]. However, there are marked differences depending on the tumor type. It has been shown that the 10-year survival rate for papillary, follicular, insular and anaplastic thyroid cancer is 89%, 68%, 20%, and 2%, respectively. The 10-year survival rate for non-hereditary medullary cancer lies between 50% and 70%. These survival rates demonstrate the prognostic value of the histologic diagnosis.

For clinical purposes, different staging systems have been developed to divide patients into low- and high-risk cases. For differentiated (papillary and follicular) thyroid cancer,

Table 5.1. TNM classification of thyroid cancer

pTX	Primary tumor is not assessable
pT0	No evidence of primary tumor
pT1	Tumor < 2 cm, limited to the thyroid
pT2	Tumor > 2 cm and < 4 cm, limited to the thyroid
pT3	Tumor > 4 cm, limited to the thyroid or any tumor with minimal extrathyroid extension (e.g., extension to sternothyroid muscle or perithyroid soft tissue)
pT4a	Tumor extends over the thyroid capsule and invades any of the following structures: subcutaneous soft tissue, larynx, trachea, esophagus, recurrent laryngeal nerve
pT4b	Tumor invades prevertebral fascia, mediastinal vessels, or encases carotid artery
pNX	Regional lymph nodes cannot be assessed
pN0	No regional lymph node metastasis
pN1a	Lymph node metastasis of the central compartment
pN1b	Lymph node metastasis of the ipsilateral or contralateral cervical compartment, mediastinal lymph node metastasis
pMX	Distant metastasis cannot be assessed
pM0	No distant metastasis
pM1	Distant metastasis

a widely accepted system is the already mentioned TNM-based concept of the UICC that is shown in Table 5.2. It was demonstrated that age is one of the most important prognostic factors. Therefore, in this staging system, patients are grouped in a section with either below or equal/over 45 years. Surprisingly, patients under 45 years of age enjoy the favorable status of stage II even when distant metastases are present. This results from the experience that pulmonary metastatic disease is curable by high-dose iodine therapy in younger patients. Especially in younger patients with diffuse

pulmonary spread which can be visualized by scintigraphy but not by radiography or CT of the chest [19], prognosis is still good when sufficient iodine uptake is present. The 10-year survival for stage II patients is estimated at a level of 87%. However, it must be mentioned that some of these patients might demonstrate recurrent pulmonary disease even after a time interval of 20 years. Furthermore, patients with bone metastases cannot be cured but stabilized over a long period. Bone metastases are a rare finding in differentiated thyroid cancer and are more frequently found in less differentiated cancers.

The prognostic relevance of lymph node metastases is an issue of discussion because some studies have shown a prognostic relevance of lymph nodes but others have not. However, it seems to be generally accepted that lymphatic disease is of low prognostic impact at least in patients with differentiated thyroid cancer aged under 45 years. In patients over 45 years, the presence of pre- and peritracheal (cervicocentral, N1a) and cervicolateral or mediastinal (N1b) lymph node metastases is grouped as stage III and stage IVa in the UICC system, indicating a higher risk. This is especially true

Table 5.2. TNM stage classification for differentiated thyroid cancer

Stage	< 45 years	DTC > 45 years or medullary cancer
I	Any T, any N, M0	T1 N0 M0
II	Any T, any N, M1	T2 N0 M0
III	–	T3 N0 M0 or T1–3 N1a M0
IV	–	T1–3 N1b M0 or T4 any N M0 or any T any N M1

for medullary thyroid cancer. The 10-year survival rate of stages I, II, III, and IV is estimated at a level of approximately 98%, 87%, 65%, and 31%, respectively.

In patients older than 45 years, the size of the tumor also presents a significant risk factor. In particular, the infiltration of the thyroid capsule and invasive growth in the surrounding tissue with angioinvasion is of relevant prognostic significance leading to a stage IV diagnosis. Finally, patients over 45 years bearing distant metastases are also grouped into stage IV with the worst prognosis. The criteria of this over-45-years section can also applied to the entity of medullary thyroid cancer. There are other scoring systems for differentiated thyroid cancer such as the EORTC, the AMES or the AGES scoring systems. In these systems, age, tumor grading, invasion of perithyroid tissue, and the presence of distant metastases are taken into account as the major prognostic factors.

In the primary diagnosis of thyroid cancer, the standard procedures, besides physical examination, are sonography, scintigraphy, and fine needle aspiration cytology. In a region with a high prevalence of multinodular goitre like Germany, often all three mentioned diagnostic modalities are used. Sonography can identify nodules with hypoechogenicity. However, the positive predictive value is only 10%–20%. In nodules larger than 1 cm, scintigraphy is recommended to rule out autonomously functioning tissue. It is known that scintigraphically cold nodules indicate an increased risk of having thyroid cancer in comparison with hot nodules. However, this risk is only 5%–10%, meaning that 90% of these patients have benign lesions. Therefore, fine needle aspiration (FNA) cytology is needed to further specify thyroid nodules. Sensitivity and specificity of FNA lies in the range of 30%–90% and 70%–90%, respectively. One major limitation of FNA is that a malignant tumor cannot be ruled out in case of a negative cytology. Therefore, multiple prognostic and diagnostic factors are taken into account in deciding whether the patient must be operated on. In most patients, the histological results by operative resection of the thyroid are necessary before the diagnosis

of thyroid cancer can be made. FDG-PET does not play a role in the preoperative work-up of patients suspected of having thyroid cancer. However, it should be kept in mind that a focal FDG accumulation in a thyroid nodule demonstrated a risk of up to 60% for the presence of thyroid cancer in some studies.

If thyroid cancer is present total thyroidectomy is the treatment of choice [28]. One exception is the highly differentiated papillary cancers of stage pT1 N0 M0. In this case, hemithyroidectomy is considered sufficient as a complete treatment. Generally, lymph node dissection of the central compartment completes the procedure. If additional lymph node metastases are suspected in patients with differentiated cancers, lateral lymph node dissection, in most cases a modified neck dissection, on the tumor side and possibly also on the contralateral side is performed. In medullary cancers, lateral neck dissection of at least one side is necessary. In patients with anaplastic cancers, palliative resection of tumor tissue under palliative aspects is the therapy of choice.

In differentiated carcinomas, the aim of total thyroidectomy is not only to remove tumor tissue (that might show multifocal growth) but also to create the optimal preconditions for the following treatment with radioiodine. Except for the above-mentioned unifocal, papillary T1 tumors, all patients receive iodine-131 at a dosage of 30–100 mCi (1.1–3.7 GBq), which is called ablative radioiodine therapy. One aim is to destroy the remaining malignant tumor cells. Another goal is the total elimination of normal thyroid tissue so as to optimize patient follow-up. During therapy, whole body scintigraphy with I-131 is performed for staging purposes.

The therapeutic effect of iodine-131 is based on the emission of electrons with a maximal energy of 0.61 MeV. Provided that the uptake mechanism via sodium-iodine symporter into the cell is intact, iodine-131 leads to a relatively homogenous radiation dose within the follicles and their cells. Since the mean range of electrons is below 1 mm, the surrounding tissue is not exposed to a significant radiation dose. Gamma radiation of iodine-131 is used to perform whole-body scintigraphy 3–6 days after I-131 application. This way the amount of remnant thyroid tissue can be determined. Furthermore, the presence of iodine-positive metastases can be excluded or confirmed. Radioiodine therapy should be performed at maximal TSH-stimulation, with a value generally greater than 30 mU/l. This is generally achieved by withdrawal of thyroid hormones for 4 weeks before the application of the activity. In patients with metastatic disease, such as pulmonary metastases that have a residual hormone production, a lower TSH value must be accepted. Pituitary insufficiency might also be a rare reason for low TSH values. Alternatively, recombinant TSH (rTSH) might be used instead of withdrawal of hormones. Two intramuscular injections of rTSH are given starting 2 days before iodine treatments. It seems that under rTSH, the maximal uptake is lower but the effective half-life is increased in comparison to withdrawal.

Generally, one or two treatments of radioiodine (at an interval of 3 months) are sufficient to eliminate the remnant thyroid tissue. Additionally, the thyroglobulin value should be below 1 ng/ml under TSH stimulation. This is one of the main therapy goals of ablative radioiodine therapy resulting in the optimal preparation of the patients for the follow-up by TG measurements, sonography, and whole-body scintigraphy. Making the decision on whether another ablative radioiodine therapy is necessary also depends on the individual risk of the patient. Hürthle cell carcinomas are frequently not diagnosed by whole-body scintigraphy because their iodine uptake is very low or completely missing.

If metastatic disease is present higher activities with single doses up to 300 mCi (11.1 GBq) are administered [12]. Whether surgical intervention can reduce the volume of the tumor should be investigated, a procedure that should be favored because the radiation effect of radioiodine is better in smaller volumes. Small lymph node and pulmonary metastases can be very effectively treated with radioiodine therapy [19, 24] with curative intention. Tumors with tracheal infiltration or bone metastases do not have a curative treatment with radioiodine therapy, but stable disease for a longer time interval is achievable. Percutaneous irradiation should be preserved for inoperable tumors in the thyroid bed without radioiodine uptake or for metastases to bone that has a risk of fracturing. There is no evidence that prophylactic external beam irradiation is advantageous for patients with extended pT4 tumors. Chemotherapy can be proposed in patients with undifferentiated carcinomas or in patients with progression of multiple metastases after radioiodine therapy. A further option is treatment with radioiodine after application of retinoic acid for several weeks, aiming to redifferentiate tumor cells and to re-induce their ability to accumulate iodine [15]. Scintigraphically, in approximately one-third of cases after redifferentiation treatment, a new iodine accumulation in the tumor can be demonstrated. However, the following radioiodine therapy does not always lead to significant tumor reduction. The rate of response has been described at a level of roughly 30%.

5.2   FDG-PET

Since thyroid carcinomas are generally a slowly growing and well-differentiated tumor entity, they have the ability to take up iodine into the tumor cell via sodium-iodine symporter (NIS) and to subsequently perform organification. This mechanism is used to perform whole-body scintigraphy and therapy of local and distant tumor disease by application of radioactive iodine.

It is known that fluorine-18 deoxyglucose is accumulated in high concentration in tumor cells with low differentiation and marked proliferative activity. In this state of tremendous growth, the cell tries to compensate the missing delivery of energy by increasingly metabolizing glucose via glycolysis. Under hypoxemic conditions, which frequently occur in less differentiated tumors, a high amount of glucose is necessary to supply sufficient energy for the cell because without the aerobic metabolism in form of citrate cycle and respiratory chain, the energy gain per molecule glucose is very low.

As stated in the background section, prognosis of differentiated tyroid cancer is favorable and treatment consisting of primary surgery and ablative radioiodine administration achieves a 10-year survival rate between 80% and 90% [10]. However, there are subgroups of patients who demonstrate a less favorable course of disease with much lower survival rates. Besides the above-mentioned classic risk factors (e.g., age over 45 years, histopathological grading), poor radioiodine accumulation in the tumor is of prognostic relevance [1, 31]. Patients without sufficient radioiodine uptake in the tumor cells have a significantly lower survival rate if distant metastases are present.

Low expression of the sodium-iodine symporter seems to be one main reason for the lack of iodine uptake that may be present at primary diagnosis or that develops during the further course of disease [5]. Patients with differentiated thyroid cancer may have only iodine-negative tumor lesions or both iodine-negative and iodine-positive tumor tissue [13]. Consequently, the presence of iodine negative-tumor tissue decreases the accuracy of iodine scintigraphy, which is routinely used for staging and restaging patients. This can lead to the situation where tumor tissue is not detected by iodine scintigraphy and will remain without further treatment [14].

Positron emission tomography (PET) with FDG has been able to improve the diagnostic work-up of these patients with iodine-negative differentiated thyroid cancer [14]. Studies on the value of FDG-PET for differentiated thyroid cancer have concentrated on the cases where radioiodine scintigraphy is negative but metastatic spread is associated with an increase in thyroglobulin level or unclear morphological findings. It has been shown that FDG-PET is the most accurate method in this situation and sensitivities and specificities range between 85% and 94% [4, 8, 27, 36]. Advantages of FDG-PET over the currently used morphological imaging methods such as sonography, CT, and MRI are the whole-body imaging procedure and the fact that an anatomically altered situation after surgery, for example thyroidectomy or neck dissection, does not aggravate the interpretation of PET scans. For the detection of local disease, principally sonography is performed to detect enlarged lymph nodes and to look at the thyroid bed. However, it is difficult to diagnose tumor tissue in the operated thyroid bed and in soft tissue. Also, small lymph node metastases less than 1 cm and lymph node metastases located in the deeper cervical region can be easily missed by sonography. MRI can give additional information in some of these cases, but the limitations mentioned for sonography also exist. CT as a whole body technique is mainly performed without iodine-containing contrast agent because further radioiodine therapy might be necessary. This leads to a marked decrease in the diagnostic accuracy of CT. Many studies have shown that FDG-PET has a high sensitivity over 90% if a patient has a negative-iodine whole-body scintigraphy [7, 8, 14]. Interesting is the observation that a tumor lesion very often takes up either only radioiodine or only FDG. In one patient, both radioiodine-positive and FDG-positive tumor lesions can be present due to a varying differentiation grade of the lesions in comparison with the original tumor cell clone. Therefore, it is clear that the diagnostic information of iodine scintigraphy and of FDG-PET can complement each other and that, in special cases, both imaging modalities must be performed.

Other tumor-seeking agents that have been used instead of FDG are technetium-99m methoxyisobutylisonitrile (Tc-99m MIBI) and technetium-99m tetrofosmin [3, 9, 21]. These agents are single photon-emitting tracers and therefore, a gamma camera and the SPECT technique is used. Sensitivities of MIBI and tetrofosmin whole-body scintigraphy were described at a level between 80% and 90%. However, because of the better spatial resolution of PET (5 mm) in comparison with SPECT (10 mm), FDG-PET is recently favored. Another advantage of FDG-PET over tumor scintigraphy with MIBI is the trapping mechanism into the cell and the resulting plateau phase of FDG after injection that is not observed after MIBI injection [22].

Also in patients with medullary thyroid cancer, FDG-PET has been shown to be a sensitive method for the detection of local recurrence and metastases [2]. A multicentric trial has shown that sensitivity and specificity of FDG-PET in medullary thyroid cancer is about 80%. Sensitivity of PET did not depend on the level of calcitonin elevation. This means that tumor lesions can also be detected with good sensitivity in patients with slightly elevated calcitonin levels. In comparison with CT and MRI, PET showed better diagnostic accuracy.

The FDG-PET scan can be performed in the euthyroid as well as the hypothyroid state. However, the results of several studies have shown that more FDG-positive lesions are detected by PET if the patient is investigated under TSH stimulation. In comparison with TSH suppression, up to 30% of lesions and up to 20% of patients were FDG-positive only in the hypothyroid state in some studies [20, 34]. On the one hand, it is understandable that glucose metabolism of the tumor cell is increased by TSH-receptor stimulation leading to a higher detectability. On the other hand, hypothyroidism itself results in a reduced glucose metabolism throughout the organism [18]. However, thyroid tumor cells might not be affected in the same way as normal body cells are. In this situation, the application of recombinant TSH could be advantageous.

After radioiodine therapy or operative procedures, it is helpful to keep a time interval of 2 months until FDG-PET is performed. This will reduce the rate of false-positive findings. After FDG injection, the patient should be instructed not to talk and to rest in a relaxed position to avoid false-positive findings.

The indications for FDG-PET in thyroid cancer are shown in Table 5.3. In the year 2000, a German multidisciplinary consensus conference established the indications of FDG-PET for different tumor entities [25]. The indications were listed with a score from 1 to 4 (see Table 5.3). The most important indication for differentiated thyroid cancer, the 1a classification, is the case of a patient with a negative radioiodine scintigraphy in whom tumor recurrence or persisting tumor is suspected due to elevated thyroglobulin values and/or to an unclear or suspicious finding in anatomical imaging. Also in patients with positive radioiodine scintigraphy, FDG-PET can be performed (1b indication) because it is crucial to know if additional low differentiated tumor lesions are present that cannot be treated by radioiodine. In this type of patient, further treatment options such as surgical resection of the FDG-positive and iodine-negative tumor lesions must be considered. In patients with medullary thyroid cancer, FDG-PET can be helpful in individual cases in the pre- and postoperative situation when calcitonin or CEA levels are elevated and tumor recurrence is suspected. There is no indication for FDG-PET in the preoperative work-up of patients suspected of having thyroid cancer. Specificity and sensitivity in this situation are too low to justify its use.

5.3   PET/CT

Patients with differentiated thyroid cancer have a less favorable prognosis if radioiodine negative tumor tissue, especially in distant metastases, is present [26]. One major reason for this may be that these cancers are not detected by routine diagnostic work-up with I-131 scintigraphy and that they cannot be treated efficiently by radioiodine therapy. Therefore tumor cells will continue to grow undetected and the chance of cure decreases significantly. The presence of tumor tissue with no I-131 accumulation is suspected at the time of primary diagnosis if histopathology reveals the so-called Hürthle cell tumor. More often, the suspicion for iodine-negative tumor cells arises later during the course of disease after the ablative treatment with radioiodine has been completed. In this case, thyroglobulin level

Table 5.3. Indications for FDG-PET in thyroid cancer

Staging in radioiodine-negative lesions	1a
Staging in radioiodine-positive lesions	1b
Therapy monitoring	3
Differential diagnosis of primary tumor	4
Medullary thyroid cancer	3

re rising in spite of I-131 scintigraphy that aises no suspicions.

One limitation of FDG-PET, especially in the egion of the neck, is the possibility of false-ositive FDG accumulations leading to the diagnosis of lymph node metastases, for example, nd consequently to the potential scheduling of a futile operation [30]. It is known that ontumorous cervical muscular uptake and aryngeal accumulation can occur. Also physiological uptake in salivary glands, lymphatic issue of the oropharynx such as the base of he tongue or the thymus must be considered. These findings lower specificity of the imaging modality. Furthermore, a focal FDG-positive sion cannot be precisely localized because ET only contains rough anatomical information. However, the correlation of PET results with anatomical imaging is crucial to achieve maximal diagnostic accuracy and to be able to lan surgical interventions. New cameras have een developed integrating sensitive PET and igh-resolution spiral CT. These PET/CT cameras allow for image fusion in such a way that recise anatomical location of a FDG-positive sion is possible.

Integrated PET/CT might have advantages ver the diagnostic work-up by PET alone or by eparate PET and morphological imaging. We onducted a study in 40 patients hypothesizing hat the diagnostic accuracy of integrated PET/ T would be significantly higher than that of ET alone or of side-by-side PET and CT [23]. he more accurate definition of tumor location by PET/CT should also result in a better ecision in terms of therapy with an impact on atient management.

We investigated patients with a negative raioiodine whole-body scintigraphy who were suspected of having thyroid tumor tissue beause of elevated TG levels or morphological maging. FDG-PET/CT was performed under SH stimulation. Data analysis evaluated the iagnostic accuracy and the ability of localizing a lesion of PET alone, side-by-side PET and T, PET/CT (Table 5.4).

In our study, specificity for detecting lymph ode metastases could be increased by PET/CT comparison to PET alone and side-by-side ET and CT from 76% to 91%. Three patients

Table 5.4. Probabilities for the different imaging modalities (on a per-patient basis)

	PET	CT	Side-by-side	PET-CT
Sensitivity (%)	79	79	95	95
Specificity (%)	76	71	76	91
Positive predictive value (%)	75	71	78	86
Negative predictive value (%)	80	79	94	95
Accuracy (%)	78	75	85	93

(60% of the cervical false-positives) were identified by PET/CT as having a physiologic or nontumoral cervical FDG accumulation that was classified as lymph node metastases by PET alone and side-by-side PET and CT (Fig. 5.1).

Whereas sensitivity on a per-patient basis for lymph node metastasis detection was equal for PET and PET/CT, sensitivity for M-staging was increased from 84% to 100% by PET/CT. This was achieved by the detection of small and miliary lung metastases in three patients with PET/CT which were not diagnosed by PET alone. This confirms the findings of previous studies demonstrating that FDG-PET is not able to adequately assess miliary lung metastases smaller than 6 mm. It is not clear whether this is generated from motion artifacts by inhalation and exhalation or from a lower metabolic activity of the lung metastases [7].

One important aspect of our study was the evaluation of the therapeutic relevance of PET/CT. In clinical routine, treatment of differentiated thyroid cancer is dominated by the combination of surgical tumor removal and subsequently application of radioiodine [16]. Whereas this approach is almost optimal for patients with iodine-accumulating tumors, it is not appropriate if only iodine-negative tumors are present. In this case, complete surgical removal of iodine-negative tissue is the only curative treatment option. Furthermore, it seems important to diagnose and remove iodine-negative tumor tissue as early as possible because prognosis of this tumor subgroup is essentially worse than that of most differentiated

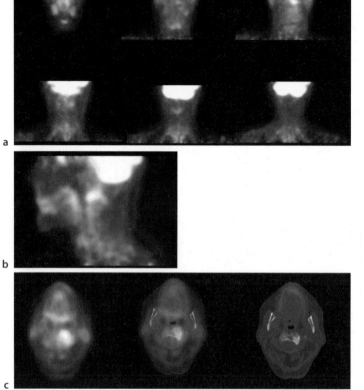

Fig. 5.1a–c. A 73-year-old patient with follicular thyroid cancer (with oxyphilic parts) pT2 at primary diagnosis. Eighteen months after thyroidectomy and ablative radioiodine therapy, the patient presented with slightly elevated Tg-level of 2 ng/ml and indeterminable lymph nodes at sonography. Coronal and sagittal PET slices (**a,b**) show a focal accumulation with suspected malignancy. PET/CT fusion image (**c**) shows that FDG uptake is caused by degenerative disease in the cervical vertebral column

thyroid cancers [26]. Therefore, it is crucial to be able to exactly localize an iodine-negative and FDG-PET-positive tumor to enhance complete resection and curing the patient [11, 29, 35, 37]. For this purpose, additional morphological imaging is necessary to help localize a FDG-positive focus.

To determine if PET/CT would be helpful in the afore-mentioned situation, we performed a second analysis comparing PET/CT results to a side-by-side interpretation of PET and CT images. This side-by-side interpretation revealed that 57% (73/127) of all scored lesions in different anatomical regions were discordant. One main reason for this is a positive PET finding without a corresponding CT finding, for example when the lymph nodes of the affected area are not enlarged or if CT images show an abnormality at a different anatomical region. In this situation, it is not possible to exactly localize the suspected tumor tissue for surgical resection. In our study, this situation was observed in 17 patients (74% of suspicious PET patients) in whom PET/CT could correctly localize the tumor as confirmed by histopathology and follow-up. In this group, three patients could be identified as having benign findings which prevented futile surgical treatment in all cases. In ten FDG-positive tumor patients, the surgical resection of iodine-negative tumor tissue was extended to additional regions after PET/CT truly identified the location of tumor lesions that were not localized by side-by-side PET and CT (Fig. 5.2). This resulted in an efficient tumor volume reduction by surgery (Tables 5.5, 5.6). If only standard lymph node resection of the lateral and central compartment of the neck had been performed in this group, a relevant amount of FDG-positive tumor tissue would have been unnecessarily left

Summarizing the results, integrated PET/CT hanged the treatment in 48% of patients with a rue positive FDG-PET finding. Additionally, an unnecessary operation was prevented in three patients. We consider these results as highly relevant for the therapeutic decision making of patients with thyroid cancer and, therefore, would recommend a diagnostic algorithm as shown in Figures 5.3 and 5.4. Thereafter, integrated PET/CT would be proposed in all patients in who iodine-negative tumor tissue is suspected. Alternatively, separated PET and CT could first be performed followed by integrated PET/CT only in cases with discordant findings.

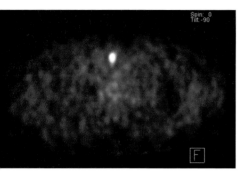

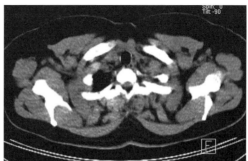

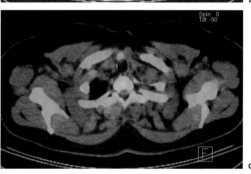

Fig. 5.2a–c. A 53-year-old patient with follicular thyroid cancer (pT3 N0 M0 after thyroidectomy and ablative radioiodine therapy) who presented with elevated TG-levels but negative sonography 2 years later (patient no. 6, Table 5.5). Whole-body scintigraphy with iodine was also negative. PET slices (a) show a focal accumulation indicating recurrence but CT slices (b) are not diagnostic. To localize the FDG focus preoperatively, PET/CT images were used showing that the recurrence must be in the right supraclavicular region (c). A wire-guided operation was performed and histology revealed 4-mm and 3-mm lymph node metastases (in direct vicinity to each other)

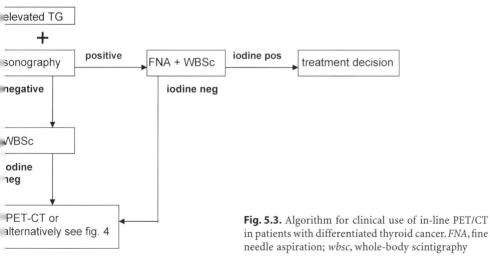

Fig. 5.3. Algorithm for clinical use of in-line PET/CT in patients with differentiated thyroid cancer. *FNA*, fine needle aspiration; *wbsc*, whole-body scintigraphy

Table 5.5. Data of ten PET- and tumor-positive patients in whom PET/CT led to a change in therapy (but not side by-side PET and CT) (from Palmedo [23] 2006)

Patient	PET	Therapy change by PET/CT	Histology
1	Cervical lateral left Lateral trachea	Wire-guided extension of surgery to retrotracheal	Lymph node metastasis cervical lateral Lymph node metastasis lateral trachea 5 mm
2	Supraclavicular left Supraclavicular right	Extension of surgery to supraclavicular right	Lymph node metastasis supraclavicular left Lymph node metastasis supraclavicular right 9 mm
3	Cervical lateral left Supraclavicular right and left Upper mediastinal	Extension of surgery to mediastinal and supracla- vicular right and left	Lymph node metastasis cervical Lymph node metastasis supraclavicular left and right Lymph node metastasis mediastinal 10 mm
4	Cervical left	Extension of surgery parapharyngeal	Lymph node metastasis cervical (1×9 mm)
5	Upper cervical right Lower cervical right Upper mediastinal	Extension of surgery to upper cervical and mediastinal	Lymph node metastasis upper cervical right Lymph node metastasis cervical r Lymph node metastasis mediastinal (8 mm)
6	Supraclavicular right	Wire-guided surgery, supraclavicular right	Lymph node metastasis supraclavicular right 3+4 mm
7	Cervical dorsal left	Extension of surgery to left neck	Lymph node metastasis left neck 6 mm
8	Cervical lateral right Lateral trachea	Extension of surgery, retrotracheal	Lymph node metastasis Lymph node metastasis lateral trachea
9	Supraclavicular left Lateral trachea	Extension of surgery, supraclavicular left	Lymph node metastasis supraclavicular left Local recurrence paratracheal
10	Mediastinal Lateral trachea	Extension of surgery, mediastinal	Lymph node metastasis mediastinal Local recurrence paratracheal

Table 5.6. Data of ten PET- and tumor-positive patients in whom PET/CT led to a change in therapy (but not side-by-side PET and CT) (from Palmedo 2006)

Patient	TG levels ng/ml Pre-/postoperative	Reduction of tumor volume
1	11.2/< 1.0	100%
2	5.6/< 1.0	100%
3	27.3/4.39	80%
4	16.7/6.2	80%
5	74/3.8	90%
6	3.3/< 1.0	100%
7	5.2/< 1.0	100%
8	2.9/< 1.0	100%
9	20.5/7.8	60%
10	167/25.9	50%

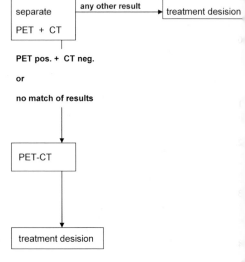

Fig. 5.4. Alternative imaging modality to PET/C referring to algorithm in Figure 5.3

References

1. Akslen LA (1993) Prognostic importance of histologic grading in papillary thyroid carcinoma. Cancer 72:2680–2685
2. Brandt-Mainz K, Muller SP, Gorges R, Saller B, Bockisch A (2000) The value of fluorine-18 fluorodeoxyglucose PET in patients with medullary thyroid cancer. Eur J Nucl Med 27:490–496
3. Briele B, Hotze A, Kropp J, Bockisch A, Overbeck B, Grunwald F, Kaiser W, Biersack HJ. A comparison of 201Tl and 99mTc-MIBI in the follow-up of differentiated thyroid carcinomas (in German). Nuklearmedizin 30:115–124
4. Chung JK, So Y, Lee JS et al (1999) Value of FDG PET in papillary thyroid carcinoma with negative I-131 whole-body scan. J Nucl Med 40:986–992
5. Dai G, Levy O, Carrasco N (1996) Cloning and characterization of the thyroid iodide transporter. Nature 379:458–460
6. Diehl M, Risse JH, Brandt-Mainz K, Dietlein M, Bohuslavizki KH, Matheja P, Lange H, Bredow J, Korber C, Grunwald F (2001) Fluorine-18 fluorodeoxyglucose positron emission tomography in medullary thyroid cancer: results of a multicentre study. Eur J Nucl Med 28:1671–1676
7. Dietlein M, Scheidhauer K, Voth E et al (1997) Fluorine-18 fluorodeoxyglucose positron emission tomography and iodine-131 whole-body scintigraphy in the follow-up of differentiated thyroid cancer. Eur J Nucl Med 24:1342–1348
8. Feine U, Lietzenmayer R, Hanke JP et al (1996) Fluorine-18-FDG and iodine-131-iodide uptake in thyroid cancer. J Nucl Med 37:1468–1472
9. Gallowitsch HJ, Kresnik E, Mikosch P, Pipam W, Gomez I, Lind P (1996) Tc-99m-tetrofosmin scintigraphy: an alternative scintigraphic method for following differentiated thyroid carcinoma–preliminary results. Nuklearmedizin 35:230–235
10. Gilliland FD, Hunt WC, Morris DM et al (1997) Prognostic factors for thyroid carcinoma. A population-based study of 15,698 cases from the Surveillance, Epidemiology and End Results (SEER) program 1973–1991. Cancer 79:564–573
11. Grebe SK, Hay ID (1996) Thyroid cancer nodal metastases: biologic significance and therapeutic considerations. Surg Oncol Clin N Am 5:43–63
12. Grünwald F, Ruhlmann J, Ammari B, Knopp R, Hotze A, Biersack HJ (1988) Experience with a high-dose therapy concept in metastatic differentiated thyroid cancer (in German). Nuklearmedizin 27:266–271
13. Grünwald F, Schomburg A, Bender H et al (1996) Fluorine-18 fluorodeoxyglucose positron emission tomography in the follow-up of differentiated thyroid cancer. Eur J Nucl Med 23:312–319
14. Grünwald F, Menzel C, Bender H et al (1997) Comparison of F-18 FDG-PET with iodine-131 and Tc-99m-sestamibi scintigraphy in differentiated thyroid cancer. Thyroid 7:327–335

15. Grünwald F, Menzel C, Bender H, Palmedo H, Otte R, Fimmers R, Risse J, Biersack HJ (1998) Redifferentiation therapy-induced radioiodine uptake in thyroid cancer. J Nucl Med 39:1903–1906
16. Hay ID, Grant CS, Bergstralh EJ et al (1998) Unilateral total lobectomy: is it sufficient surgical treatment for patients with AMES low-risk papillary thyroid carcinoma? Surgery 124:958–964
17. Lardinois D, Weder W, Hany TF, Kamel EM, Korom S, Seifert B, von Schulthess GK, Steinert HC (2003) Staging of non-small-cell lung cancer with integrated positron-emission tomography and computed tomography. N Engl J Med 348:2500–2507
18. Matthaei S, Trost B, Hamann A, Kausch C, Benecke H, Greten H, Hoppner W, Klein HH (1995) Effect of in vivo thyroid hormone status on insulin signalling and GLUT1 and GLUT4 glucose transport systems in rat adipocytes. J Endocrinol 144:347–357
19. Menzel C, Grunwald F, Schomburg A, Palmedo H, Bender H, Spath G, Biersack HJ (1996) "High-dose" radioiodine therapy in advanced differentiated thyroid carcinoma. J Nucl Med 37:1496–1503
20. Moog F, Linke R, Manthey N, Tiling R, Knesewitsch P, Tatsch K, Hahn K (2000) Influence of thyroid-stimulating hormone levels on uptake of FDG in recurrent and metastatic differentiated thyroid carcinoma. J Nucl Med 41:1989–1995
21. Nemec J, Nyvltova O, Blazek T, Vlcek P, Racek P, Novak Z, Preiningerova M, Hubackova M, Krizo M, Zimak J, Bilek R (1996) Positive thyroid cancer scintigraphy using technetium-99m methoxyisobutylisonitrile. Eur J Nucl Med 23:69–71
22. Palmedo H, Hensel J, Reinhardt M, Von Mallek D, Matthies A, Biersack HJ (2002) Breast cancer imaging with PET and SPECT agents: an in vivo comparison. Nucl Med Biol 29:809–815
23. Palmedo H, Bucerius J, Joe A, Strunk H, Hortling N, Meyka S, Roedel R, Wolff M, Wardelmann E, Biersack HJ, Jaeger U (2006) Integrated PET/CT in differentiated thyroid cancer: diagnostic accuracy and impact on patient management. J Nucl Med 47:616–624
24. Reiners C (1993) Radiojodtherapie – Indikation, Durchführung und Risiken. Dtsch Ärztebl 90:2217–2221
25. Reske SN, Kotzerke J (2001) FDG-PET for clinical use. Results of the 3rd German Interdisciplinary Consensus Conference, "Onko-PET III", 21 July and 19 September 2000. Eur J Nucl Med 28:1707–1723
26. Schlumberger M, Challeton C, De Vathaire F et al (1996) Radioactive iodine treatment and external radiotherapy for lung and bone metastases from thyroid carcinoma. J Nucl Med 37:598–605
27. Scott GC, Meier DA, Dickinson CZ (1995) Cervical lymph node metastasis of thyroid papillary carcinoma imaged with fluorine-18-FDG, technetium-99m-pertechnetate and iodine-131-sodium iodide. J Nucl Med 36:1843–1845
28. Simon D (1997) Von limitierter bis erweiterter Radikalität der Operation beim Schilddrüsenkarzinom.

In: Roth et al (eds) Klinische Onkologie. Huber, Bern, pp 347–357

29. Simon D, Goretzki PE, Witte J, Röher HD (1996) Incidence of regional recurrence guiding radicality in differentiated thyroid carcinoma. World J Surg 20:860–866

30. Sisson JC, Ackermann RJ, Meyer MA, Wahl RL (1993) Uptake of 18-fluoro-2-deoxy-D-glucose by thyroid cancer: implications for diagnosis and therapy. J Clin Endocrinol Metab 77:1090–1094

31. Sisson JC, Giordano TJ, Jamadar DA, Kazerooni EA, Shapiro B, Gross MD, Zempel SA, Spaulding SA (1996) 131-I treatment of micronodular pulmonary metastases from papillary thyroid carcinoma. Cancer 78:2184–2192

32. Sobin LH, Wittekind C (2002) TNM classification of malignant tumours, 6th edn. Wiley, New York, p 52

33. Stewart BW, Kleihues P (2003) Thyroid cancer. In: Stewart BW, Kleihues P (eds) World cancer report. IARC Press, Lyon, pp 257–260

34. Van Tol KM, Jager PL, Piers DA, Pruim J, de Vries EG, Dullaart RP, Links TP (2002) Better yield of (^{18})fluorodeoxyglucose-positron emission tomography in patients with metastatic differentiated thyroid carcinoma during thyrotropin stimulation. Thyroid 12:381–387

35. Vassilopoulou-Sellin R, Schultz PN, Haynie TP (1996) Clinical outcome of patients with papillary thyroid carcinoma who have recurrence after initial radioactive iodine therapy. Cancer 78:493–501

36. Wang W, Macapinlac H, Larson SM et al (1999) [^{18}F]-2-fluoro-2-deoxy-D-glucose positron emission tomography localizes residual thyroid cancer in patients with negative diagnostic (^{131})I whole body scans and elevated serum thyroglobulin levels. J Clin Endocrinol Metab 84:2291–2302

37. Wang W, Larson SM, Fazzari M et al (2000) Prognostic value of F-18 fluorodeoxyglucose positron emission tomographic scanning in patients with thyroid cancer. J Clin Endocrinol Metab 85:1107–1113

6 Esophageal Cancer

H. A. Wieder, A. Stahl, F. Lordick, and K. Ott

Recent Results in Cancer Research, Vol. 170
© Springer-Verlag Berlin Heidelberg 2008

6.1 Introduction

Esophageal cancer ranks among the ten most common malignancies in the world and is a frequent cause of cancer-related death. However, carcinomas of the esophagus are a heterogeneous group of tumors in terms of etiology, histopathology, and epidemiology. In the upper two-thirds of the esophagus squamous cell carcinomas (SCC) predominate, with alcohol and smoking being the main risk factors. Carcinomas of the distal esophagus/esophagogastric junction, on the other hand, are mostly adenocarcinomas. The primary etiological factors for adenocarcinomas are gastroesophageal reflux disease and obesity, whereas alcohol and smoking seem to play no major roles. Adenocarcinomas arise from metaplastic epithelial cells at the esophagogastric junction, which have been transformed into an intestinal type mucus layer in response to prolonged irritation from gastric juice. In Western countries, the incidence and prevalence of esophageal adenocarcinomas have increased since the past 25 years in parallel with a shift from SCCs to adenocarcinomas. Adenocarcinomas of the esophagus (-gastric junction, AEG) are among the carcinomas with the highest increase in incidence per year

Depending on the tumor stage, the available therapeutic approaches for esophageal cancer are endoscopic mucosal resection, primary esophagectomy, neoadjuvant or palliative chemotherapy/radiotherapy followed by surgery and palliative resection. Most of the therapeutic modalities are associated with substantial morbidity and mortality. Accurate pretherapeutic staging is crucial to select the appropriate type of therapy. The first step is to distinguish between patients with locoregional and systemic disease, because for patients with distant lymph node metastasis or organ metastasis there is no curative therapeutic approach available; these patients are candidates for palliative treatment regimens. After exclusion of distant metastasis, the choice of the therapeutic approach depends on the T-stage. In case of a localized stage (T1/T2) there is a high probability of complete (R0) resection. In these cases, patients are mostly offered primary esophagectomy as the most important and frequently only therapeutic procedure

Patients with T3 and T4 tumors may undergo preoperative chemotherapy or chemoradiotherapy. These therapy modalities have been introduced in an attempt to increase the rate of complete resections by downsizing the primary tumor in order to improve local tumor control and to prevent distant metastasis. However, so far, clinical trials have not shown any improvement in survival by preoperative chemotherapy compared with surgery alone. Nevertheless, numerous studies have found that patients undergoing neoadjuvant treatment and showing an objective tumor response have a better prognosis than those undergoing surgical treatment alone. The problem of neoadjuvant therapy is that only

30%–40% of the patients respond to preoperative chemotherapy. Sixty percent or even more undergo several months of toxic therapy without obvious benefit, which in turn may compromise overall survival due to delayed surgery, therapy-associated side effects, or even selection of biologically more aggressive tumor cells. In line with these considerations, in a neoadjuvant setting, prognosis for patients with nonresponding tumor seems to be even worse than for patients treated by surgery alone. Therefore, a diagnostic test that allows prediction of response is considered to be crucial for the use of preoperative chemotherapy in patients with esophageal cancer

For recurrent esophageal cancer, the available therapeutic approaches are radical and palliative re-resection, stenting, laser thermocoagulation, brachytherapy, chemotherapy, and/or radiotherapy. The choice of the specific therapeutic modality depends on the location and the extent of the recurrence. In 30% of patients, the recurrence is located in the prior surgical bed. However, the majority of the recurrences are distant metastasis, underlining the systemic character of the disease

6.2 Initial Staging

6.2.1 Primary Cancer and Regional Lymph Node Involvement

Several studies report a high sensitivity of FDG-PET for staging SCC and adenocarcinomas of the esophagus (Fig. 6.1). Detection rates for the primary tumor range from 69% to 100% [1–7]. In most studies, FDG-PET is more sensitive than CT. Rasanen et al. investigated 42 patients who had undergone FDG-PET and CT before esophagectomy [8]. They found that the primary tumor was correctly detected in 35 (83%) of 42 patients by FDG-PET and in 28 (67%) patients by CT. Furthermore, Heeren et al. reported that the primary tumor was visualized in 95% (70/74 patients) with FDG-PET but only in 84% (62/74 patients) with CT [7]. False negative FDG-PET findings in squamous cell carcinoma are often due to a small tumor size. This is a consequence of the limited spatial resolution of FDG-PET which is approximately 5–8 mm in studies of the chest or abdomen. A small percentage of adenocarcinomas shows a limited or absent FDG accumulation regard

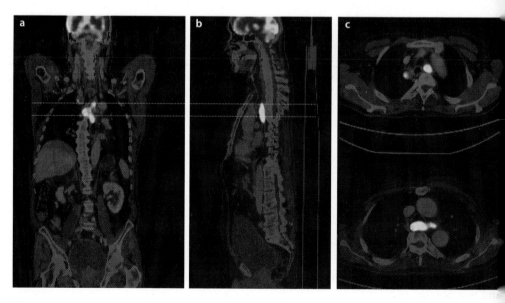

Fig. 6.1a–c. Coronal (a), sagittal (b), and axial (c) PET/CT fusion images of a patient with squamous cell carcinoma of the esophagus with multiple locoregional lymph node metastases. The primary tumor as well as lymph node metastases show a high FDG-uptake

ess of tumor size. This seems to be related to the growth type: limited or absent FDG-uptake has been found in diffusely growing and/or mucus producing subtypes

Locoregional lymph node metastasis is one of the most important prognostic factors in patients with esophageal cancer. Not only the number and location of regional metastatic lymph nodes, but also the lymph node size is predictive of the patient's outcome. Table 6.1 summarizes the results of studies evaluating the diagnostic accuracy of CT and FDG-PET for the detection of regional lymph node metastasis. Despite the importance of regional lymph node staging, noninvasive staging is still less than ideal for this purpose. Depending on the criteria used for detection of regional lymph node involvement, the values for sensitivity and specificity vary substantially between different studies

Table 6.1. Detection of patients with locoregional lymph-node metastasis with FDG-PET

Author	Year	Patients	Sensitivity	Specificity
Flamen et al.	2000	39	39%	97%
Lerut et al.	2000	42	22%	91%
Kim et al.	2001	53	52%	95%
Kato et al.	2002	32	78%	93%
Yoon et al.	2003	81	30%	82%
Heeren et al.	2004	74	55%	71%

In a meta-analysis, Westreenen et al. investigated 12 studies concerning the diagnostic accuracy of FDG-PET in staging locoregional lymph node status [9]. The pooled sensitivity and specificity of FDG-PET in detecting locoregional lymph node involvement was 51% and 84%, respectively

Flamen et al. prospectively studied 74 patients with esophageal cancer with regard to lymph node staging [3]. Endoscopic ultrasound (EUS) was more sensitive (81% vs 33%) but less specific (67% vs 89%) than FDG-PET for the detection of regional lymph node metastasis. Compared with the combined use of CT and EUS, FDG-PET had a higher specificity (98% vs 90%) and a similar sensitivity (43% vs 46%) for the assessment of regional and distant lymph node involvement. Choi et al. compared the diagnostic accuracy of FDG-PET and CT/EUS in 61 consecutive patients [10]. Forty-eight patients (13 excluded because of nonsurgical treatment) underwent transthoracic esophagectomy with lymph node dissection, with 382 lymph nodes dissected, 100 of which in 32 patients were malignant on histologic examination. On a patient basis, N-staging was correct in 83% of the patients on FDG-PET, whereas it was correct in 60% on CT and in 58% by using EUS (p < 0.05). However, in the neighborhood of the primary tumor, the authors report a low sensitivity of PET in detecting metastatic lymph nodes owing to the limited spatial resolution of the PET scanners and scatter effects arising from FDG accumulation in the primary tumor. In contrast to other tumor types, regional lymph node metastases in esophageal cancer are frequently located very close to the primary tumor making it difficult to differentiate lymph node metastasis from the primary tumor on FDG-PET

Lerut et al. prospectively included 42 patients in a staging study of esophageal carcinoma [11]. All patients underwent FDG-PET, CT, and EUS. For the diagnosis of regional lymph node metastasis FDG-PET was considered not useful because of a lack of sensitivity which was 22% compared to 83% for CT and EUS. The authors explain the low sensitivity of FDG-PET through difficulties in discriminating regional lymph nodes from the primary tumor

6.2.2 Distant Metastasis

CT of the chest and the abdomen currently present the standard noninvasive test for evaluating distant metastasis with a sensitivity of 37%–66%. However, CT is entirely dependent on structural characteristics for diagnosis. However, in esophageal cancer, metastatic involvement is often found in normal-sized nodes (limitations in diagnostic sensitivity) and, on the other hand, unspecific lymph node enlargement is commonly encountered in the cervical and mediastinal area (limitations in diagnostic specificity). FDG-PET has the advantage over CT that, unspecific lymph node enlargement does not lead to increased FDG-uptake by size alone and the FDG uptake may already increase in metastatic lymph nodes that are not enlarged

Van Westreenen et al. included 12 studies in a meta-analysis in patients with newly diagnosed cancer of the esophagus [9]. Pooled sensitivity and specificity of FDG-PET for detection of distant metastasis were 67% and 97%, respectively. Flamen et al. evaluated 74 patients with potentially respectable esophageal cancer in a prospective study and compared the diagnostic accuracy for FDG-PET, CT, and EUS [3]. For detecting distant metastases the sensitivity for FDG-PET, CT, and EUS were 74%, 41%, and 42% and the corresponding specificities were 90%, 83%, and 94%, respectively. The diagnostic accuracy of FDG-PET was 82% while it was only 64% for a combination of CT and EUS mainly by virtue of a superior sensitivity. These findings changed patient management in 22% of the studied patients by upstaging 11 patients (15%) and downstaging five patients (7%). In two patients, FDG-PET falsely understaged disease because of false-negative PET findings with regard to supradiaphragmatic lymph nodes

Heeren et al. compared FDG-PET with a combination of CT/EUS in the pretherapeutic staging for distant node metastasis and distant organ metastasis in 74 patients [7]. FDG-PET was able to identify distant nodal disease in 17 of 24 (71%) of the patients while this ratio was only 7 of 24 patients (29%) for CT/EUS. The sensitivity for detection of distant metastasis was also significantly higher for FDG-PET (70%) than for the combined use of CT and EUS (30%). PET correctly upstaged 15 patients (20%) who were missed on CT/EUS and correctly downstaged four patients (5%). However, in this study, PET also misclassified eight of the 74 patients (11%) by false upstaging in five patients (7%) and false downstaging in thee patients (4%)

There are several sources for false-positive findings in FDG-PET: inflammatory reactions (e.g., inflammatory infiltrates in the lung) benign tumors (e.g., benign thyroid adenoma or Warthin's tumor of the parotid gland), and increased FDG uptake in brown adipose tissue or skeletal muscles. However, all these causes are rare in patients with esophageal cancer. In all studies published so far, the diagnostic accuracy of FDG-PET in detection of distant metastasis of esophageal cancer has been found to be higher than that of morphological imaging techniques such as CT or EUS. This seems to apply to both the detection of distant lymph node metastases and organ metastases. FDG-PET excels by an outstanding sensitivity for bone metastases and appears to have a higher specificity than CT for detection of lung metastases and liver metastases. CT, on the other hand appears to have a higher sensitivity for lung metastases

Table 6.2 summarizes the results of studies evaluating the diagnostic accuracy of FDG-PET and CT for detection of distant metastasis in patients with esophageal cancer. In summary, the value of FDG-PET for staging esophageal carcinoma mainly resides in better characterization of distant metastases (lymph nodes and organs). However, FDG-PET should be regarded a supplemental procedure (e.g., in addition to CT), as it does not accurately determine the local tumor extent and locoregional lymph node involvement

6.3   Therapy Monitoring

In general, response rates to chemotherapy and/or radiotherapy in esophageal cancer are below 50% for all carcinoma types as measured by histopathological examination of the surgical specimen (after termination of therapy e.g., in a neoadjuvant setting). A common criterion for histopathological response to therapy is the presence of no or only scattered tumor cells (< 10% viable tumor cells) in the resected specimen [12–14]. In a neoadjuvant (preoperative) setting, the overall survival of patients is strongly dependent on whether his

Table 6.2. Detection of distant metastasis with FDG-PET and CT

Author	Year	Patients	Patients$_m$	FDG-PET		CT	
				Sensitivity	Specificity	Sensitivity	Specificity
Block et al.	1997	58	17	100%	–	29%	–
Luketich et al.	1999	91	39	69%	93%	46%	74%
Flamen et al.	2000	74	34	74%	90%	41%	83%
Rasanen et al.	2003	42	15	47%	89%	33%	96%
Heeren et al.	2004	74	27	78%	98%	37%[a]	87%[a]
Lowe et al.	2005	75	26	81%	91%	81%	82%

Patients$_m$, number of patients with distant metastasis. [a]CT/EUS

opathological response is achieved or not [12]. However, because of the tumor heterogeneity after neoadjuvant therapy, small biopsies of the tumor tissue are not representative of the whole tumor mass. A complete tumor resection and a histopathological examination of the whole tumor including adjoining areas is needed to definitely determine the histopathological tumor response

In contrast to pre- or posttherapeutic biopsies used for histopathologic analysis, the whole tumor mass can be analyzed noninvasively by imaging techniques such as contrast-enhanced CT or EUS. However, morphological changes are not always representative of tumor response, as large tumor masses may remain despite response or therapy-induced fibrosis, or edema may mimic residual tumor, and shrinking tumors may still contain vital tumor cells. The overall accuracy for response assessment is relatively low when determining posttherapeutic T-stage or comparing pre- and posttherapeutic T-stage by using morphological imaging. Thus, following chemotherapy or chemoradiotherapy, tumor response cannot reliably be assessed by computed tomography or endoscopic ultrasound

Despite these limitations, changes in tumor size have been used to assess tumor response in patients with esophageal cancer. According to criteria of the World Health Organization (WHO), the size of the tumor is to be measured in two perpendicular diameters. Tumor response is defined as a therapy-induced reduc-

tion of the product of these two diameters by at least 50%. Previous studies have shown that mean changes in tumor size of 50% and more are seen in esophageal cancer at the end of chemotherapy. However, these changes show no strong correlation with histopathologic response. It is well known that the esophageal wall often shows pathological thickening and irregularities regardless of the degree of therapy response. Therefore, anatomical imaging modalities usually are not able to distinguish residual tumor from therapy-related changes such as inflammatory reaction, edema, and scar tissue

The reproducibility of the PET signal arising from FDG accumulation in tumors has been shown to be rather stable at repeated examinations [15]. The interstudy variability of repeated FDG measurements within 3 weeks is less than 20% [15]. In other words, during therapy, any change in tumor FDG uptake greater than ± 20% between baseline PET and follow-up PET must be considered a true one. For example, a decrease of more than 20% can be seen as a therapeutic effect

The metabolic effects of a neoadjuvant chemotherapy/radiochemotherapy can be assessed during and after treatment. Evaluation late in the course of treatment and after completion of treatment may predict the amount of residual viable tumor cells, histopathological tumor response, and survival. However, the therapeutic relevance of this prognostic information is limited, as it is obtained too late for alteration of therapeutic strategy. Therefore, it is considered important to differentiate between responding and nonresponding tumors early in the course of neoadjuvant therapy

6.3.1 Late Response Assessment

In 2001, Brucher et al. were the first to report a study evaluating FDG-PET for the assessment of a late metabolic response after completion of chemoradiotherapy in 27 patients with advanced SCC of the esophagus [16]. The patients underwent a PET scan prior to therapy and 3–4 weeks after completion of therapy. Therapy-induced reduction of tumor FDG uptake was significantly higher for histopathologic responders (72% ± 11%) than for nonresponders (42% ± 22%). At a threshold of 52% decrease of metabolic activity, sensitivity to detect response was 100%, with a corresponding specificity of 55%. Metabolic tumor response was also a strong prognostic parameter. Responders to PET scanning had a median survival of 23 months, whereas it was only 9 months in PET nonresponders

Similar results were obtained by Flamen et al. who studied 36 patients with esophageal cancer before and 3–4 weeks after completion of chemoradiotherapy [17]. In contrast to Brucher et al, PET response was assessed using a visual analysis. Patients were classified as PET responders if they showed a complete or almost complete normalization of the FDG uptake at the primary site of the tumor together with a complete normalization of all lymph node metastases seen on the first PET scan before therapy. Histopathologic response was detected with a sensitivity of 78% and a specificity of 82% by FDG-PET. However, the sensitivity and the positive predictive value of the PET scan for the diagnosis of a complete histopathologic response was only 67% and 50%, respectively. The authors stated that the underestimation of complete histopathological response by PET was mainly based on false-positive findings at the primary tumor site. An influx of leukocytes and macrophages due to inflammatory immune and scavenging reactions may increase the FDG uptake, resulting

in an underestimation of therapeutic efficacy. Again, metabolic response was also correlated with overall survival. The median overall survival for patients without a PET response was 6.4 months, whereas it was 16.4 months for patients classified as PET responders

6.3.2 Early Response Assessment

Using quantitative measurements of tumor FDG uptake, it is feasible not only to assess tumor response late after onset of therapy but also to predict response early during chemotherapy

In a study by Weber et al, 40 consecutive patients with an AEG had a PET scan prior to chemotherapy and on day 14 of the first chemotherapy cycle [14]. The reduction of tumor FDG uptake after 14 days of therapy was significantly different between tumors that showed a clinical and histopathological response and those which showed no response (Fig. 6.2) Optimal differentiation was achieved by a cut-off value of 35% reduction of initial FDG uptake. Applying this cut-off value as a criterion for a metabolic response predicted clinical response with a sensitivity and specificity of 93% and 95%, respectively. Histopathologically complete or subtotal tumor regression was observed in 53% of the patients with a metabolic response but only in 5% of the patients without a metabolic response. Patients with a metabolic response were also characterized by a significantly longer time to progression/recurrence and longer overall survival

Radiotherapy/chemoradiotherapy often causes local inflammatory reactions in the esophagus. Uptake of FDG in inflammatory lesions is a commonly known phenomenon Increased FDG uptake due to radiation-induced inflammation may limit the use of FDG-PET for metabolic monitoring of esophageal carcinomas as observed in late response assessment with FDG-PET (see above). Therefore, it has been recommended that FDG-PET should be further postponed and only be performed several weeks or even months after completion of radiotherapy in order to assess tumor response However, these recommendations are not based

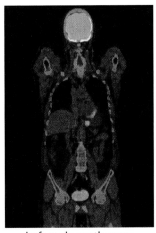 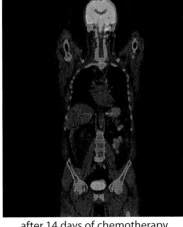

Fig. 6.2. Coronal PET/CT fusion images of a patient with a locally advanced adenocarcinoma of the esophagus. Already 14 days after initiation of neoadjuvant chemotherapy, there is a marked decrease in tumor metabolic activity (>35%). After completion of chemotherapy, no viable tumor cells were found in the resected specimen

before chemotherapy
SUV: 7.3

after 14 days of chemotherapy
3.1

on systematic clinical data, but only on theoretical considerations and a few case reports

Wieder et al. studied the time course of changes in tumor FDG uptake in 38 patients with locally advanced squamous cell carcinomas of the esophagus during preoperative chemoradiotherapy [13]. Patients underwent PET scans prior to chemoradiotherapy 2 weeks after the initiation of therapy and 3–4 weeks after completion of chemoradiotherapy, i.e., before surgery. None of the serial PET scans demonstrated a relevant increase in tumor FDG uptake, indicating that radiation-induced inflammation is too small to outweigh the decrease in FDG uptake due to therapy-induced loss of viable tumor cells. Furthermore, radiation-induced esophagitis often involves a long segment of the esophagus and, in most cases, is markedly different from than in esophageal cancer. Therefore, it is mostly possible to differentiate between residual tumor tissue and radiation-induced inflammation

The reduction of tumor FDG uptake after 14 days of chemoradiotherapy was significantly higher in histopathologic responding tumors (44% ± 15%) than in nonresponders (21% ± 14%). The ROC analysis demonstrated that the highest accuracy for differentiation of subsequently responding and nonresponding tumors was achieved by applying a cut-off of a 30% decrease in tumor FDG uptake from baseline values. Applying this cut-off value as

a criterion for metabolic response allowed for prediction of histopathologic response with a sensitivity and a specificity of 93% and 88%, respectively. Patients with a metabolic response were also characterized by a significantly longer overall survival. The median overall survival for patients with a decrease in FDG uptake by more than 30% was more than 38 months, while it was 18 months for patients with a decrease by less than 30%. Thus, response prediction is clearly feasible with FDG-PET early in the course of chemoradiotherapy. This is the basis for individualizing therapy, i.e., continuing therapy in patients with tumor response and intensifying or aborting ineffective therapy in cases without response

6.4 Recurrence

Kato et al. studied 55 patients with thoracic SCC who had undergone radical esophagectomy [18]. Twenty-seven of the 55 patients had recurrent disease in a total of 37 organs. The accuracy of FDG-PET and CT in detecting recurrences during follow-up was calculated by always using the first images that suggested the presence of recurrent disease. FDG-PET showed 100% sensitivity, 75% specificity, and 84% accuracy for detecting locoregional recurrence. The corresponding values for CT were

84%, 86%, and 85% respectively. The specificity of FDG-PET was lower because of unspecific FDG uptake in the gastric tube and in thoracic lymph nodes of the lung hilum or the pretracheal region. Distant recurrence was observed in 15 patients in 18 organs. Most of the recurrences were located in liver, lung, and bone. The sensitivity, specificity and accuracy for FDG-PET were 87%, 95%, and 93% v-s 87%, 98%, and 95%, respectively, for CT. The diagnostic accuracy of FDG-PET for distant recurrence was similar to that of CT. The sensitivity of FDG-PET in detecting bone metastasis was higher than that of CT. The sensitivity for lung metastasis was higher on CT going back to the excellent spatial resolution and high tumor-to-tissue contrast in the lung. Similar sensitivities for FDG-PET and CT were observed for both liver and distant lymph node metastasis

Flamen et al. used FDG-PET in 41 symptomatic patients for diagnosis and staging of recurrent disease after radical esophagectomy [19]. All patients underwent a whole-body FDG-PET and a conventional diagnostic workup including a combination of CT and EUS. Recurrent disease was present in 33 patients (40 locations). Nine lesions were located at the anastomotic site, 12 at regional and 19 at distant sites. For the diagnosis of a recurrence at the anastomotic site, no significant difference between PET and CT/EUS was found. The sensitivity, specificity, and accuracy of FDG-PET were 100%, 57%, and 74% vs 100%, 93%, and 96%, respectively, for conventional diagnostic workup. A reason for the high incidence of false-positive PET findings at the perianastomic region might have been progressive benign anastomotic strictures in these patients, requiring repetitive endoscopic dilatation. Probably the dilatation-induced trauma resulted in an inflammatory reaction. For the diagnosis of regional and distant recurrence, FDG-PET showed 94% sensitivity, 82% specificity, and 87% accuracy vs 81%, 84%, and 81% for CT/EUS, respectively. On a patient basis, PET provided additional information in 27% (11/41) of the patients.

In summary, FDG-PET is associated with a similar clinical benefit in restaging esophageal carcinoma as in primary staging (Fig. 6.3). However, the perianastomotic site often remains equivocal, as an unspecific increase of metabolic activity may be present owing to inflammatory or reparative processes

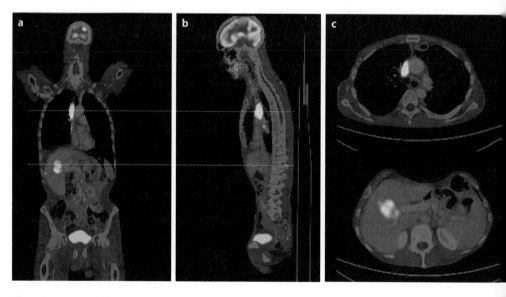

Fig. 6.3a–c. Coronal (a), sagittal (b), and axial (c) PET/CT fusion images of a patient after esophagectomy of a squamous cell carcinoma of the esophagus. The FDG-PET scan shows locoregional recurrent cancer and liver metastasis

References

1. Kato H, Kuwano H, Nakajima M et al (2002) Usefulness of positron emission tomography for assessing the response of neoadjuvant chemoradiotherapy in patients with esophageal cancer. Am J Surg 184:279–283

2. McAteer D, Wallis F, Couper G et al (1999) Evaluation of 18F-FDG positron emission tomography in gastric and oesophageal carcinoma. Br J Radiol 72:525–529

3. Flamen P, Lerut A, Van Cutsem E et al (2000) Utility of positron emission tomography for the staging of patients with potentially operable esophageal carcinoma. J Clin Oncol 18:3202–3210

4. Meltzer CC, Luketich JD, Friedman D et al (2000) Whole-body FDG positron emission tomographic imaging for staging esophageal cancer comparison with computed tomography. Clin Nucl Med 25:882–887

5. Kim K, Park SJ, Kim BT et al (2001) Evaluation of lymph node metastases in squamous cell carcinoma of the esophagus with positron emission tomography. Ann Thorac Surg 71:290–294

6. Yoon YC, Lee KS, Shim YM et al (2003) Metastasis to regional lymph nodes in patients with esophageal squamous cell carcinoma: CT versus FDG PET for presurgical detection prospective study. Radiology 227:764–770

7. Heeren PA, Jager PL, Bongaerts F et al (2004) Detection of distant metastases in esophageal cancer with (^{18})F-FDG PET. J Nucl Med 45:980–987

8. Rasanen JV, Sihvo EI, Knuuti MJ et al (2003) Prospective analysis of accuracy of positron emission tomography, computed tomography, and endoscopic ultrasonography in staging of adenocarcinoma of the esophagus and the esophagogastric junction. Ann Surg Oncol 10:954–960

9. van Westreenen HL, Westerterp M, Bossuyt PM et al (2004) Systematic review of the staging performance of ^{18}F-fluorodeoxyglucose positron emission tomography in esophageal cancer. J Clin Oncol 22:3805–3812

10. Choi JY, Lee KH, Shim YM et al (2000) Improved detection of individual nodal involvement in squamous cell carcinoma of the esophagus by FDG PET. J Nucl Med 41:808–815

11. Lerut T, Flamen P, Ectors N et al (2000) Histopathologic validation of lymph node staging with FDG-PET scan in cancer of the esophagus and gastroesophageal junction: a prospective study based on primary surgery with extensive lymphadenectomy. Ann Surg 232:743–752

12. Mandard A, Dalibard F, Mandard J et al (1994) Pathologic assessment of tumor regression after preoperative chemoradiotherapy of esophageal carcinoma. Clinicopathologic correlations. Cancer 73:2680–2686

13. Wieder HA, Brucher BL, Zimmermann F et al (2004) Time course of tumor metabolic activity during chemoradiotherapy of esophageal squamous cell carcinoma and response to treatment. J Clin Oncol 22:900–908

14. Weber WA, Ott K, Becker K et al (2001) Prediction of response to preoperative chemotherapy in adenocarcinomas of the esophagogastric junction by metabolic imaging. J Clin Oncol 19:3058–3065

15. Weber WA, Ziegler SI, Thodtmann R et al (1999) Reproducibility of metabolic measurements in malignant tumors using FDG PET. J Nucl Med 40:1771–1777

16. Brücher B, Weber W, Bauer M et al (2001) Neoadjuvant therapy of esophageal squamous cell carcinoma: response evaluation by positron emission tomography. Ann Surg 233:300–309

17. Flamen P, Van Cutsem E, Lerut A et al (2002) Positron emission tomography for assessment of the response to induction chemotherapy in locally advanced esophageal cancer. Ann Oncol 13:361–368

18. Kato H, Miyazaki T, Nakajima M et al (2004) Value of positron emission tomography in the diagnosis of recurrent oesophageal carcinoma. Br J Surg 91:1004–1009

19. Flamen P, Lerut A, Van Cutsem E et al (2000) The utility of positron emission tomography for the diagnosis and staging of recurrent esophageal cancer. J Thorac Cardiovasc Surg 120:1085–1092

20. Kato H, Kuwano H, Nakajima M et al (2002) Comparison between positron emission tomography and computed tomography in the use of the assessment of esophageal carcinoma. Cancer 94:921–928

21. Block MI, Patterson GA, Sundaresan RS et al (1997) Improvement in staging of esophageal cancer with the addition of positron emission tomography. Ann Thorac Surg 64:770–776; discussion 776–777

22. Luketich JD, Friedman DM, Weigel TL et al (1999) Evaluation of distant metastases in esophageal cancer: 100 consecutive positron emission tomography scans. Ann Thorac Surg 68:1133–1136; discussion 1136–1137

23. Lowe VJ, Booya F, Fletcher JG et al (2005) Comparison of positron emission tomography, computed tomography, and endoscopic ultrasound in the initial staging of patients with esophageal cancer. Mol Imaging Biol 7:1–9

7 Lung Cancer

H. C. Steinert

Recent Results in Cancer Research, Vol. 170
© Springer-Verlag Berlin Heidelberg 2008

7.1   Introduction

Lung cancer is the most common type of cancer and is the leading cause of cancer deaths worldwide for both women and men. The common types of lung cancer are non-small cell lung cancer (NSCLC) and small cell lung cancer (SCLC). Accurate tumor staging is essential for choosing the appropriate treatment strategy in lung cancer. In NSCLC, surgical resection offers the best chance for cure. However, curable surgical resection is only possible for early stages of NSCLC (no contralateral mediastinal lymph node metastases, no distant metastases). Patients with SCLC are treated with chemotherapy and radiation treatment. Malignant pleural mesothelioma (MPM) is the most common cancer of the pleura. MPM usually develops at least 20–30 years after asbestos exposure. The treatment consists of a tri-modality therapy, including chemotherapy, radical surgery, and radiation treatment. Even though the 5-year survival rate of patients with lung cancer and pleural cancer remains low, treatments are improving and newer agents appear promising. Therefore, the accurate assessment of the extent of disease is critical to determine whether the patient is treated by surgical resection, chemotherapy, radiation therapy, or a combination of these therapies.

Computed tomography (CT) has an import role in the initial determination of the stage of disease in lung cancer. CT provides excellent morphologic information but has limited ability to differentiate between benign and malignant lesions in lymph nodes or in organs such as the adrenal glands, the liver, or bone. Whole-body positron emission tomography (PET) using [18F]fluoro-2-deoxy-D-glucose (FDG) has a higher rate of detection of mediastinal lymph node metastases as well as extrathoracic metastases (Steinert et al. 1997; Weder et al. 1998). It has also proved effective in the management of patients with NSCLC (Dietlein et al. 2000; van Tinteren et al. 2002). Since commercial PET scanners provide nominal spatial resolution of 4.5–6.0 mm in the center of the axial field of view, even lesions that are less than 1 cm in diameter can be detected on the basis of an increased accumulation of FDG.

However, FDG is not specific for malignant tissue but is also taken up in muscles and inflammatory processes (Engel et al. 1996; Strauss 1996). Furthermore, PET provides imprecise information on the exact location of focal abnormalities. Thus, even if the results of PET and CT are visually correlated, the precise location of lesions is sometimes difficult to determine.

Recently, several groups have shown that integrated positron emission tomography imaging and computed tomography imaging (PET/CT) improves the diagnostic accuracy of the staging of patients with lung cancer (Lardinois et al. 2003; Antoch et al. 2003; Shim et al. 2005).

In this chapter, the role of PET imaging and PET/CT imaging in patients with NSCLC, SCLC, and MPM is discussed.

7.2 PET Imaging and Integrated PET/CT Imaging

By far the most widely used radiopharmaceutical for the staging of lung cancer with PET is 18F fluorodeoxyglucose (FDG), which is an analog of glucose. FDG is transported across cell membranes by glucose transporter proteins and is phosphorylated by hexokinase, like glucose. Once phosphorylated, FDG-6-phosphate is metabolically trapped. Thus FDG labels cellular glucose uptake and metabolism.

The efficacy of PET in detecting emitted photons is by far higher than that for single photon imaging such as SPECT (single photon emission computed tomography). However, the fraction of all emitted photon pairs that are detected is small (< 1%). Even with the low detection efficacy, PET imaging is the most sensitive way to detect small concentrations of tracers in the body. The system resolution of a modern PET scanner for patient imaging is 4–5 mm.

Attenuation, the loss of true events through absorption, influences the quality of PET images. In order to obtain homogeneous images, an attenuation correction of the PET data, which are called emission data, must be done. In conventional PET scanners, attenuation is measured by using photons from a rotation radioactive source. The photons are registered by the detectors of the PET scanner. However, the photon flux of these sources is very low and attenuation correction scans are therefore lengthy procedures. In clinical routine, an emission PET scan lasts approximately 30 min. For an attenuation correction scan, called a transmission scan, additional 15 min are needed. The attenuation data are introduced into the image reconstruction process of the emission images, resulting in attenuation-corrected PET images.

Today, PET (positron emission tomography) and CT (computed tomography) are combined into a single in-line imaging system, where the patient is moved from the CT to the PET gantry by table motion. The integrated PET/CT devices offer several advantages over a PET scanner alone. The attenuation correction can be performed more accurately by CT data, resulting in better quality PET images. Since CT imaging takes only a few seconds, the total imaging time is shortened. The PET (metabolic) and CT (morphologic) information are perfectly co-registered. This is of major importance because PET scans provide little anatomic information. Several studies have demonstrated that the diagnostic accuracy of integrated PET/CT imaging is higher compared to conventional visual correlation of PET and CT on separate units in staging lung cancer (Lardinois et al. 2003; Antoch et al. 2003; Shim et al. 2005). It is likely that the synergistic effects obtained when adding CT to PET are responsible for the almost explosive growth of PET/CT imaging worldwide.

At our institution, the following PET/CT protocol is used: patients fast for at least 4 h before the scanning procedure. Oral CT contrast agent is given 15 min before the injection of a standard dose of 350–400 MBq of FDG. After the FDG injection, patients rest at least 45 min. Patients are examined in the supine position. An intravenous contrast agent is not given routinely. After bladder voiding just prior to scanning, we first perform a low-dose CT scan at 80 mA, 140 kV, 0.5 s/tube rotation, slice thickness 4.25 mm, scan length 867 mm, and data-acquisition time 22.5 s. Our CT scanner is a state-of-the-art sixteen-slice MDCT. Patients are instructed to exhale and hold their breath when the CT scanner scans this body region. Immediately following the CT acquisition, a PET emission scan is acquired with an acquisition time of 3 min per cradle position with a one-slice overlap. The six to seven cradle positions from the upper legs to the head result in an acquisition time of approximately 24–27 min. Starting PET scanning in the upper legs rather than the head avoids a potential major PET/CT mismatch in the bladder region. This is due to bladder filling between CT data acquisition and the relatively lengthy PET scan, if started at the head.

After this baseline PET/CT data acquisition, additional standard CT protocols can be performed depending upon the clinical requirements. In patients with central lung tumors, we also perform a CT scan enhanced with an intravenous contrast agent, which can better delineate the tumor in relation to the vessels. Other groups have advocated the use of contrast-enhanced CT scans from the beginning and as the only CT scan. We believe that contrast-enhanced CT should not be performed routinely for PET/CT imaging. In many settings, CT contrast is not needed, as FDG is mostly a much better contrast agent for the tumor than the contrast agents used in CT. The additional radiation burden to a patient with a low-dose CT at 40 mAs is in the range of 2–3 mSv, and that of PET around 8–9 mSV. Thus, a PET/CT examination with the above protocol has a lower radiation dose compared to a standard CT.

The CT data is used for the attenuation correction and the images are reconstructed using a standard iterative algorithm (OSEM). The acquired images are viewed with software providing multiplanar reformatted images of PET alone, CT alone, and fused PET/CT with linked cursors.

7.3 Non-small Cell Lung Cancer

There are four main histologic types of NSCLC: adenocarcinoma, squamous cell carcinoma, large cell carcinoma, and mixed carcinoma. Adenocarcinomas typically develop in the periphery of the lung and are most common in women and in nonsmokers. Adenocarcinomas have a high incidence of early metastases and tend to grow more rapidly than squamous cell carcinomas. Bronchioalveolar cell carcinoma (BAC) is a subtype of adenocarcinoma. BACs typically grow along the alveolar spaces without invasion of the stroma. BAC can appear as a solitary pulmonary nodule, a pneumonia-like consolidation or as multiple nodules throughout the lung. Squamous cell carcinomas are strongly associated with smoking. In general, they have the best prognosis because of their slow growth rate and their low incidence of distant metastases. They tend to become large and develop a central necrosis. Metastases to regional lymph nodes are common. Squamous cell carcinoma is the most common cause of Pancoast tumors. These occur typically at the apex of the lung and are associated with Horner's syndrome and bone destruction.

Large cell carcinomas are also strongly associated with smoking. They tend to grow rapidly, metastasize early, and are associated with a poor prognosis. Staging of NSCLC is based on the TNM system and requires accurate characterization of the primary tumor (T stage), regional lymph nodes (N stage), and extrathoracic metastases (M stage).

NSCLC is also classified into four stages. Only patients with stage I to stage IIIA can benefit from radical surgery. Stages IIIB and IV are no longer considered resectable. Stage IV includes patients with distant metastases or an intrapulmonary metastasis in non-primary-tumor lobes of the lung. A tumor invading the mediastinum, the great vessels, or the vertebral body, or a contralateral mediastinal lymph node metastasis is classified as stage IIIB. At our institution, all patients with a non-invading primary-tumor combined with an ipsilateral mediastinal lymph node metastasis (stage IIIA) will receive neoadjuvant chemotherapy before surgery.

It has been shown that FDG PET is highly accurate in classifying lung nodules as malignant or benign. Whole-body PET improves the rate of detection of mediastinal lymph-node metastases as well as extrathoracic metastases when compared to CT, MRI, ultrasound, or bone scanning. Since modern PET scanners have a fairly high resolution (< 6 mm), even small lesions less than 1 cm can be detected. This is a critical advantage of PET over CT and MR. It has been shown that integrated PET/CT provides more than the sum of PET and CT (Lardinois et al. 2003; Antoch et al. 2003; Shim et al. 2005). Given the precise CT correlation with the extent of FDG uptake, the location of even small lesions can be exactly defined. The information of a PET/CT scan guides the surgeons to the lesions.

7.3.1 Solitary Pulmonary Nodule

A solitary pulmonary nodule (SPN) is a circumscribed round or oval lesion in the lung parenchyma less than 3 cm in diameter. About 60% of SPNs are benign and 40% are malignant. Benign SPNs represent infectious or inflammatory nodules, adenomas, and hamartomas. In 20%–30% of patients, a SPN is the initial presentation of a lung cancer (Erasms et al. 2000). Therefore, the early definitive diagnosis of a SPN is important for treatment management. Traditionally, a benign diagnosis for a SPN is made through a series of conventional radiographs or CT. If a SPN resolves or remains stable over time, it is considered to be a benign finding. The major drawback to the follow-up examinations is the time needed to establish the diagnosis. At least one follow-up study after 3–6 months is necessary to rule out growth of the SPN. Invasive transbronchial or transthoracic needle aspiration biopsy can be performed to clarify the diagnosis. The complications include pneumothorax and hemorrhage. Another limitation is that biopsies can miss the lesion or be nondiagnostic.

Many studies have demonstrated that FDG-PET or PET/CT is a useful method to distinguish between benign and malignant SPN. PET was found to be 97% sensitive and 78% specific for malignancy (Gould et al. 2001; Hellwig et al. 2001). The standardized uptake value (SUV) is a semiquantitative measurement of the intensity of the FDG accumulation. A SUV cut-off of 2.5 is used for distinguishing between benign and malignant lesions. Particularly in SPN with indeterminate radiographic findings, FDG-PET and PET/CT have a high clinical impact. PET and PET/CT are also useful in patients with SPN, where biopsy may be risky. If PET or PET/CT does not show an increased FDG accumulation, then the lesion is monitored using CT to definitely establish whether it is benign. It must be recognized that FDG-PET or PET/CT may show negative results for pulmonary carcinoid tumors, bronchiolo-alveolar lung carcinomas, and mucinous tumors (Higashi et al. 1998; Yap et al. 2002). Lesions with increased FDG accumulation should be considered malignant, although false-positive results have been reported in cases of inflammatory and infectious processes, such as histoplasmosis, aspergillosis, tuberculosis, or occult lung infarction after pulmonary thromboembolism (Kamel et al. 2005). However, most FDG active SPNs are malignant and should be resected (Figs. 7.1, 7.2).

7.3.2 Staging of the Primary Tumor

Surgical resection is the only treatment for cure in patients with NSCLC. The infiltration of the primary tumor into the chest wall, the mediastinum, or great vessels may limit the resectability. Without image fusion, the use of PET in the diagnosis of a tumor invasion in the surrounding tissue is limited (Fig. 7.1). It has been shown that integrated PET/CT is superior to CT alone, PET alone, and visual correlation of PET and CT in T staging of patients with non-small cell lung cancer (Lardinois et al. 2003; Shim et al. 2005). Because of the exact anatomic correlation of the extent of FDG uptake, the primary tumor can be delineated precisely. Therefore, the diagnosis of chest wall infiltration and the mediastinal invasion by the tumor is improved. Lesions with chest wall infiltration are classified as stage T3 and are potentially resectable. Surgical treatment requires en bloc resection of the primary tumor and the contiguous chest wall. Particularly in patients with poor cardiopulmonary reserve, the preoperative determination of chest wall infiltration is desirable in order to avoid extended en bloc resection. Integrated PET/CT provides important information on mediastinal infiltration as well. However, PET/CT imaging is unable to distinguish contiguity of tumor with the mediastinum from the direct invasion of the walls of mediastinal structures. It has been shown that FDG-PET is a useful tool for the differentiation between tumor and peritumoral atelectasis. This is particularly important for the planning of radiotherapy in patients with lung cancer associated with an atelectasis. The information provided by FDG-PET results in a change in the radiation field in approximately 30%–40% of patients (Nestle et al. 1999).

7.3.3 Mediastinal Lymph Node Staging

Accurate mediastinal staging is essential for therapy management of patients with NSCLC. Patients with ipsilateral mediastinal lymph node metastases (N2 disease) are considered to have potentially resectable disease. In case

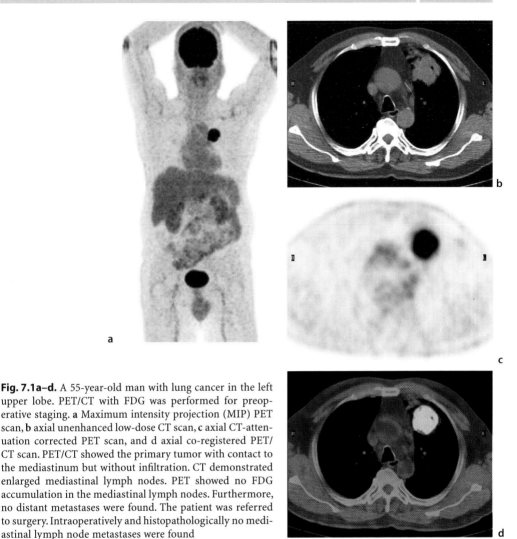

Fig. 7.1a–d. A 55-year-old man with lung cancer in the left upper lobe. PET/CT with FDG was performed for preoperative staging. **a** Maximum intensity projection (MIP) PET scan, **b** axial unenhanced low-dose CT scan, **c** axial CT-attenuation corrected PET scan, and **d** axial co-registered PET/CT scan. PET/CT showed the primary tumor with contact to the mediastinum but without infiltration. CT demonstrated enlarged mediastinal lymph nodes. PET showed no FDG accumulation in the mediastinal lymph nodes. Furthermore, no distant metastases were found. The patient was referred to surgery. Intraoperatively and histopathologically no mediastinal lymph node metastases were found

of ipsilateral bulky mediastinal metastases or contralateral mediastinal lymph node metastases (N3 disease), surgery is generally not indicated. CT and MRI have substantial limitations in depicting mediastinal lymph node metastases. Normal-sized lymph nodes may prove to have metastases upon histologic examination, and nodal enlargement can be due to reactive hyperplasia or other nonmalignant conditions. The sensitivity and specificity of determining lymph node metastases for non-small cell lung cancer by CT is 60%–70% (Webb et al. 1991; McLoud et al. 1992). Thus, in 30%–40% of cases, CT scanning will erroneously suggest the presence of mediastinal lymph node metastases and will miss lymph node metastases in 30%–40% of cases.

Multiple studies have demonstrated that FDG-PET is significantly more accurate than CT in determining nodal status (Steinert et al. 1997; Vansteenkiste et al. 1998; Pieterman et al. 2000) (Figs. 7.1, 7.3). With modern PET, even small lesions (< 1 cm) with an increased FDG accumulation can be detected. This is a critical advantage of PET over CT and MRI. Several meta-analyses comparing PET and CT

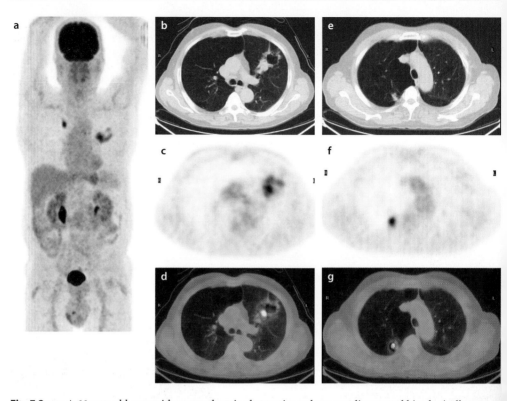

Fig. 7.2a–g. A 66-year-old man with severe chronic obstructive pulmonary disease and histologically proven lung cancer in the left upper lobe. PET/CT with FDG was performed for preoperative staging. **a** Maximum intensity projection (MIP) PET scan, **b, e** axial unenhanced low-dose CT scans (lung window), **c, f** axial CT-attenuation corrected PET scans, and **d, g** axial co-registered PET/CT scans. PET/CT showed the necrotic primary tumor in the left upper lobe. In addition, another lesion was found in the right upper lobe. This lesion was interpreted as second lung cancer or a lung metastasis of the primary tumor in the contralateral lung. No mediastinal lymph node metastases and no extrathoracic metastases were found. Histopathological correlation revealed two separate lung cancers. A lobectomy of both lesions was performed

in the mediastinal staging of NSCLC have been conducted. Dwamena et al. (1999) calculated a mean sensitivity and specificity of 0.79 and 0.91, respectively, for PET, and 0.60 and 0.77, respectively, for CT. These results were confirmed in another meta-analysis including more than 1,000 patients (Hellwig et al. 2001).

However, inflammatory mediastinal lymph nodes which accumulate FDG may occur and lead to false-positive results. Thus, histopathological correlation of FDG accumulating mediastinal lymph nodes is recommended. With the information of PET and PET/CT, the surgeon is guided to the suspicious lymph node. The site of lymph node metastases should be recorded according to the lymph node station-map-

ping system of the American Thoracic Society (Mountain and Dresler 1997).

In our experience, integrated PET/CT imaging will become the new standard of mediastinal staging. Still, microscopic foci of metastases within normal sized lymph nodes cannot be detected with any imaging modality. It must be recognized that FDG-PET or PET/CT up to 4 weeks after induction therapy is less accurate in mediastinal staging than in staging of untreated NSCLC because of inflammatory lymph nodes or microscopic nodal tumor involvement (Akhurst et al. 2002). For restaging after chemotherapy, PET or PRT/CT imaging should be performed after an interval of 4–8 weeks.

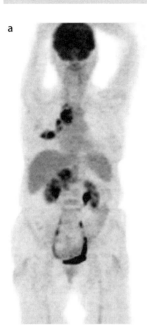

Fig. 7.3a–j. An 82-year-old woman with lung cancer in the middle lobe. PET/CT with FDG was performed for preoperative staging. **a** Maximum intensity projection (MIP) PET scan, **b, e** axial unenhanced low-dose CT scans, **h** axial enhanced low-dose CT scan, **c, f, i** axial CT-attenuation corrected PET scans, and **d, g, j** axial co-registered PET/CT scans. PET/CT showed the primary tumor with contact to the pleura but without infiltration of the thoracic wall. CT demonstrated a lung effusion. PET/CT demonstrated an ipsilateral hilar lymph node metastasis and precarinal lymph node metastases. In the duodenum, another tumor was found, which was proven as a metastasis of the lung cancer. The patient was referred to chemotherapy

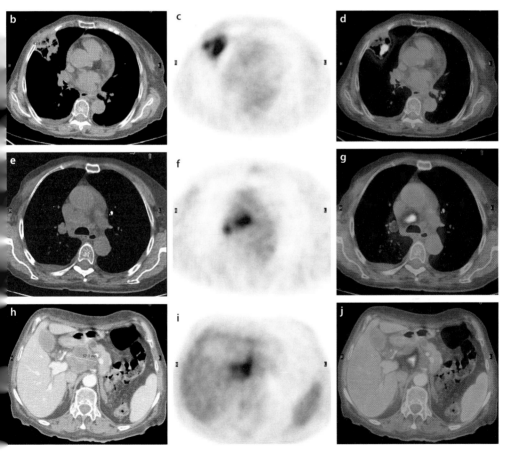

7.3.4 Staging of Distant Metastases

Whole-body PET or PET/CT are excellent methods to screen for extrathoracic metastases. Our group has shown that whole-body PET or PET/CT detects in 15% of patients with NSCLC previously unknown and unsuspected extrathoracic metastases (Weder et al. 1998). In a meta-analysis of 581 patients, sensitivity, specificity, and accuracy of FDG PET were 94%, 97%, and 96%, respectively (Hellwig et al. 2001). Because of the detection of unknown metastases, PET and PET/CT changes therapeutic management in approximately 20% of patients. The most common sites of distant metastases are the liver, adrenal glands, bone, and the brain. With the exception of the brain, PET or PET/CT are more accurate than current imaging modalities for M staging of patients (Erasmus et al. 1997; Marom et al. 1999).

However, FDG is not tumor-specific but is also taken up in lymphoid tissue or inflammatory cells. Recently, our group analyzed 350 PET/CT examinations in patients with NSCLC for single extrapulmonary lesions (Lardinois et al. 2005). In 72 patients (21%), a solitary extrapulmonary lesion with an increased FDG accumulation were found. Histopathological confirmation was performed in 69 of these patients: 50% of the lesions were metastases of NSCLC, 25% of lesions were unknown secondary cancer, and 25% of lesions were benign, for example acute fracture, colon adenoma, or Warthin's tumor.

It is well known that active muscles accumulate FDG. In some patients with lung cancer, an intense focal FDG accumulation is seen in the lower anterior neck just lateral to the midline. Co-registered PET/CT images revealed that this focal FDG uptake is frequently localized in the internal laryngeal muscles (Kamel et al. 2002). This finding is a result of compensatory laryngeal muscle activation caused by contralateral recurrent laryngeal nerve palsy due to direct nerve invasion by lung cancer of the left mediastinum or lung apices. The knowledge of this finding is important to avoid false-positive PET results.

7.3.5 Recurrent Lung Cancer

Despite radical therapy, the overall 5-year survival rate for patients with NSCLC remains low. Progression of disease may occur as intrathoracic recurrence or metastases. The differentiation of recurrent lung cancer and posttherapeutic changes remains a problem for radiological imaging. Therefore, some patients may undergo a biopsy to determine tumor viability, although invasive procedures including transthoracic needle biopsy and open lung biopsy carry associated risks. Furthermore, because of sampling errors, these procedures do not always provide a definitive answer. High accuracy of FDG-PET and PET/CT in distinguishing recurrent disease from benign treatment effects has been reported (Patz et al. 1994; Inoue et al. 1995; Hicks et al. 2001; Keidar et al. 2004). PET/CT is helpful to select biopsy sites to confirm recurrent disease. Patients should be evaluated a minimum of 2 months after completion of therapy. Otherwise posttherapeutic healing processes or radiation pneumonitis may result in false-positive FDG findings. These abnormal findings return to normal at variable times without further intervention.

7.3.6 Therapy Monitoring

The early prediction of tumor response is of high interest in patients with advanced NSCLC. Tumor progression during first-line chemotherapy occurs in approximately one-third of patients, with a significant percentage of patients undergoing several weeks of toxic and costly therapy without benefit. It has been shown that effective chemotherapy causes a rapid reduction of the SUV in the primary tumor during the course of therapy (Weber et al. 2003) (Fig. 7.4). In patients without metabolic response, the drug regimen may be changed to second-line therapy, thereby reducing the morbidity and costs from ineffective therapy. PET has also been evaluated to assess the response after radiation treatment in patients with NSCLC (MacManus et al. 2003). In this study, PET scans were performed at a median of 70 days after completion of radiation treat-

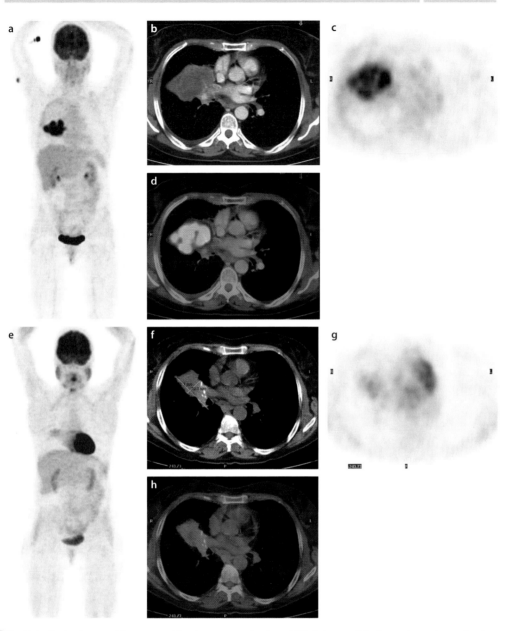

Fig. 7.4a–h. A 58-year-old woman with a lung cancer in the middle lobe. **a, e** Maximum intensity projection (MIP) PET scans, **b** axial enhanced low-dose CT scan, **f** axial unenhanced low-dose CT scan, **c, g** axial CT attenuation-corrected PET scans, and **d, h** axial co-registered PET/CT scans. **a–d** In the baseline examination, PET/CT showed the lung cancer with an extensive contact to the A. pulmonalis. The patient was referred to chemotherapy. **e–h** Two months after the last chemotherapy, PET/CT was performed for restaging. CT demonstrated a decrease in the size of the primary tumor. PET showed an excellent response to chemotherapy. No increased FDG accumulation in the tumor was found

ment. PET imaging differentiated viable tumor from fibrotic tissue. The PET response was significantly associated with survival duration. PET and PET/CT may have a wide application in measuring treatment response in patients with NSCLC. Because prognostic information can be obtained at a early time point, therapies can be modified depending on the PET response.

7.3.7 Effectiveness

Several studies have shown the effectiveness of PET imaging in patients with NSCLC. It has been demonstrated that a combined CT- and PET-based strategy is cost-effective in the staging of NSCLC (Gambhir et al. 1996). In this study, the expected costs and projected life expectancy were evaluated. The combined CT and PET strategy showed savings of more than US $1,000 per patient without loss of life expectancy compared with the alternate strategy using CT alone. The major advantage of FDG-PET is the cost savings that result from a patient with unresectable disease not undergoing unnecessary surgery. The cost savings are the result of improved staging of lung carcinoma before deciding on surgery.

In a subsequent study, five decision strategies of selecting potential surgical candidates were compared (Scott et al. 1998): one was based on thoracic CT alone, while the other four used chest CT plus PET. For all possible outcomes of each strategy, the expected cost and projected life expectancy were compared. A strategy that uses PET after a negative CT study was shown to be a cost-effective alternative to the CT-alone strategy (US $25,286 per life-year saved). The implementation of whole-body FDG-PET imaging using a dedicated PET scanner in the preoperative staging of patients with NSCLC and normal-sized lymph nodes is clearly cost-effective (Dietlein et al. 2000). However, patients with nodal-positive PET results should not be excluded from biopsy.

A randomized controlled trial in patients with suspected NSCLC, who were scheduled for surgery after conventional workup, was conducted to test whether FDG-PET reduces the numbers of thoracotomies (van Tinteren et al. 2002). Patients were followed up for 1 year. Thoracotomy was regarded as futile if the patient had benign disease, exploratory thoracotomy, pathological stage IIIA/IIIB, or postoperative relapse or death within 12 months of randomization. The investigators found that adding PET to standard workup in routine clinical practice improved selection of surgically curable patients and prevented unnecessary surgery in 20% of patients with suspected NSCLC.

7.4 Small Cell Lung Cancer

Small cell lung cancer (SCLC) is the most aggressive lung cancer. SCLC is characterized by rapid growth and early metastases, which are present in 60%–80% at the time of diagnosis. The staging procedures for SCLC do not differ from those for NSCLC. The primary role for imaging is to separate limited disease (LD) from extended disease (ED) accurately. In patients with disease confined to the thorax, radiation treatment is performed. Patients with extended disease are managed with chemotherapy. Integrated PET/CT imaging is an accurate method for the assessment of the total tumor extent and plays an important role in the planning of radiation treatment (Kamel et al. 2003). It is useful for accurate target definition by reducing the probability of overlooking involved areas. FDG-PET is superior to conventional staging in the detection of all involved sites, and particularly in the assessment of mediastinal lymph node metastases.

7.5 Malignant Pleural Mesothelioma

Malignant pleural mesothelioma (MPM) is the most common neoplasm of the pleura and directly linked to asbestos exposure. MPM usually develops at least 20–30 years after asbestos exposure. Imaging is particularly helpful in preoperative staging of MPM. Similarly to lung cancer, excellent FDG uptake in malignant pleural mesothelioma (MPM) has been previously described (Schneider et al. 2000). Our first experience suggests that PET/CT imaging is a promising method for MPM, as the extent of the tumor can be precisely defined. Integrated PET/CT imaging is helpful to identify the optimal biopsy site, thereby increasing diagnostic accuracy of the histological examination.

References

Akhurst T, Downey RJ, Ginsberg MS et al (2002) An initial experience with FDG-PET in the imaging of residual disease after induction therapy for lung cancer. Ann Thorac Surg 73:259–266

Antoch G, Stattaus J, Nemat AT et al (2003) Non-small cell lung cancer: dual modality PET/CT in preoperative staging. Radiology 229:526–533

Dietlein M, Weber K, Gandjour A et al (2000) Cost-effectiveness of FDG-PET for the management of potentially operable non-small cell lung cancer: priority for a PET-based strategy after nodal-negative CT results. Eur J Nucl Med 27:1598–1609

Dwamena BA, Sonnad SS, Angobaldo JO, Wahl RL (1999) Metastases from non-small cell lung cancer: mediastinal staging in the 1990s – meta-analytic comparison of PET and CT. Radiology 213:530–536

Engel H, Steinert H, Buck A et al (1996) Whole-body PET: physiological and artifactual fluorodeoxyglucose accumulations. J Nucl Med 37:441–446

Erasmus JJ, Patz EF, Mc Adams HP et al (1997) Evaluation of adrenal masses in patients with bronchogenic carcinoma using ^{18}F-fluorodeoxyglucose positron emission tomography. AJR 168:1357–1362

Erasmus JF, Connolly JE, McAadms HP (2000) Solitary pulmonary nodules: Part 1. Morphologic evaluation for differentiation of benign and malignant lesions. Radiographics 20:43–58

Gambhir SS, Hoh CK, Phelps ME et al (1996) Decision tree sensitivity analysis for cost-effectiveness of FDG-PET in the staging and management of non-small-cell lung carcinoma. J Nucl Med 37:1428–1436

Gould MK, Maclean CC, Kuschner WG et al (2001) Accuracy of positron emission tomography for diagnosis of pulmonary nodules and mass lesions: a meta-analysis. JAMA 285:914–924

Hellwig D, Ukena D, Paulsen F et al (2001) Meta-analysis of the efficacy of positron emission tomography with F-18-fluorordeoxyglucose in lung tumors. Pneumologie 55:367–377

Hicks RJ, Kalff V, MacManus MP et al (2001) The utility of ^{18}F-FDG PET for suspected recurrent non-small

cell lung cancer after potentially curative therapy: impact on management and prognostic stratification. J Nucl Med 42:1605–1613

Higashi K, Ueda Y, Seki H et al (1998) Fluorine-18-FDG PET imaging is negative in bronchoalveolar lung carcinoma. J Nucl Med 39:1016–1020

Inoue T, Kim E, Komaki R et al (1995) Detecting recurrent or residual lung cancer with FDG-PET. J Nucl Med 36:788–793

Kamel E, Goerres GW, Burger C, von Schulthess GK, Steinert HC (2002) Detection of recurrent laryngeal nerve palsy in patients with lung cancer using PET-CT image fusion. Radiology 224:153–156

Kamel EM, Zwahlen D, Wyss MT et al (2003) Whole-body (^{18})F-FDG PET improves the management of patients with small cell lung cancer. J Nucl Med 44:1911–1917

Kamel EM, McKee TA, Calcagni ML et al (2005) Occult lung infarction may induce false interpretation of ^{18}F-FDG PET in primary staging of pulmonary malignancies. Eur J Nucl Med Mol Imaging 32:641–664

Keidar Z, Haim N, Guralnik L et al (2004) PET/CT using ^{18}F-FDG in suspected lung cancer recurrence: diagnostic value and impact on patient management. J Nucl Med 45:1640–1646

Lardinois D, Weder W, Hany TF et al (2003) Staging of non-small-cell lung cancer with integrated positron-emission tomography and computed tomography. N Engl J Med 348:2500–2507

Lardinois D, Weder W, Roudas M et al (2005) Etiology of solitary extrapulmonary positron emission tomography and computed tomography findings in patients with lung cancer. J Clin Oncol 23:6846–6853

MacManus MP, Hicks RJ, Matthews JP et al (2003) Positron emission tomography is superior to computed tomography for response-assessment after radical radiotherapy or chemoradiotherapy in patients with non-small cell lung cancer. J Clin Oncol 21:1285–1292

Marom EM, McAdams HP, Erasmus JJ (1999) Staging non-small cell lung cancer with whole-body PET. Radiology 212:803–809

McLoud TC, Bourgouin PM, Greenberg RW et al (1992) Bronchogenic carcinoma: analysis of staging in the mediastinum with CT by correlative lymph node mapping and sampling. Radiology 182:319–332

Mountain CF, Dresler CM (1997) Regional lymph node classification for lung cancer staging. Chest 11:1718–1723

Nestle U, Walter K, Schmidt S, Licht N et al (1999) ^{18}F-deoxyglucose positron emission tomography (FDG-PET) for the planning of radiotherapy in lung cancer: high impact in patients with atelectasis. Int J Radiat Oncol Biol Phys 44:593–597

Patz EF, Lowe VJ, Hoffman JM et al (1994) Persistent or recurrent bronchogenic carcinoma: detection with PET and 2-[F-18]-2-deoxy-D-glucose. Radiology 191:379–382

Pieterman RM, van Putten JWG, Meuzelaar JJ et al (2000) Preoperative staging of non-small-cell lung cancer with positron-emission tommography. N Engl J Med 343:254–261

Schneider DB, Clary-Macy C, Challa S et al (2000) Positron emission tomography with F18-fluorodeoxyglucose in the staging and preoperative evaluation of malignant pleural MPM. J Thorac Cardiovasc Surg 120:128–133

Scott WJ, Shepherd J, Gambhir SS (1998) Cost-effectiveness of FDG-PET for staging non-small cell lung cancer: a decision analysis. Ann Thorac Surg 66:1876–1885

Shim SS, Lee KS, Kim BT et al (2005) Non-small cell lung cancer: prospective comparison of integrated FDG PET/CT and CT alone for preoperative staging. Radiology 236:1001–1019

Steinert HC, Hauser M, Allemann F et al (1997) Non-small cell lung cancer: nodal staging with FDG PET versus CT with correlative lymph node mapping and sampling. Radiology 202:441–446

Strauss LG (1996) Fluorine-18 deoxyglucose and false positive results: a major problem in the diagnostics of oncological patients. Eur J Nucl Med 23:1409–1415

Vansteenkiste JF, Stroobants SG, De Leyn PR et al (1998) Lymph node staging in non-small cell lung cancer with FDG PET scan: a prospective study on 690 lymph node stations from 68 patients. J Clin Oncol 16:2142–2149

Van Tinteren H, Hoekstra OS, Smit EF et al (2002) Effectiveness of positron emission tomography in the preoperative assessment of patients with suspected non-small-cell lung cancer: the PLUS multicentre randomised trial. Lancet 359:1388–1393

Webb WR, Gatsonis C, Zerhouni E et al (1991) CT and MR imaging in staging non-small cell bronchogenic carcinoma: report of the Radiology Diagnostic Oncology Group. Radiology 178:705–713

Weber WA, Peterson V, Schmidt B et al (2003) Positron emission tomography in non-small cell lung cancer: prediction of response to chemotherapy by quantitative assessment to glucose use. J Clin Oncol 21:2651–2657

Weder W, Schmid R, Bruchhaus H, Hillinger S, von Schulthess GK, Steinert HC (1998) Detection of extrathoracic metastases by positron emission tomography in lung cancer. Ann Thorac Surg 66:886–893

Yap CS, Schiepers C, Fishbein MC et al (2002) FDG-PET imaging in lung cancer: how sensitive is it for bronchioloalveolar carcinoma? Eur J Nucl Med Mol Imaging 29:1166–1173

8 FDG-PET and PET/CT in Malignant Lymphoma

S. N. Reske

Recent Results in Cancer Research, Vol. 170
© Springer-Verlag Berlin Heidelberg 2008

FDG-PET and FDG PET/CT have been developed as sophisticated functional imaging methods for evaluating important aspects of the biology and clinical management of malignant tumors in patients, particularly of patients with malignant lymphoma. Due to highly increased glycolysis in most malignant lymphomas, FDG is the mostly preferred radiopharmaceutical for PET imaging of lymphomas. Interestingly, however, one of the earliest reports of PET imaging in lymphoma used C-11-methionine for assessment of viability of a residual mass in non-Hodgkin's lymphoma (NHL) after radiation therapy [1]. In a letter to The Lancet, Leskinnen-Kallio and colleagues made the far-sighted statement that "PET may be a new way of detecting viable malignant tissue" [1]. Since that time, many reports have shown use and value of PET and more recently of PET/CT imaging of malignant lymphomas for pretherapeutic staging, therapy control, interim response assessment of various combinations of radio-, chemo-, immuno- and radioimmunotherapy [2–5] and evaluation of prognosis [6–8]. Several excellent recent reviews covering these issues have been published [6, 8–11]. This article will briefly summarize use of FDG-PET and PET/CT for:

- Initial pretherapeutic staging
- Relevance of response monitoring
- Technical considerations
- Treatment remission assessment
  - Evaluation after completion of chemotherapy and/or radiotherapy
  - Early response assessment

- Discuss some novel functional imaging approaches in malignant lymphoma.

8.1 Staging

The Ann Arbor classification can be used both for Hodgkin's disease (HD) and NHL and differentiates malignant lymphoma distribution into four stages.
- Stage I: Disease limited to a single lymph node or a single lymph node group;
- Stage II: Two or more noncontiguous nodal groups or the spleen on the same side of the diaphragm;
- Stage III: Two or more nodal groups or the spleen on both sides of the diaphragm;
- Stage IV: Disease in extranodal sites (bone marrow, liver, lung, bone or other organs/tissues).

Extension from a nodal manifestation into extranodal tissue (S) such as the lung, pleura, pericardium, skin etc. may occur in stage I–III and does not increase the stage into stage IV, but is designated by the involved tissue/organ with the subscript E. Nodal disease greatze10 cm in the largest diameter is defined as bulky and designated with a suffix X to the numeric stage [10].

There are several preferred sites of NHL involvement: compared to HD, Waldyer's ring is involved in 5%–10% of patients with NHL and is extremely rare in HD. Waldyer's ring involvement by NHL may be associated with involvement of the gastrointestinal tract and stomach or bowel. Mesenteric lymph node involvement is quite common in NHL, but is only rarely seen (< 5%) in HD. Bone marrow involvement is present in 15%–40% of patients with NHL [9].

Stage is an important component of a predictive model for untreated patients with intermediate or high-grade NHL [12]. The five important factors at presentation are age (≤ 60 years vs > 60 years, serum low-density lipoprotein concentration (≤ 1 × normal vs > 1 × normal), performance status (0 or 1 vs 2–4), stage (I or II vs III or IV), and extranodal involvement (≤ 1 site vs >1 site).

FDG PET or more recently FDG-PET/CT can be used both for nodal and extranodal staging [5, 13–18]. Fast and convenient imaging of the whole body or more practically the trunk within about 30 min in conjunction with contrast-enhanced CT provides excellent and precise imaging of virtually all organs and tissues potentially involved by HD or NHL (Fig. 8.1). This approach offers the advantage of both diagnostic CT with the added benefit of the functional imaging of FDG-PET with high technical quality and devoid of the restriction of size

criteria limiting sensitivity of nodal staging of CT. Thus, increased FDG uptake can be easily measured with FDG-PET or FDG-PET/CT in nodes smaller than 1 cm in diameter. In addition, it has been shown that focal involvement of bone marrow can be accurately detected with FDG-PET or PET/CT, but is limited with CT. Virtually all nodal groups can be imaged with the FDG-PET/CT approach in high- and intermediate-grade lymphoma.

Practically all studies comparing FDG-PET to CT reported a 10%–20% higher accuracy of FDG-PET for staging of lymphoma resulting in treatment changes in 10%–20% of cases (see [5] for review). Improved staging in HD with FDG-PET/CT compared to CT was recently demonstrated by Hutchings [19].

The limitations of FDG-PET- or FDG-PET/CT-based staging are diffuse from bone marrow involvement by NHL, with less than 10% infiltration of bone marrow with NHL [16], and a reduced sensitivity of FDG-PET or probably also FDG-PET/CT in indolent (low-grade) lymphoma [20]. FDG uptake in lymphoma manifestations varies depending on histology [21]. In a recent study, the sensitivity of FDG-PET was excellent (~95%) in grade I–III follicular lymphoma, moderate (74%) in mantle cell lymphoma, and limited (~50%) in B-cell small

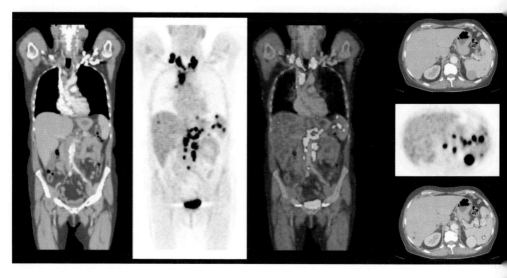

Fig. 8.1. FDG PET/CT staging in NHL. Supra- and infradiaphragmatic nodal disease as well as multifocal involvement within the spleen

cell lymphocytic lymphoma (SCL/CLL) [21]. A study by Jerusalem et al. reported that FDG-PET identified 40% more abnormal lymph node sites than conventional staging in 24 patients with follicular histology, but less than 58% of abnormal nodal sites compared to CT in 11 patients with small lymphocytic lymphoma [20]. As suggested by studies in small patient series, performance of FDG PET is rather poor in patients with MALT lymphoma [22]. Sensitivity is probably dependent on histology and limited in low-grade MALT lymphoma [23]. With regard to a false-negative case of bronchial wall involvement by NHL reported by Bangerter et al. [24], it is clear that microscopic involvement in any tissue is beyond the detection capabilities of FDG-PET or FDG-PET/CT. Unspecific nodal or extranodal FDG uptake due to focal inflammatory disease may be a cause of false-positive results, but rarely causes problems in the context of initial staging of malignant lymphomas.

8.2   Relevance of Response Monitoring

As recently reviewed by Mikhaeel [8], lymphoma is generally a curable disease, but its treatment is associated with significant short-and long-term toxicity. In the treatment of curable lymphoma (HD) and aggressive high-grade NHL, the goal of treatment is to achieve a complete response (CR), which is a prerequisite for cure. Patients who do not achieve a CR by the end of treatment are offered various salvage treatment regimens. Accurate remission assessment after the completion of a planned course of treatment is therefore essential, to improve the prognosis of patients who do not achieve CR and to avoid unnecessary treatment-related toxicity and treatment-associated short- and long-term morbidity in those patients who achieve CR. FDG-PET or PET/CT has been very successfully employed for this post-treatment remission assessment. Another comparable interesting and potentially more important form of assessment is early response assessment. The main goal of this approach is

to adjust the intensity and type of treatment to the individual patient's prognosis. Response of treatment is probably the most important single factor determining the prognosis of the individual patient. Response-adjusted treatment aims to optimize the balance between the chance of cure and potential toxicity for the individual patient. Early response assessment provides a strategy by minimizing treatment for good prognosis patients and intensifying treatment for patients with a poor prognosis [8].

8.3   Technical Considerations

The best time for end-of-treatment evaluation remains unknown, but most investigators suggest waiting at least 1 month after the last day of chemotherapy and 3 months after the last dose of radiotherapy [6, 8]. It must be kept in mind that F-18 FDG-PET or PET/CT cannot exclude minimal residual disease and it may be indicated to repeat F-18 FDG-PET or PET/CT during routine follow-up to overcome insecurities regarding the potential of residual tumor at the end of treatment [6]. Residual lymphoma may also be missed or its extent underestimated because of the low grade of lymphoma is not FDG-avid or has very low uptake. This is, however, relatively uncommon (see previous section). On the other hand, positive findings in PET/CT do not necessarily represent residual disease. Meticulous evaluation of PET images is mandatory to avoid false-positive findings associated with muscle tension or normal intestinal structures. Brown fat can avidly incorporate FDG, frequently seen in young slim women. Because FDG is not a tumor-specific radiotracer and acute inflammation stimulates glycolytic flux in leukocytes [25], inflammatory lesions may show up as intense FDG uptake. Documented causes of false-positive PET studies in response assessment of lymphoma are shown in Table 8.1).

Although not studied in detail in lymphoma, it is well known from studies in various solid tumors that diabetes mellitus and increased blood sugar concentration can reduce sensitivity of FDG-PET considerably [26, 27]. Therefore, it is our institutional practice to examine patients only with a blood sugar concentration below 150 mg/dl and to keep patients fastened at least 5, and better 8 h before the examination. Intravenous furosemide before the PET study to flush the renal collecting system and thus to avoid reconstruction artifacts is not used since powerful iterative reconstruction algorithms and CT-based attenuation correction have greatly improved the image quality of PET scans.

Table 8.1. Documented causes of false-positive ^{18}F-FDG PET studies in response evaluation (modified from [8])

Second primary
Thyroid adenoma
Rebound thymic hyperplasia
Infectious process
Toxoplasmosis
Tuberculosis
Pneumonia
Radiotherapy-induced pneumonia/pneumonitis
Inflammatory lung process
Pleural inflammation
Histiocytic reaction
Benign follicular lymph node hyperplasia
Unspecific lymphadenitis
Granulomatous lymphadenitis
Sarcoidosis and sarcoid-like reaction
Epithelioid cell granuloma
Eosinophilic granuloma
Erythema nodosum
Fracture at the site of lymphoma infiltration before treatment
Fistula
Granulation tissue
Nonviable scar tissue
Talc granuloma

8.4　Treatment Remission Assessment

Remission status assessment commonly involves clinical examination, a blood test, CT scanning, and in some cases histopathological examination of bone marrow and other imaging modalities such as MRT [8, 28]. Criteria for response assessment and response categories have been established for lymphoma and are commonly known as the International Workshop Classification (IWC) [28]. The IWC predominantly relies on anatomical imaging modalities such as CT scanning or MRT. Response assessment criteria have recently been revised and PET or PET/CT has been implemented [12]. The reason for revision was that it has long been recognized that lymphoma masses, especially when bulky on presentation, may not disappear completely if the disease has been eradicated completely (Fig. 8.2). These residual masses are formed mainly of necrotic or fibrotic tissue and may continue to shrink during follow-up [8, 29]. Only approximately 20% of residual masses harbor residual viable malignant cells. Therefore, offering more treatment to all patients with residual masses would involve overtreating many patients unnecessarily [8] (Fig. 8.3). Follow-up of these masses to treat only the progressing ones may waste valuable time and compromise the chances of cure (Fig. 8.3).

Against this background, the introduction of functional metabolic imaging using FDG-PET or PET/CT has proven to be helpful in the accurate assessment of remission after treatment and in characterizing residual masses. In particular, the role of FDG-PET in assessing residual masses has been widely accepted [12].

From the published literature, some general conclusions can be drawn [8]:

- FDG-PET is more accurate than CT in virtually all studies.
- The accuracy of PET is high enough to be used as a standard measure of revision assessment, either supplementing or in combination with PET/CT replacing the CT-only study.

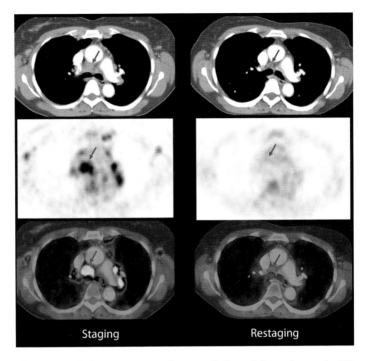

Fig. 8.2. Remission assessment after completion of chemotherapy in HD with FDG PET/CT. All nodal manifestations with increased FDG uptake (axillary nodes right and left, mammary internal nodes left, mediastinal nodes) show complete normalization, i.e., no residual FDG uptake, 4 weeks after completion of chemotherapy. Residual mediastinal mass without FDG uptake in CT (*arrow*) indicative of scar tissue

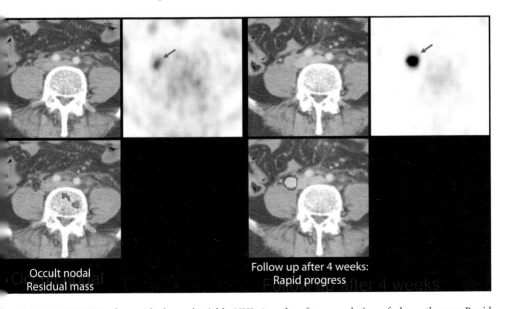

Fig. 8.3. FDG-PET/CT of a residual occult viable NHL 8 weeks after completion of chemotherapy. Rapid progression at 4-week follow-up

8.5 Evaluation After Completion of Chemotherapy and/or Radiotherapy

Achieving a complete remission is a major objective in patients with HD or NHL, because it is usually associated with a longer progression-free survival than a partial remission (see [6] for review). However, in as many as 64% of all HD cases and in 30%–60% of all NHL cases, CT or MRT show abnormalities during restaging [8]. Residual masses are observed more frequently in patients with an aggressive NHL and with a large tumor mass at diagnosis as well as in patients suffering from HD of a nodular sclerosis histologic subtype [6]. Unfortunately, conventional imaging cannot differentiate between benign fibrous tissue and an inflammatory process or persistent malignant disease. Only a maximum of 20% of residual masses at the completion of treatment are reported to be positive for lymphoma on biopsy and eventually relapse [28, 30]. If the tumor is easily accessible, such as an enlarged peripheral lymph node, the questionable lesion should be excised and histologically analyzed.

If the anatomical access is difficult, non invasive imaging with FDG-PET or PET/CT i of major importance (Fig. 8.4). Several recen studies demonstrate the value of FDG PET o PET/CT for end of treatment response assess ment [6]. Jerusalem et al. compiled 17 selec tive studies with a total of 752 patients [6]. Th overall accuracy of PET was 88%–91% [6]. I particular, PET had a better positive predictiv value (PPV) for NHL (100%) than for HD (74% and a better negative predictive value (NPV fo HD 93%) than for NHL (83%). As indicated b Mikhael [8], a positive PET after NHL treat ment is strongly predictive of residual diseas but less so in HD. A negative PET after HD treatment is predictive of freedom of residua disease, but slightly less in NHL. This possibl reflects the presence of inflammatory cellula infiltrate in HD and the higher relapse rate o NHL [8] (Tables 8.2, 8.3).

Since FDG uptake is not specific for tumo tissue, it may be advisable to carefully chec lesions occurring outside of normal FDG up take of initially involved sites, because infec tious or inflammatory lesions are much mor abundant in these lesions.

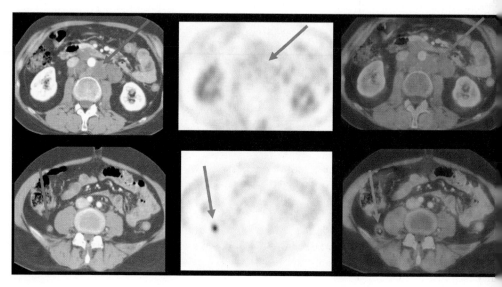

Fig. 8.4. Residual FDG-PET/CT negative left paraaortic mass 6 months after completion of chemotherapy i NHL (*upper row, arrows*). Simultaneous abdominal relapse (*arrow*) in a lymph node near right M. iliopso (*lower row, arrow*)

Table 8.2. Predictive value of whole-body ^{18}F-FDG for posttreatment evaluation in NHL (from [6])

Authors	Median follow-up (months)	Sensitivity	Specificity	Positive predictive value	Negative predictive value	Accuracy
Mikhaeel et al. [30]	30	60% (9/15)	100% (30/30)	100% (9/9)	83% (30/36)	87% (39/45)
Spaepen et al. [31]	21	70% (26/37)	100% (56/56)	100% (26/26)	84% (56/67)	88% (82/93)
Overall		67% (35/52)	100% (86/86)	100% (35/35)	83% (86/103)	88% (121/138)

Table 8.3. Predictive value of whole body ^{18}F-FDG PET for posttreatment evaluation in HD (from [6])

Authors	Median follow-up (months)	Sensitivity	Specificity	Positive predictive value	Negative predictive value	Accuracy
de Wit et al. [32]	26	100% (10/10)	78% (18/23)	67% (10/15)	100% (18/18)	85% (28/33)
Dittmann et al. [33]	6	87% (7/8)	94% (17/18)	87% (7/8)	94% (17/18)	92% (24/26)
Spaepen et al. [34]	32	50% (5/10)	100% (50/50)	100% (5/5)	91% (50/55)	92% (55/60)
Weihrauch et al. [35]	28	67% (6/9)	80% (16/20)	60% (6/10)	84% (16/19)	76% (22/29)
Guay et al. [36]	16	79% (11/14)	97% (33/34)	92% (11/12)	92% (33/36)	92% (44/48)
Friedberg et al. [37]	24	80% (4/5)	85% (23/27)	50% (4/8)	96% (23/24%)	84% (87/32)
Panizo et al. [38]	28	100% (9/9)	85% (17/20)	75% (9/12)	100% (17/17)	90% (26/29)
Overall		80% (52/65)	91% (174/192)	74% (52/70)	93% (174/187)	88% (226/257)

8.6 Early Response Assessment

About 30%–40% of aggressive NHL patients fail to achieve CR with initial standard chemotherapy, which is a prerequisite for cure. Overall long-term cure is achieved only in 40%–60%. This means that a substantial portion of patients may not respond to their initial treatment. Early response assessment is usually performed with CT after three to four cycles of chemotherapy. PET has been investigated for potentially improving accuracy of early response assessment through functional metabolic imaging [6, 8, 9].

The results of several recent studies have been summarized by Jerusalem [6] (Table 8.4).

Despite the limitations of some studies, some general conclusions can be drawn [8]:

- CR is evident on a repeated PET or PET/CT after one to three cycles of chemotherapy, much earlier than size reduction of lymphoma masses seen on the CT scan.
- This early CR on PET, presumably reflecting high chemosensitivity, correlates with better prognosis.
- Early PET is a more accurate predictor of outcome than posttreatment PET.

Mikhaeel et al. introduced the concept of minimal residual uptake (MRU) [44, 45]. These authors studied 121 patients with high-grade NHL with FDG-PET after two to three cycles of chemotherapy [44] for prediction of progression-free survival (PFS) and overall survival (OS). They reported that early interim PET was an accurate and independent predictor of PFS and OS [44]. They also identified a subgroup of patients with NHL and MRU and an intermediate prognosis between those patients with a negative PET and an excellent prognosis as shown by a PFS of 89% and those with a positive PET, a poor prognosis, and a PFS of only 16% [44]. It was concluded from this study that early interim FDG-PET is an accurate and independent predictor of PFS and OS in NHL [44]. This study also shows that early interim PET has the potential to improve individualized management of patients with NHL, providing a basis for early identification of nonresponding patients to whom an alternative second-line therapy may be offered.

As the authors of the above-cited study state, the three-group classification system of FDG uptake as:

● Class(1): negative
● Class (2): MRU
● Class (3): positive

suffers from the limitations of the subjectivity of the MRU designation, which needs a definition producing objective and reproducible results [44] (Fig. 8.5).

The same investigators also studied the value of early interim PET, i.e., after two to three cycles of chemotherapy, in 85 patients with HD [45]. After a median follow up of 3 years three of 63 patients with a negative PET and one of 13 patients with MRU relapsed [45]. In contrast, nine of 13 patients with a positive PET progressed and two patients died [45]. Survival analysis showed a highly significant association between early interim PET and PFS (p<0.0001) as well as OS (p<0.03). All advanced-stage patients with a positive early interim PET scan relapsed within 2 years [45].

In particular, the time from early interim PET to recognition of progression with conventional methods was 1–21 months (mean, 9 months) for eight PET-positive patients and 12–33 months (mean, 24.3 months) for three PET-negative patients [45] (Fig. 8.6).

The results of a recent prospective study conducted by Hutchins et al. in 77 patients with HD confirm these observations [46]. For prediction of PFS, interim PET was as accurate after two cycles as later during treatment and superior to CT at all time points [46]. In regression analysis, interim PET was stronger than the established prognostic factors. Other significant prognostic factors for progression were advanced stage and extranodal disease [46].

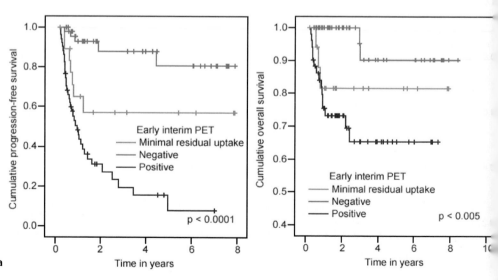

Fig. 8.5a,b. Kaplan-Meier plots depicting (a) progression-free survival and (b) overall survival according to the outcome of early interim FDG PET [44]

Table 8.4 Predictive value of whole-body ^{18}F-FDG PET for early response assessment (from [6])

Authors	No. of cycles before evaluation	Median follow-up (months)	Sensitivity	Specificity	Positive predictive value	Negative predictive value	Accuracy
Mikhaeel et al. [30]	2–4	30	100% (7/7)	94% (15/16)	87% (7/9)	100% (15/15)	96% (22/23)
Jerusalem et al. [39]	3-(2–5)	17	42% (5/12)	100% (14/14)	100% (5/5)	67% (14/21)	73% (19/26)
Kostakoglu et al. [40]	1	19	87% (13/15)	87% (13/15)	87% (13/15)	87% (13/15)	87% (26/30)
Spaepen et al. [41]	3–4	36	85% (33/39)	100% (31/31)	100% (33/33)	84% (31/37)	91% (64/70)
Zijlstra et al. [42]	2	25	64% (9/14)	75% (9/12)	75% (9/12)	64% (9/14)	69% (18/26)
Torizuka et al. [43]	1–2	24	87% (14/16)	50% (2/4)	87% (14/16)	50% (2/4)	80% (16/20)
Friedberg et al. [37]	3	24	80% (4/5)	94% (16/17)	80% (4/5)	94% (16/17)	91% (20/22)
Overall			**79% (85/108)**	**92% (100/109)**	**90% (85/94)**	**81% (100/123)**	**85% (185/217)**

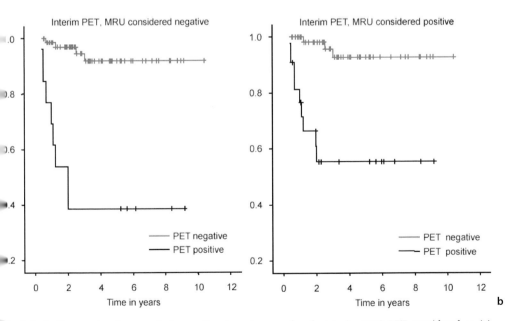

Fig. 8.6a,b. Progression-free survival according to outcome of early interim FDG PET considered as (a) negative and (b) positive [45]

8.7 Novel Functional Imaging Approaches in Malignant Lymphoma

Current molecular targets for PET imaging may be divided into principles relying on overexpression of key proteins of important pathways of intermediary metabolism upregulated in malignant lymphomas and receptors or antigens overexpressed at the cell membrane of lymphoma cells. Glucose transporters and key enzymes of glycolysis are certainly the most abundantly used molecular targets for diagnostic PET imaging in lymphoma. These are discussed elsewhere in this volume.

Amino acid (AA) utilization is increased in malignant lymphoma as well as in many other malignant tumors or tumor cell lines [47]. The molecular targets for this imaging approach are a variety of AA transporters, facilitating AA cellular influx. Most investigators assume that increased tumoral uptake of, for example, C-11 methionine mainly reflects transmembrane AA transport and not protein synthesis [48]. Our group found highly increased L-type AA transporter expression on the DOHH2 lymphoma cell line [49].

Proliferation may be increased in HD and NHL, depending on histologic subtype, stage, and biological aggressiveness. Increased proliferation has been linked to an impaired prognosis in NHL. The major metabolic target for assessment of proliferation in vivo with PET are key enzymes of the thymidine salvage pathway [50], particularly thymidine kinase 1 (TK1) and probably also DNA-dependent polymerases, overexpressed in many malignant tumors including malignant lymphoma [51].

Several authors reported mildly overexpressed somatostatin (sst) receptors, predominantly subtype 2 and 3 [52, 53] in a subgroup of NHL, forming the basis of first imaging studies with appropriately radiolabeled sst receptor ligands [54].

CD 20, 19, 45 and many other cluster-defined antigens may be abundantly overexpressed in NHL [55]. These receptors are addressed by a variety of monoclonal antibodies, radiolabeled with therapeutic isotopes with considerable therapeutic success [55, 56]. Since the kinetics of most antibodies in blood and tissue are relatively slow and radiolabeling methods of antibodies with appropriate PET isotopes are not widely available, the exquisite antibody-mediated targeting approach is currently not used for PET imaging of malignant lymphoma.

8.8 Imaging Proliferative Activity in Malignant Lymphoma

Imaging proliferative activity of malignant lymphoma is of considerable interest because proliferative activity of lymphomas is linked to biologic proliferative activity. Imaging of proliferative activity in individual lymphoma manifestations may improve early detection of development of aggressive transformation of low-grade lymphoma [57]. 3-Deoxy-3-18F-fluorothymidine (FLT) is the radiopharmaceutical currently most widely used for imaging proliferative activity.

8.9 3-Deoxy-3-18F-Fluorothymidine

Thymidine is incorporated into DNA in close relation to cellular proliferation, and 3H-thymidine uptake in experimental systems is well established for measuring cellular or tissue proliferation rate. Since C-11-thymidine is very rapidly degraded in vivo, several C-11 or F-18 labeled thymidine analogs were developed for evaluating tissue proliferation in vivo with PET [50, 58]. FLT was first described by Shields et al. in 1998 as a PET imaging probe in a dog lymphoma [59]. FLT is taken up by the cell through passive diffusion and facilitated Na+ dependent nucleoside transporter-mediated inward transport (see Beets et al. for review [50]). Within the cell, FLT is phosphorylated by TK1 to FLT monophosphate and to a limited degree also to the di- and triphosphate. Only minor amounts of FLT are incorporated into DNA and result in DNA chain terminations. TK1 is virtually absent in quiescent cells but is upregulated severalfold in proliferating cells during the late G1 and S phase of the cell cycle [50].

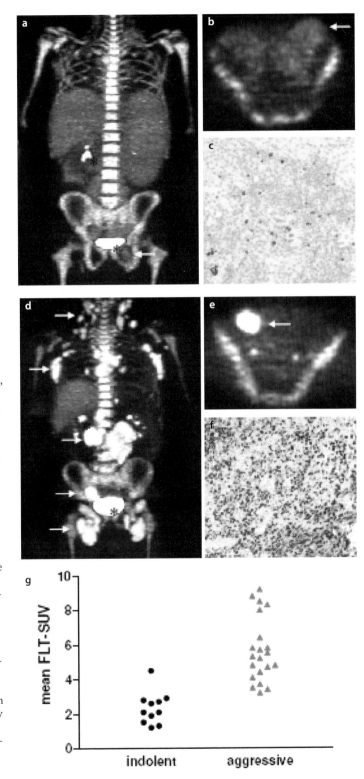

Fig. 8.7a–g. Significantly higher FLT uptake was observed in aggressive compared to indolent lymphoma. **a** FLT-PET (maximum intensity projection) of patient with indolent lymphoma. Low FLT uptake in enlarged spleen and in paraaortic, iliac, and inguinal bulky lesions (*arrow*). Physiological intense FLT uptake in proliferating bone marrow and mild FLT uptake in liver. **b** Transaxial section of the inguinal region with low FLT uptake in lymphoma (*arrow*). **c** Anti-Ki-67 immunostaining (MIB-1) indicates low proliferation fraction of < 5%. **d** FLT-PET (maximum intensity projection) of patient 14 with aggressive lymphoma. Intense uptake of FLT in cervical, axillary, mediastinal, paraaortic, iliac, and inguinal lymph nodes (*arrows*). **e** Transaxial section of inguinal region shows intense FLT uptake in lymphoma (*arrow*). **f** Anti-Ki-67 immunostaining (MIB-1) indicates high proliferation fraction (immunoreactivity in 95% of nuclei). **g** Significantly higher standardized uptake value (SUV) of FLT in aggressive compared to indolent lymphoma [57]

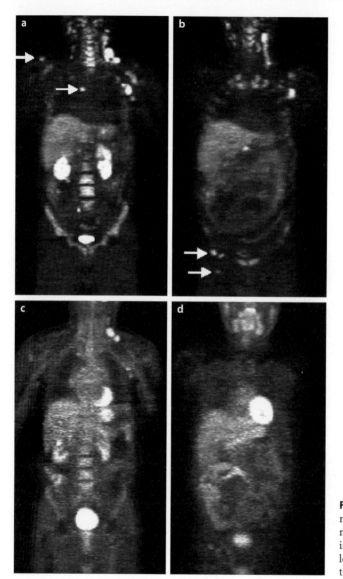

Fig. 8.8a–d. FLT PET (**a, b**) shows more extensive nodal involvement compared to FDG PET (**c, d**) in aggressive NHL. *Arrows* mark lesions not detected with conventional imaging [57]

8.10 Proliferation Imaging with FLT

FLT is physiologically taken up into bone marrow and liver and excreted via the urinary tract [57]. There is no physiologic uptake of FLT in brain, myocardium, or skeletal muscle. Uptake in the liver is due to glucuronidation of FLT followed by renal excretion. Recent studies from our group comparing FDG and FLT in patients with NHL indicated that both tracers detected

a comparable number of lesions [60]. A close correlation was observed in eight of the nine patients. We observed a significant correlation of Ki-67 labeling index and the SUV of FLT in lymphoma manifestations in another study in 26 patients with NHL (r = 0.76, p < 0.01) [57] (Fig. 8.7).

An attractive approach is the use of in vivo markers of lymphoma proliferative activity, the presumed true measure of malignancy grade o malignant lymphoma [7]. Using FLT, our group demonstrated excellent separation between aggressive and indolent lymphoma with a high correlation observed the SUV of FLT and proliferative activity of lymphomas [57] (Fig. 8.8). As stated by Juweid et al. in a recent review in the Journal of Clinical Oncology, the use of FLT might obviate the need of quantitative tracer kinetic methods potentially required when other radiotracers such as FDG are used for grading NHL [7]. In fact, lymphoma grading could turn out to become the predominant indication in lymphoma PET imaging [7].

Beyond this diagnostic approach, novel proliferation markers are currently being developed, which are incorporated into DNA and can be used as molecular carriers for Auger electron-mediated cell kill. Preliminary experimental results of our group indicate that this targeted nano-irradiation of DNA is highly effective in triggering apoptosis in DOHH-2 cells with radiation doses as low as 0.1 Gy.

References

1. Leskinen-Kallio S, Minn H, Joensuu H (1990) PET and [^{11}C]methionine in assessment of response in non-Hodgkin lymphoma. Lancet 336(8724):1188
2. Friedberg JW, Chengazi V (2003) PET scans in the staging of lymphoma: current status. Oncologist 8:438–447
3. Reske SN (2003) PET and restaging of malignant lymphoma including residual masses and relapse. Eur J Nucl Med Mol Imaging 30 [Suppl 1]:S89–S96
4. Israel O, Keidar Z, Bar-Shalom R (2004) Positron emission tomography in the evaluation of lymphoma. Semin Nucl Med 34:166–179
5. Hicks RJ, Mac Manus MP, Seymour JF (2005) Initial staging of lymphoma with positron emission tomography and computed tomography. Semin Nucl Med 35:165–175
6. Jerusalem G, Hustinx R, Beguin Y, Fillet G (2005) Evaluation of therapy for lymphoma. Semin Nucl Med 35:186–196.
7. Juweid ME, Cheson BD (2005) Role of positron emission tomography in lymphoma. J Clin Oncol 23:4577–4580
8. Mikhaeel NG (2006) Use of FDG-PET to monitor response to chemotherapy and radiotherapy in patients with lymphomas. Eur J Nucl Med Mol Imaging 33 [Suppl 13]:22–26
9. Jhanwar YS, Straus DJ (2006) The role of PET in lymphoma. J Nucl Med 47:1326–1334
10. Lu P (2005) Staging and classification of lymphoma. Semin Nucl Med 35:160–164
11. Schröder H, Larson SM, Yeung HWD (2004) PET/CT in oncology: integration into clinical management of lymphoma, melanoma, and gastrointestinal malignancies. J Nucl Med 45:72–81
12. Juweid ME, Wiseman GA, Vose JM, Ritchie JM, Menda Y, Wooldridge JE et al (2005) Response assessment of aggressive non-Hodgkin's lymphoma by integrated international workshop criteria and fluorine-18-fluorodeoxyglucose positron emission tomography. J Clin Oncol 23:4652–4661
13. Buchmann I, Moog F, Schirrmeister H, Reske SN (2000) Positron emission tomography for detection and staging of malignant lymphoma. Recent Results Cancer Res 156:78–89
14. Moog F, Kotzerke J, Reske SN (1999) FDG PET can replace bone scintigraphy in primary staging of malignant lymphoma. J Nucl Med 40:1407–1413
15. Moog F, Bangerter M, Diederichs CG, Guhlmann A, Kotzerke J, Merkle E et al (1997) Lymphoma: role of whole-body 2-deoxy-2-[F-18]fluoro-D-glucose (FDG) PET in nodal staging. Radiology 203:795–800
16. Moog F, Bangerter M, Kotzerke J, Guhlmann A, Frickhofen N, Reske SN (1998) ^{18}F-fluorodeoxyglucose-positron emission tomography as a new approach to detect lymphomatous bone marrow. J Clin Oncol 16:603–609
17. Moog F, Bangerter M, Diederichs CG, Guhlmann A, Merkle E, Frickhofen N et al (1998) Extranodal malignant lymphoma: detection with FDG PET versus CT. Radiology 206:475–481
18. Jerusalem F, Beguin Y, Fassotte MF, Najjar F, Paulus P, Rigo P et al (2001) Whole-body positron emission tomography using ^{18}F-fluorodeoxyglucose compared to standard procedures for staging patients with Hodgkin's disease. Haematologica 86:266–273
19. Hutchings M, Loft A, Hansen M, Pedersen LM, Berthelsen AK, Keiding S et al (2006) Position emission tomography with or without computed tomography in the primary staging of Hodgkin's lymphoma. Haematologica 91:482–489
20. Jerusalem G, Beguin Y, Najjar F, Hustinx R, Fassotte MF, Rigo P et al (2001) Positron emission tomography (PET) with 18F-fluorodeoxyglucose (^{18}F-FDG) for the staging of low-grade non-Hodgkin's lymphoma (NHL). Ann Oncol 12:825–830
21. Karam M, Novak L, Cyriac J, Ali A, Nazeer T, Nugent F (2006) Role of fluorine-18 fluoro-deoxyglucose positron emission tomography scan in the evaluation and follow-up of patients with low-grade lymphomas. Cancer 107:175–183
22. Hoffmann M, Kletter K, Diemling M, Becherer A, Pfeffel F, Petkov V et al (1999) Positron emission tomography with fluorine-18-2-fluoro-2-deoxy-D-glucose (F18-FDG) does not visualize extranodal B-cell lymphoma of the mucosa-associated lymphoid tissue (MALT)-type. Ann Oncol 10:1185–1189

23. Rodriguez M, Ahlstrom H, Sundin A, Rehn S, Sundstrom C, Hagberg H et al (1997) [18F] FDG PET in gastric non-Hodgkin's lymphoma. Acta Oncol 36:577–584

24. Bangerter M, Griesshammer M, Binder T, Hafner M, Heimpel H, Reske SN et al (1996) New diagnostic imaging procedures in Hodgkin's disease. Ann Oncol 7 [Suppl 4]:55–59

25. Jones HA, Cadwallader KA, White JF, Uddin M, Peters AM, Chilvers ER (2002) Dissociation between respiratory burst activity and deoxyglucose uptake in human neutrophil granulocytes: implications for interpretation of 18F-FDG PET images. J Nucl Med 43:652–657

26. Diederichs C, Staib L, Glatting G, Beger H, Reske S (1998) FDG-PET: elevated plasma glucose reduces both uptake and detection rate of pancreatic malignancies. J Nucl Med 39:1030–1033

27. Langen KJ, Braun U, Rota-Kops E, Herzog H, Kuwert T, Nebeling B et al (1993) The influence of plasma glucose levels on fluorine-18-fluorodeoxyglucose uptake in bronchial carcinomas. J Nucl Med 34:355–359

28. Cheson BD, Horning SJ, Coiffier B, Shipp MA, Fisher RI, Connors JM et al (1999) Report of an international workshop to standardize response criteria for non-Hodgkin's lymphomas. NCI Sponsored International Working Group. J Clin Oncol 17:1244

29. Canellos GP (1988) Residual mass in lymphoma may not be residual disease. J Clin Oncol 6:931–933

30. Mikhaeel NG, Timothy AR, O'Doherty MJ, Hain S, Maisey MN (2000) 18FDG-PET as a prognostic indicator in the treatment of aggressive non-Hodgkin's lymphoma: comparison with CT. Leuk Lymphoma 39:543–553

31. Spaepen K, Stroobants S, Dupont P, Van-Steenweghen S, Thomas J, Vandenberghe P et al (2001) Prognostic value of positron emission tomography (PET) with fluorine-18 fluorodeoxyglucose ([18F]FDG) after first-line chemotherapy in non-Hodgkin's lymphoma: is [18F]FDG-PET a valid alternative to conventional diagnostic methods? J Clin Oncol 19:414–419

32. De Wit M, Bohuslavizki KH, Buchert R, Bumann D, Clausen M, Hossfeld DK (2001) 18FDG-PET following treatment as valid predictor for disease-free survival in Hodgkin's lymphoma. Ann Oncol 12:29–37

33. Dittmann H, Sokler M, Kollmannsberger C, Dohmen BM, Baumann C, Kopp A et al (2001) Comparison of 18FDG-PET with CT scans in the evaluation of patients with residual and recurrent Hodgkin's lymphoma. Oncol Rep 8:1393–1399

34. Spaepen K, Stroobants S, Dupont P, Thomas J, Vandenberghe P, Balzarini J et al Can positron emission tomography with (18F)-fluorodeoxyglucose after first-line treatment distinguish Hodgkin's disease patients who need additional therapy from others in whom additional therapy would mean avoidable toxicity? Br J Haematol 115:272–278

35. Weihrauch MR, Re D, Scheidhauer K, Ansen S, Dietlein M, Bischoff S et al (2001). Thoracic positron emission tomography using 18F-fluorodeoxyglucose for the evaluation of residual mediastinal Hodgkin disease. Blood 98:2930–2934

36. Guay C, Lepine M, Verreault J, Benard F (2003) Prognostic value of PET using 18F-FDG in Hodgkin disease for posttreatment evaluation. J Nucl Med 44:1225–1231

37. Friedberg JW, Fischman A, Neuberg D, Kim H, Takvorian T, Ng AK et al (2004) FDG-PET is superior to gallium scintigraphy in staging and more sensitive in the follow-up of patients with de novo Hodgkin lymphoma: a blinded comparison. Leuk Lymphoma 45:85–92

38. Panizo C, Perez-Salazar M, Bendandi M, Rodriguez-Calvillo M, Boan JF, Garcia-Velloso MJ et al (2004) Positron emission tomography using 18F-fluorodeoxyglucose for the evaluation of residual Hodgkin's disease mediastinal masses. Leuk Lymphoma 45:1829–1833

39. Jerusalem G, Beguin Y, Fassotte MF, Najjar F, Paulus P, Rigo P et al (2000) Persistent tumor 18F-FDG uptake after a few cycles of polychemotherapy is predictive of treatment failure in non-Hodgkin's lymphoma. Haematologica 85:613–618

40. Kostakoglu L, Coleman M, Leonard JP, Kuji I, Zoe H, Goldsmith SJ (2002) PET predicts prognosis after 1 cycle of chemotherapy in aggressive lymphoma and Hodgkin's disease. J Nucl Med 43:1018–1027

41 Spaepen K, Stroobants S, Dupont P, Vandenberghe P, Thomas J, De Groot T et al (2002) Early restaging positron emission tomography with 18F-fluorodexoxyglucose predicts outcome in patients with aggressive non-Hodgkin's lymphoma. Ann Oncol 13:1356–1363

42. Zijlstra JM, Hoekstra OS, Raijmakers PG, Comans EF, van der Hoeven JJ, Teule GJ et al (2003) 18FDG positron emission tomography versus 67Ga scintigraphy as prognostic test during chemotherapy for non-Hodgkin's lymphoma. Br J Haematol 123:454–462

43. Torizuka T, Nakamura F, Kanno T, Futatsubashi M, Yoshikawa E, Okada H et al Early therapy monitoring with FDG-PET in aggressive non-Hodgkin's lymphoma and Hodgkin's lymphoma. Eur J Nucl Med Mol Imaging 31:22–28

44. Mikhaeel NG, Hutchings M, Fields PA, O'Doherty MJ, Timothy AR (2005) FDG-PET after two to three cycles of chemotherapy predicts progression-free and overall survival in high-grade non-Hodgkin lymphoma. Ann Oncol 16:1514–1523

45 Hutchings M, Mikhaeel NG, Fields PA, Nunan T, Timothy AR (2005) Prognostic value of interim FDG-PET after two or three cycles of chemotherapy in Hodgkin lymphoma. Ann Oncol 16:1160–1168

46. Hutchings M, Loft A, Hansen M, Pedersen LM, Buhl T, Jurlander J et al (2006) FDG-PET after two cycles of chemotherapy predicts treatment failure and progression-free survival in Hodgkin lymphoma. Blood 107:52–59

47. Chillaron J, Roca R, Valencia A, Zorzano A, Palacin M (2001) Heteromeric amino acid transporters: biochemistry, genetics, and physiology. Am J Physiol Renal Physiol 281:F995–F1018.

48. Jacobs AH, Thomas A, Kracht LW, Li H, Dittmar C, Garlip G et al (2005) ^{18}F-Fluoro-L-thymidine and 11C-methylmethionine as markers of increased transport and proliferation in brain tumors. J Nucl Med 46:1948–1958

49. Reske SN (2006) PET assessment of lymphoma: beyond ^{18}F-fluorodeoxyglucose. PET Clin 1:275–281

50. Been LB, Suurmeijer AJH, Cobben DCP, Jager PL, Hoekstra HJ, Elsinga PH (2004) [^{18}F]FLT-PET in oncology: current status and opportunities. Eur J Nucl Med Mol Imaging 31:1659–1672

51. Toyohara J, Wakib A, Takamatsub S, Yonekurab Y, Magatac Y, Fujibayashi Y (2002) Basis of FLT as a cell proliferation marker: comparative uptake studies with [^{3}H]thymidine and [^{3}H]arabinothymidine, and cell-analysis in 22 asynchronously growing tumor cell lines. Nucl Med Biol 29:281–287

52. Reubi JC, Waser B, Schaer JC, Laissue JA (2001) Somatostatin receptor sst1-sst5 expression in normal and neoplastic human tissues using receptor autoradiography with subtype-selective ligands. Eur J Nucl Med 28:836–846

54. Reubi JC (2003) Peptide receptors as molecular targets for cancer diagnosis and therapy. Endocr Rev 24:389–427

55. Ferone D, Semino C, Boschetti M, Cascini GL, Minuto F, Lastoria S (2005) Initial staging of lymphoma with octreotide and other receptor imaging agents. Semin Nucl Med 35:176–185

55. Press O, Leonard J, Coiffier B, Levy R, Timmerman J (2001) Immunotherapy of non-Hodgkin's lymphomas. In: Hematology. Orlando: American Society of Hematology, pp 221–240

56. Witzig TE (2004) Yttrium-90-ibritumomab tiuxetan radioimmunotherapy: a new treatment approach for B-cell non-Hodgkin's lymphoma. Drugs Today (Barc) 40:111–119

57. Buck A, Bommer M, Stilgenbauer S, Juweid M, Mottaghy F, Glatting G et al (2006) Molecular imaging of proliferation in malignant lymphoma. Cancer Res 66:11055–11061

58. Toyohara J, Hayashia A, Sato M, Gogamia A, Tanakab H, Haraguchib K, et al. Development of radioiodinated nucleoside analogs for imaging tissue proliferation: comparisons of six 5-iodonucleosides. Nucl. Med. Biol. 2003;30:687–696.

59. Shields AF, Grierson JR, Dohmen BM, Machulla HJ, Stayanoff JC, Lawhorn-Crews JM et al (1998) Imaging proliferation in vivo with [F-18]FLT and positron emission tomography. Nat Med 4:1334–1336

60. Buchmann I, Neumaier B, Schreckenberger M, Reske SN (2004) (^{18}F)3'-deoxy-3'-fluorothymidine-PET in NHL patients. whole-body biodistribution and imaging of lymphoma manifestations – a pilot study. Cancer Biother Radiopharm 19:436–442

9 PET in Colorectal Cancer

S. Dresel and P. M. Schlag

Recent Results in Cancer Research, Vol. 170
© Springer-Verlag Berlin Heidelberg 2008

9.1 Introduction

The incidence of colorectal cancer is approximately 400,000 new cases per year in Western Europe and the United States [1–3]. This tumor entity represents the second most malignant disease, and colorectal cancer ranks second as a cause of cancer death in the United States. Nearly 57,000 patients died of colorectal cancer in 2004 [4]. Early diagnosis is the key to long-term survival. The American Cancer Society screening guidelines suggest yearly fecal occult blood test plus flexible sigmoidoscopy every 5 years beginning at age 50 for asymptomatic individuals with no risk factors. All positive tests are followed up with colonoscopy and biopsy if needed. Surgical resection is the optimal treatment for colorectal cancer, which is a highly curable disease if detected in its early stages. Preoperative imaging with abdominal computed tomography (CT) and endorectal ultrasound is the standard of care for rectal carcinomas to determine the need for neoadjuvant treatment although it has limited sensitivity [5]. This approach is largely attributable to the fact that most patients will benefit from surgical resection of the tumor to prevent colonic obstruction or bleeding. Additionally, accurate staging can take place intraoperatively with excision of pericolonic and mesenteric lymph nodes along with peritoneal exploration. However, the assessment of tumor involvement of regional lymph nodes

with anatomical imaging is solely based on size and number of nodes present, limiting its diagnostic accuracy.

Several studies have shown the ability of FDG-PET imaging in the detection of primary carcinomas of the large bowel [6–9]. Sensitivity is highly dependent on both the size of the lesion and the grade of dysplasia [9]. There is a wide range of nonmalignant conditions in which increased FDG uptake is observed in the colon, such as inflammatory bowel disease, diverticulitis, and physiologic uptake in colonic mucosa, lymphoid tissue, and smooth muscle. Differentiation between benign and malignant uptake is predominantly based on the focal nature of hypermetabolism and also on semi-quantitative measurements. Inflammatory bowel disease and physiologic uptake tend to be diffuse or segmental, whereas the accumulation of FDG in premalignant and malignant lesions is focal. Despite a low positive predictive value for malignancy, focally increased uptake of FDG in the large bowel should not be ignored, particularly in light of the high incidence of premalignant adenomas and colorectal cancer in the age group that typically undergoes FDG-PET imaging. Focally increased uptake in the colon should lead to further investigation with colonoscopy and, when necessary, biopsy and polypectomy.

There is an urgent need for advanced imaging methods since despite modern strategies in the therapeutic surgical and nonsurgical approaches, recurrence will occur in 30%–40% of patients within 2 years [10, 11]. At primary diagnosis 10%–20% of all patients present with liver metastases, 25% of which can be resected. After curative resection, approximately 50% of patients will develop liver metastases in 5 years' time. If the recurrent disease is confined to the liver, resection of the liver metastases is the treatment of choice and can result in a 5-year survival rate of 35%–40% [12–14]. However, after partial hepatic resection, 60%–65% of patients will develop recurrent tumor. Thus, a significant proportion of these patients is found to have extrahepatic metastases at surgery [15, 16]. The unnecessary surgery contributes significantly to morbidity and must be considered a failure of diagnostic imaging. There is converging evidence that the conventional staging modalities consisting of abdominal ultrasound, CT scan, and colonoscopy may not be sufficient for appropriate staging of the disease either for primary stating or in the course of follow-up [17]. Intraoperative ultrasound additionally improves the detection rate for liver metastases, but cannot contribute to preoperative planning [18].

Follow-up of the disease may also be difficult. Repeated measurements of the concentration of carcinoembryonic antigen (CEA) as a blood test is the usual means to diagnose asymptomatic recurrences. However, sensitivity (59%) and specificity (84%) are rather low [19]. Postoperative screening with CT proved to be of little value due to limited sensitivity and specificity [17, 20]. A diagnostic dilemma remains when elevated CEA levels are documented without any hints of a tumor lesion in conventional imaging.

Thus, [F-18]FDG-PET was introduced as an functional imaging modality with picomolar sensitivity and high resolution [21]. The first study on [F-18]FDG-PET in colorectal cancer patients was published in 1982 [22]. In the above-mentioned context, the weaknesses of conventional imaging appear to be the strength of [F-18]FDG-PET [23, 24].

9.2 Primary Tumor Diagnosis and Staging

Few studies have focused on the usefulness of FDG-PET scanning in the initial staging of colorectal carcinomas [25–27]. In studies with small patient numbers, FDG-PET is reported to be helpful in unclear situations and in patients with symptoms other than those caused by the local tumor spread [27–29]. Rigo et al. [30] report that false-positive findings may increase in patient groups with a low incidence for rectal carcinoma, which prevents this tool from becoming a screening method. Overall, the sensitivity for detection of nodal metastasis is poor and is not significantly different from CT imaging. These results are not surprising because of the inability of FDG-PET to identify micrometastases and the resolution capabilities of the scanners currently used. The degree of uptake in lymph nodes smaller than 1 cm is often underestimated because of intrinsic resolution limitations of the PET systems. The observed accumulation of FDG in small lesions (measuring less than twice the full width at the scanner's half maximum) is not representative of their true metabolic activity. This decreases the sensitivity of the test in detecting early tumor spread to regional lymph nodes. The use of FDG-PET imaging in the preoperative staging of colorectal cancers has been advocated [26], but a substantial impact on clinical management has not been demonstrated. It is unlikely that initial treatment decision making will be significantly altered on the basis of PET imaging. Today, there is no established role for the systematic use of PET in the preoperative staging of colorectal cancer. It often helps the oncologic surgeon decide against operation when distant metastases are found, especially in patients with increased surgical risk because of significant comorbidities. FDG-PET imaging also can serve as a baseline scan for patients who present with advanced stage disease before chemotherapy. Assessment of the overall tumor burden and degree of FDG uptake before starting chemotherapy is a powerful tool to determine appropriate response to treatment on follow-up scans.

FDG-PET has been shown to reliably detect additional lesions, as shown by Falk et al. [31]. In this study, 16 patients were reported with 15 lesions (12 colorectal, two in the liver and one in the mesenterium) with FDG-PET superior to CT (positive predictive value 93%, negative predictive value 50% vs 100% and 27% for CT). Figure 9.1 shows a patient suffering from rectal carcinoma and liver metastases with no extra-hepatic disease. Another study [25] revealed a positive predictive value of 90% and a negative predictive value of 100% for the FDG PET in a study with 48 patients. Sensitivity for lymph node involvement was similar to CT in only 29% of cases. However, sensitivity for detecting liver metastases was better with FDG-PET than with CT (88% vs 38%).

9.3 Recurrent Disease

Most recurrences after surgical resection for colorectal cancer occur within the first 4 years. The likelihood of tumor recurrence is related to several factors, including tumor penetration through the bowel wall into the pericolic fat, poorly differentiated histology, tumor extension to adjacent organs or vessels, number of involved lymph nodes, and a preoperative elevation of carcinoembryonic antigen levels [4]. Accurate restaging of patients with colorectal carcinoma plays a pivotal role in guiding further treatment. Barium studies have been used for detection of local recurrence with accuracy in the range of 80%. However, barium studies have been

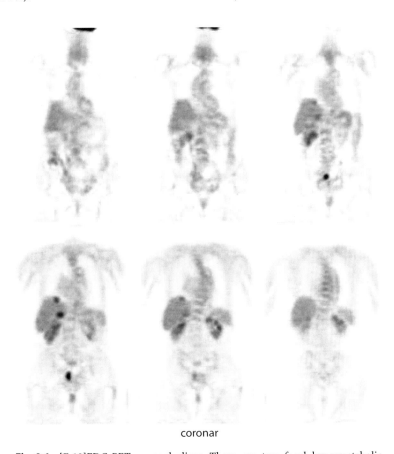

coronar

Fig. 9.1. [F-18]FDG-PET, coronal slices. There are two focal hypermetabolic lesions in the liver representing two liver metastases. Furthermore, uptake in the area of previously operated rectal tumor can be seen, which was histopathologically confirmed as local recurrence

reported to be only 49% sensitive and 85% specific for overall recurrence [32]. CT has been the conventional imaging modality used to localize recurrence, with an accuracy of 25%–73%, but it fails to demonstrate hepatic metastases in up to 7% of patients and underestimates the number of lobes involved in up to 33% of patients. In addition, metastases to the peritoneum, mesentery, and lymph nodes are commonly missed on CT, and the differentiation of postsurgical changes from local tumor recurrence is often equivocal [33–37]. Among the patients with negative CT, 50% will be found to have nonresectable lesions at the time of exploratory laparotomy. CT portography (superior mesenteric arterial portography) is more sensitive (80%–90%) than CT (70%–80%) for detection of hepatic metastases, but has a considerable rate of false-positive findings, lowering the positive predictive value [38–41]. In patients undergoing exploration for recurrent colorectal cancer, the presence of adhesions or the limitations of surgical exposure (transverse upper abdominal incision for liver resection) often preclude a detailed operative staging. Approximately 25% of recurrences are isolated to the liver [42] and curative resection is feasible, but it is highly dependent on the number, size, and location of the hepatic metastases. The presence of extrahepatic disease typically precludes surgery. Ultrasound of the upper abdomen is an inexpensive and valuable screening tool for detecting liver metastasis and identifying patients who are not eligible for curative treatment. Some parts of the liver may not be well visualized with ultrasound, and its overall sensitivity is poor. CT commonly is used as a first-line imaging modality for the detection of colorectal tumor recurrence. Its diagnostic accuracy, however, is far from ideal. CT often underestimates the number of liver lesions, and postsurgical changes can be difficult to distinguish from local tumor recurrence.

Elevated serum CEA levels are detected in two-thirds of patients with colorectal carcinoma. Abnormal CEA levels can be observed in a variety of benign conditions, but an increase in CEA levels is strongly associated with tumor recurrence, with a reported specificity of 70%–84% [19, 43]. Frequent monitoring of CEA postoperatively may allow identification of patients with disease recurrence in whom curative surgical resection or other localized therapy might be attempted. Serial CEA measurements appear to be more effective than clinical evaluation to detect recurrent disease from colorectal cancer. Its sensitivity is not as high for locoregional recurrence or pulmonary metastases as it is for liver metastases. Patients with rising CEA levels but no detectable disease on anatomical imaging pose a clinical challenge. It takes on average 3 to 9 months for conventional methods to localize disease relapse after elevation of CEA levels has been documented [19, 44, 45].

Several studies have described the additional value of FDG-PET imaging over anatomical imaging in recurrent colorectal cancer [21, 46–54]. Metabolically active tumors can be detected before a morphologic change is noted on anatomical imaging. A number of studies have demonstrated the role of FDG-PET as a functional imaging modality for detecting recurrent or metastatic colorectal carcinoma [24, 29, 31, 47, 55–60]. Overall, the sensitivity of FDG-PET imaging is in the 90% range and the specificity greater than 70%, both superior to CT. However, false-negative FDG-PET findings have been reported with mucinous adenocarcinoma. Whiteford and co-workers [54] reported that the sensitivity of FDG-PET imaging for detection of mucinous adenocarcinoma is significantly lower than the nonmucinous adenocarcinoma, 58% and 92%, respectively (p=0.005). They suspect that the low sensitivity of FDG-PET for detection of mucinous adenocarcinoma is due to the relative hypocellularity of these tumors. Similar findings (41% sensitivity) were reported in a subsequent series of 22 patients [61]. Several studies have compared FDG-PET and CT for differentiation of scar from local recurrence [23, 24, 31, 55, 59, 60]. CT was equivocal in most cases and the accuracy of FDG-PET imaging was greater than 90%. In the largest study (76 patients) [24], the accuracy of FDG-PET and CT were 95% and 65%, respectively.

Flanagan and co-workers [62] reported the use of FDG-PET in 22 patients with unexplained elevation of serum CEA level after resection of colorectal carcinoma, and no abnormal findings on conventional workup, including CT. Sensitivity and specificity of FDG-PET for tumor recurrence were 100% and 71%, respectively. Valk and co-workers [21] reported sensitivity of 93% and specificity of 92% in a similar group of 18 patients. In both studies, PET correctly demonstrated tumor in two-thirds of patients with rising CEA levels and negative CT scans. Valk and co-workers [21] compared the sensitivity and specificity of FDG-PET and CT for specific anatomic locations and found that FDG-PET was more sensitive than CT in all locations except the lung, where the two modalities were equivalent. The largest difference between PET and CT was found in the abdomen, pelvis, and retroperitoneum, where over one-third of PET-positive lesions were negative by CT. PET was also more specific than CT at all sites except the retroperitoneum, but the differences were smaller than the differences in sensitivity. In their study of 34 patients, Lai and co-workers [51] found that FDG-PET was especially useful for detecting retroperitoneal and pulmonary metastases. Delbeke and co-workers [47] concluded that outside the liver, FDG-PET was especially helpful in detecting nodal involvement, differentiating local recurrence from postsurgical changes, and evaluating the malignancy of indeterminate pulmonary nodules – indications for which CT has known limitations. In addition, since it is a whole-body technique, FDG-PET imaging allowed identification of distant metastatic disease in the chest, abdomen, or pelvis, which might not be in the field of view of routine CT staging exams. A comprehensive review of the PET literature (2,244 patient's studies) has reported a weighted average for FDG-PET sensitivity and specificity of 94% and 87%, respectively, compared with 79% and 73% for CT [63]. A meta-analysis of 11 studies with 577 patients [64] showed an overall sensitivity of 97% and specificity of 76% for FDG-PET detecting recurrent colorectal cancer. A more recent meta-analysis of 61 studies evaluating colorectal liver metastases [46] showed that FDG-PET had a sensitivity

of 95% on a per-patient basis, significantly better than CT (65%) and magnetic resonance imaging (MRI) (76%). Few studies have demonstrated the value of FDG-PET in patients with rising CEA levels and no identifiable lesions on conventional imaging. Flanagan and co-workers [62] reported a positive predictive value of 89% (15/17) and a negative predictive value of 100% (5/5) in patients with CEA measurements of 10–45 ng/ml. Valk and co-workers [21] showed a positive predictive value of 95% (18/19) and a negative predictive value of 85% (11/13).

The positive impact of PET on management decisions in this clinical scenario is evident. Curative therapy may be attempted for patients with localized disease, whereas unnecessary surgery may be prevented in patients with advanced-stage disease. FDG-PET imaging has been shown to significantly alter patient management when compared with conventional imaging modalities. A prospective study by Ruers and co-workers [65] demonstrated a change in clinical management in 20% of patients being evaluated for resection of colorectal liver metastasis. A change in patient management based on FDG-PET findings was determined to be 29% in a meta-analysis of 11 articles with 577 patients [64]. In a prospective study of 102 patients with suspected or confirmed regional recurrence of colorectal cancer [49], FDG-PET influenced management decisions in 59% of cases. The high impact on treatment planning in this particular study was predominantly avoiding surgery in patients with widespread disease. In a subset of 20 patients with rising CEA levels but no obvious site of recurrence on conventional imaging, FDG-PET localized recurrence in 13 (65%).

Concurrent PET-CT imaging with an integrated system may be especially important in the abdomen and pelvis. PET images alone may be difficult to interpret owing to both the absence of anatomical landmarks (other than the kidneys and bladder), the presence of nonspecific uptake in the stomach, small bowel, and colon, and urinary excretion of FDG. If possible, images of the abdomen and pelvis should be obtained with the arms elevated to avoid artifacts due to motion and to beam-hardening artifacts on the CT transmission images. Concurrent PET-CT imaging is helpful for differentiating focal retention of urine in the ureter, for example, compared to an FDG-avid lymph node. A recent study of 45 patients with colorectal cancer referred for FDG-PET imaging using an integrated PET-CT system concluded that PET-CT imaging increases the accuracy and certainty of locating lesions [66]. In their study, the frequency of equivocal and probable lesion characterization was reduced by 50% with PET-CT compared with PET alone, the number of definite locations was increased by 25%, and the overall correct staging increased from 78% to 89%.

Most institutions acquire CT transmission images without intravenous contrast to permit optimal attenuation correction but CT images without intravenous contrast do not allow visualization of many hepatic metastases. Therefore, although hepatic metastases are commonly seen as FDG-avid on the PET images, no corresponding lesions are seen on the noncontrasted CT transmission images. A standard-of-care CT with intravenous and oral contrast needs to be performed if surgery is contemplated. Evaluation of the effects of intravenous and oral contrast agents on the attenuation correction of the PET images is ongoing. Intravenous contrast appears as regions of high contrast on CT images, especially during the arterial and arteriovenous phase of enhancement. If these CT images are used for attenuation correction, overcorrection may create artifacts of increased uptake on the FDG-PET images [67]. High-density oral contrast agents [68, 69] and metallic implants [70] can create similar artifacts. However, the administration of low-density oral contrast results in only minimal overcorrection and is not believed to interfere with accurate interpretation of the images [69]. Review of the images without attenuation correction is helpful to discriminate an overcorrection artifact from true uptake and should be performed if there is abnormal uptake in a region of the body with accumulation of contrast agents or in a region of metallic implants. Nakamoto and co-workers [71] compared standard uptake value (SUV) measurements on PET images corrected

for attenuation with transmission maps obtained using germanium source and CT. They found that CT-based attenuation correction was overestimated by 11% in the skeleton and 2% in soft tissue compared with germanium-based attenuation correction. It is important to take these differences into consideration if the SUV is used when comparing PET studies obtained with different protocols. Serosal metastases can usually be precisely localized on the surface of the liver. As in the chest, the CT transmission images must be carefully reviewed for detection of malignant lesions that may not be FDG-avid such as mucinous tumors or renal cell carcinomas.

9.4 Liver Metastases, Exclusion of Extrahepatic Disease

Approximately 70% of patients presenting with hepatic metastatic disease are resectable with curative intent, but recurrence is noted in one-third of these patients in the first 2 years after resection. Twenty-five percent of these patients have recurrence limited to one site and are potentially curable by surgical resection [42]. For example, approximately 14,000 patients per year present with isolated liver metastases as their first recurrence, and roughly 20% of these patients die with metastases exclusively to the liver [72]. Hepatic resection is the only curative therapy in these patients, but it is associated with a 2%–7% mortality rate and has the potential for significant morbidity [73]. Early detection and prompt treatment of recurrences may lead to a cure in up to 25% of patients. However, the size and number of hepatic metastases and the presence of extrahepatic disease affect the prognosis. The poor prognosis of extrahepatic metastases is believed to be a contraindication to hepatic resection. Therefore, accurate noninvasive detection of inoperable disease with imaging modalities plays a pivotal role in selecting patients who would benefit from surgery.

A large number of studies have compared the accuracy of FDG-PET and CT for detection of hepatic metastases [21, 23, 24, 47, 53]

74]. Overall, FDG-PET was more accurate than CT. However, most of these studies suffered from a major limitation: PET was performed prospectively while CT was reviewed retrospectively and performed at various institutions, resulting in variable quality. Vitola and co-workers [53] and Delbeke and co-workers [47] reported the comparison of FDG with CT and CT portography. CT portography, which is more invasive and more costly than FDG-PET or CT alone, is regarded as the most effective means of determining resectability of hepatic metastasis by imaging. FDG-PET had a higher accuracy (92%) than CT (78%) and CT portography (80%) for detection of hepatic metastases. Although the sensitivity of FDG-PET (91%) was lower than that of CT portography (97%), the specificity was much higher, particularly at postsurgical sites. A meta-analysis conducted to compare noninvasive imaging methods (US, CT, MRI, and FDG-PET) for the detection of hepatic metastases from colorectal, gastric, and esophageal cancers demonstrated that at an equivalent specificity of 85%, FDGPET had the highest sensitivity of 90% compared with 76% for MRI, 72% for CT, and 55% for US [50]. Beets et al. and Schiepers et al. [24, 55] confirm the superiority of FDG-PET in terms of sensitivity (94%) and specificity (98%) in comparison to CT and ultrasound (85% and 93%) for diagnosing liver disease. For both methods, no false-positive results were documented; false-negative findings were seen in two patients with lesions less than 1 cm in diameter, which were also not seen on CT. These results were also corroborated by Delbeke [47] and Ogunbiyi [23] in larger patient groups. The latter also found a higher accuracy for FDG-PET with respect to the number of liver lesions in comparison to CT.

The diagnosis and exclusion of extrahepatic disease is crucial for appropriate therapy planning of patients suffering from hepatic disease. The work of Lai et al. [51] and Schiepers et al. [24] shows that FDG-PET is a highly sensitive modality for staging recurrent colorectal disease. In our own study, 58 patients (Table 9.1) suffering from liver metastases were examined before surgical procedures [75]. In 46 of 58 patients, readings of conventional staging methods were in agreement with FDG-PET. All results were confirmed by histopathology or follow-up. In 43 of these 46 patients, neither conventional modalities nor FDG-PET revealed extrahepatic lesions. In 2 of 46 patients, CT and FDG-PET showed lung metastases. In another patient, false-positive results were documented in both CT and FDG-PET due to pneumonia. In 12 out of 58 patients, there was no agreement in the findings of FDG-PET and conventional staging (Fig. 9.2). In those cases, only FDG-PET established the correct diagnosis of extrahepatic disease; among those 12 cases, six recurrences, two cases with lung metastases, one case with mediastinal disease, one case with osseous lesions, one patient with supraclavicular lymph node metastases, and one patient with abdominal lymph node lesions. These results further confirm that FDG-PET is a highly attractive, complementary imaging method in patients potentially qualifying for curative resection of liver metastases.

9.5 Therapy Monitoring

The mainstay of adjuvant chemotherapy for colorectal cancer is 5-floururacil (5-FU); which is an effective palliative treatment in colorectal cancer, improving quality of life and survival [76]. The drug is usually well tolerated but response rates are only 10%–20% in patients with advanced disease. Findlay and co-workers [77] studied 18 patients with colorectal cancer liver metastases before and during the 1st month of chemotherapy. By using a 15% reduction in the pretreatment tumor-to-liver ratio by 4–5 weeks, they were able to separate responders from nonresponders with a sensitivity of 100% and specificity of 90%. The combination of 5-FU and local radiation therapy is also associated with increased survival in patients with unresectable disease. Posttherapeutic response evaluation is particularly problematic in rectal cancer patients. Endorectal ultrasound, CT, and MRI provide detailed morphological information, but functional characterization of treated lesions is poor. Radiation-induced

Table 9.1. Patients and results: FDG-PET for detecting extrahepatic disease before curative resection of liver metastases

Pat. no.	Age	Gender	Extrahepatic disease positive/negative			Localization	CSM	PET	CIM
			CSM	PET	OP/follow-up				
1	62	M	–	+	+	Local recurrence	FN	TP	CU
2	78	F	–	–	–		TN	TN	NC
3	70	F	–	–	–		TN	TN	NC
4	59	M	–	+	+	Local recurrence	FN	TP	CU
5	79	F	–	–	–		TN	TN	NC
6	69	M	–	–	–		TN	TN	NC
7	74	F	–	–	–		TN	TN	NC
8	56	M	–	–	–		TN	TN	NC
9	68	M	–	–	–		TN	TN	NC
10	65	F	–	–	–		TN	TN	NC
11	77	F	–	+	+	Local recurrence	FN	TP	CU
12	58	F	–	+	+	Bone	FN	TP	CU
13	67	M	–	–	–		TN	TN	NC
14	76	F	–	–	–		TN	TN	NC
15	75	M	+	+	+	Lung	TP	TP	NC
16	61	F	–	–	–		TN	TN	NC
17	62	F	–	+	+	Local recurrence	FN	TP	CU
18	46	W	–	–	–		TN	TN	NC
19	60	M	–	–	–		TN	TN	NC
20	80	M	–	–	–		TN	TN	NC
21	62	M	–	–	–		TN	TN	NC
22	66	M	–	–	–		TN	TN	NC
23	60	F	–	–	–		TN	TN	NC
24	61	F	–	–	–		TN	TN	NC
25	48	F	–	–	–		TN	TN	NC
26	59	M	–	–	–		TN	TN	NC
27	60	M	–	–	–		TN	TN	NC
28	55	M	–	–	–		TN	TN	NC
29	67	M	–	–	–		TN	TN	NC
30	50	M	–	–	–		TN	TN	NC
31	47	F	–	–	–		TN	TN	NC
32	68	F	–	–	–		TN	TN	NC
33	54	M	+	+	+	Lung	TP	TP	NC
34	64	M	–	–	–		TN	TN	NC
35	81	M	–	+	+	Local recurrence	FN	TP	CU
36	55	M	–	–	–		TN	TN	NC

Pat. no.	Age	Gender	Extrahepatic disease positive/negative			Localization	CSM	PET	CIM
			CSM	PET	OP/follow-up				
38	48	F	−	−	−		TN	TN	NC
39	70	M	−	−	−		TN	TN	NC
40	69	F	−	−	−		TN	TN	NC
41	33	F	+	+	−		FP	FP	NC
42	59	M	−	−	−		TN	TN	NC
43	54	M	−	−	−		TN	TN	NC
44	76	M	−	−	−		TN	TN	NC
45	71	F	−	+	+	Lung	FN	TP	CU
46	63	M	−	+	+	Lung	FN	TP	CU
47	74	M	−	−	−		TN	TN	NC
48	68	F	−	−	−		TN	TN	NC
49	62	F	−	−	−		TN	TN	NC
50	70	M	−	−	−		TN	TN	NC
51	46	M	−	−	−		TN	TN	NC
52	60	M	−	+	+	Lung	FN	TP	CU
53	57	F	−	−	−		TN	TN	NC
54	65	M	−	−	−		TN	TN	NC
55	72	F	−	+	+	Mediastinum	FN	TP	CU
56	40	M	−	+	+	Cervical	FN	TP	CU
57	62	F	−	−	−		TN	TN	NC
58	38	M	−	+	+	Peritoneum	FN	TP	CU

inflammation, necrosis, and desmoplastic reactions may induce contrast enhancement of treated lesions, making it difficult to distinguish postradiation changes from residual tumor, which hampers adequate assessment of disease status by means of anatomical imaging alone.

FDG-PET imaging can be particularly useful in patients with advanced-stage colorectal cancer who are treated with neoadjuvant chemoradiotherapy [78]. The ability to differentiate benign from malignant lesions based on their metabolic activity and biological aggressiveness allows early assessment of response to treatment. Guillem and co-workers [79] showed that FDG-PET imaging can predict long-term outcomes in patients with advanced colorectal cancer who undergo neoadjuvant chemoradiotherapy. This study prospectively included 15 patients who had FDG-PET imaging before and 4–5 weeks after chemoradiotherapy. At a median follow-up of 42 months, a metabolic tumor response of greater than 62.5% (as measured by a decrease in maximum SUV) predicted disease-specific survival and recurrence-free survival. Similarly, in a prospective study of 20 patients, Amthauer and co-workers [80] used a cut-off SUV reduction of 36.1% to differentiate responders from nonresponders. The patients were imaged before and 2–4 weeks after the completion of treatment. The cutoff value of 36.1% yielded a sensitivity of 100% (13/13), specificity of 86% (6/7), a positive predictive value of 93% (13/14), and a negative predictive value of 100% (6/6). Reliable monitoring of neoadjuvant treatment response is pivotal for risk stratification and treatment refinement. If these findings are confirmed on a larger series, FDG-PET imaging may prove useful in identifying patients at high risk for recurrence and those in whom less aggressive resection may be attempted. Standardized interval from completion of chemoradiotherapy to imaging as well as a cutoff percent decrease in SUV still need to be established to overcome transient tumor stunning and radiation-induced inflammation, optimizing the diagnostic accuracy of FDG-PET.

9.6 Minimally Invasive Interventional Therapies

Several interventional therapies have emerged in the past few years as an alternative to more invasive surgical procedures, particularly for patients with liver metastases. Radiofrequency (RF) ablation and yttrium-90 (^{90}Y) microsphere radioembolization are increasingly becoming the interventional techniques of choice for patients with unresectable liver disease. RF ablation is typically performed percutaneously and guided with CT or ultrasound. The radiofrequency generator provides current and energy that is deposited in tissues through the RF ablation probe tip. The liver tissue is destroyed

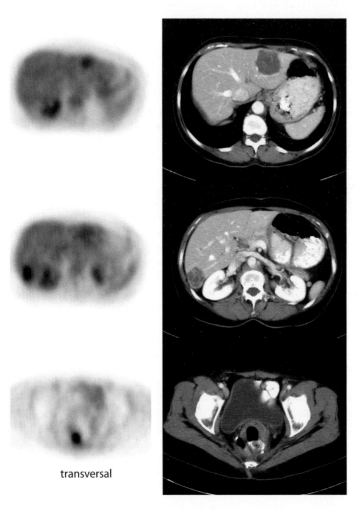

transversal

Fig. 9.2. [F-18]FDG-PET, transverse slices, computed tomography, transverse slices. Two focal lesions in the FDG-PET correlate with the CT findings of two liver metastases in the left and right liver lobe. In the previously operated area of the rectum CT only demonstrated scar, whereas the FDG-PET confirmed recurrent disease

as temperatures reach 55°C [81]. Larger tumors may require multiple sessions with repositioning of the probe. This procedure is usually indicated for patients with fewer than five liver lesions measuring less than 5 cm in diameter. RF ablation has been used with both palliative and curative intent. Median survival rates have been reported to improve with RF ablation of colorectal liver metastasis when compared with historical data [82].

Ablative treatment success depends on complete tumor destruction. Anatomical evaluation of residual tumor after the ablation procedure is limited because contrast enhancement in the periphery of the ablative necrosis may be caused by posttreatment hyperemia or tissue regeneration [83]. This decreases the specificity of ultrasound, CT, and MRI to detect residual tumor soon after RF ablation. Some authors [84, 85] propose waiting a minimum 6–12 weeks before performing anatomical imaging to decrease the false-positive rate secondary to physiologic contrast enhancement.

FDG-PET appears to have great potential in identifying residual tumor soon after RF ablation. In a prospective study of 23 patients with a mean follow-up of 16 months, Langenhoff and co-workers [86] showed that FDG-PET has a positive predictive value of 80% (4/5 lesions) and a negative predictive value of 100% (51/51 lesions) when performed soon (less than 3 weeks) after the ablative procedure (RF ablation or cryoablation). Donckier and co-workers [87] reported on the value of FDG-PET imaging when performed at 1 week and 1 month after RF ablation of 28 liver metastases from different solid tumors. Residual hypermetabolism in the periphery of ablated sites detected by FDG-PET scans correlated well with incomplete tumor destruction in 4 of 28 lesions. CT imaging performed at the same time interval failed to demonstrate residual hypervascularized tumor in these patients. After a median follow-up of 11 months, 0 of 24 lesions with negative postoperative FDG-PET scans developed local recurrence. The ideal time interval between the ablative procedure and FDG-PET imaging has not been defined. Inflammatory changes from the procedure and regenerating liver tissue in the periphery of the necrotic zone

may show increased uptake, making interpretation of the images difficult. Antoch and co-workers [88] have recently suggested that FDG-PET imaging should be performed immediately after RF ablation. None of 19 ablated liver sites in ten pigs showed increased rim of uptake within 90 min after completion of the therapy. Furthermore, no tissue regeneration was found on histopathologic examination. These results are encouraging, but prospective studies in treated patients are needed to establish the role and time of FDG-PET imaging as a first-line modality to assess adequate response to ablative procedures. A more accurate imaging modality applied soon after therapy will allow early reintervention if residual tumor is present, potentially minimizing the spread of tumor.

Intra-arterial hepatic radioembolization with ^{90}Y microspheres is a new treatment option for unresectable hepatocellular carcinoma and liver metastasis. ^{90}Y microspheres are administered by selective hepatic artery canalization under fluoroscopic guidance. The treatment strategy is based on the same principle that guides hepatic chemoembolization: liver metastases depend primarily on the hepatic arteries for their nutrition and growth. When administered intra-arterially, the microspheres (measuring approximately 30 μm in diameter) are trapped in the capillary bed and stop blood flow to the hepatic artery. ^{90}Y decays by beta emission with a half-life of 64 h and an average 2.5-mm penetration depth in soft tissue [89]. Therefore, in addition to the mechanical occlusion by the microspheres, the embolized tissues receive a substantial radiation dose from beta rays, maximizing tumor cell damage.

^{90}Y microsphere treatment is preceded by hepatic arteriography via the femoral artery on a separate day to assess the vascular anatomy of the liver and to exclude significant liver–lung shunting. The liver–lung shunt fraction is studied by administering Tc-99m-macroaggregated albumin particles in the hepatic artery with subsequent scintigraphic imaging. Since the average size of Tc-99m-macroaggregated albumin particles is similar to that of microspheres, the calculated liver–lung shunt fraction estimates the patient's potential for developing radiation pneumonitis. Radioembolization with ^{90}Y microspheres is usually contraindicated for patients with liver–lung shunt fractions greater than 20%. Larger shunt fractions are typically observed in patients with unresectable hepatocellular carcinoma when compared with patients with metastatic liver disease. Anatomical imaging appears insensitive in monitoring early response to ^{90}Y microsphere treatment when compared with metabolic imaging [90]. This is in part caused by edema, hemorrhage, and cystic/necrotic changes after therapy.

In a prospective series of eight patients with liver metastases from colorectal cancer, Wong and co-workers [90] reported on the superiority of FDG-PET over anatomical imaging (CT or MRI) to monitor response to ^{90}Y microspheres 3 months after treatment. All patients with a good metabolic response as judged by FDG-PET imaging had a drop in serum CEA levels, whereas none of these patients showed a significant anatomical response. Similar findings were again described by Wong and co-workers [91] in 27 consecutive patients. FDG-PET imaging does appear to be a promising tool for

early assessment of tumor response to 90Y microsphere radioembolization (Fig. 9.3). Larger prospective studies are needed to determine the best time interval from treatment to imaging, since it takes several days for the full radiation effect of ^{90}Y and inflammatory changes are likely to be present soon after therapy. Preliminary data suggest, however, that there are no significant changes in FDG uptake in treated vs untreated liver tissue at 4 weeks after therapy [92, 93].

9.7 Impact of FDG-PET Findings on Patient Management

The greater sensitivity of PET compared with CT in diagnosis and staging of recurrent tumor results from two factors: early detection of abnormal tumor metabolism, before changes have become apparent by anatomic imaging, and the whole body nature of PET imaging, which permits diagnosis of tumor when it occurs in unusual and unexpected sites. FDG-PET imaging allows the detection of unsuspected metastases in 13%–36% of patients and has a clinical impact

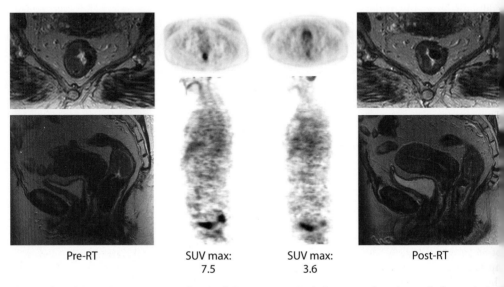

| Pre-RT | SUV max: 7.5 | SUV max: 3.6 | Post-RT |

Fig. 9.3. [F-18]FDG-PET, transverse and sagittal slices, MRI, sagittal slices. Rectal carcinoma before and after short course radiotherapy with 5×5 Gy. MRI shows relatively little response in terms of volume reduction of the tumor. FDG-PET visually and semi-quantitatively documents response at an early time point (1 week after the beginning of radiotherapy)

n 14%–65% [21, 23, 24, 49, 51, 52, 55, 56, 58, 62, 55, 94, 95]. In the study of Delbeke and co-workers [47], surgical management was altered by PET in 28% of patients, in one-third by initiating surgery and in two-thirds by avoiding surgery. In a survey-based study of 60 referring oncologists, surgeons, and generalists, FDG-PET performed at initial staging had a major impact on the management of colorectal cancer patients and contributed to a change in clinical stage in 42% (80% upstaged and 20% downstaged) and a change in the clinical management in over 60% [96]. As a result of the PET findings, physicians avoided major surgery in 41% of patients for whom surgery was the intended treatment. In a recent prospective study of 51 patients evaluated for resection of hepatic metastases, clinical management decisions based on conventional diagnostic methods were changed in 20% of patients based on the findings on FDG-PET imaging, especially by detecting unsuspected extrahepatic disease [65]. In a meta-analysis of the literature, FDG-PET imaging changed the management in 29% (102/349) patients [64]. The comprehensive review of the PET literature has reported a weighted average change of management related to FDG-PET findings in 32% of 915 patients [63]. Although survival is not an endpoint for a diagnostic test, Strasberg and co-workers [95] have estimated the survival of patients who underwent FDG-PET imaging in their preoperative evaluation for resection of hepatic metastases. The Kaplan-Meier test estimate of the overall survival at three years was 77% and the lower confidence limit was 60%. These percentages are higher than those in previously published series that ranged from 30% to 64%. In the patients undergoing FDG-PET imaging before hepatic resection, the three-year disease-free survival rate was 40%, again higher than that usually reported.

In our own study in 46 out of 58 patients, no change in management was necessary in the light of the FDG-PET findings [75]. In 12 of 58 patients (21%) FDG-PET led to a correct upstaging. The clinical management and the therapeutic strategy was altered in 21% of the cases due to the diagnosis of extrahepatic disease that was not seen in conventional staging procedures (Table 9.2).

Table 9.2. Impact of PET on clinical stage

Clinical stage	n	%
Upstaged	12	21
Downstaged	0	0
No change	46	79

9.8 Potential New PET Tracers

Besides evaluation of glucose metabolism with FDG, PET can assess various other biologic parameters such as perfusion, metabolism of other compounds, hypoxia, and receptor expression. Some of these radiopharmaceuticals are labeled with positron emitters that have a short half-life, such as O-15 (T1/2 = 2 min), N-13 (T1/2 = 10 min), and C-11 (T1/2 = 20 min). The short half-life of these radioisotopes prevents any timely distribution of the radiopharmaceuticals labeled with them and therefore, their use is restricted to institutions having a cyclotron and associated laboratories and personnel on site. Some tracers labeled with F-18, such as F-18 fluorothymidine (FLT), are being investigated for clinical use and may have applications for evaluation of patients with colorectal carcinoma.

References

1. Greenway B (1988) Hepatic metastases from colorectal cancer: resection or not. Br J Surg 75:513–519
2. Sugarbaker PH (1990) Surgical decision making for large bowel cancer metastatic to the liver. Radiology 174:621–626
3. Vauthey JN (1998) Liver imaging. A surgeon's perspective. Radiol Clin North Am 36:445–457
4. Esteves FP, Schuster DM, Halkar RK (2006) Gastrointestinal tract malignancies and positron emission tomography: an overview. Semin Nucl Med 36:169–181
5. Thoeni RF (1997) Colorectal cancer. Radiologic staging. Radiol Clin North Am 35:457–485
6. Friedland S, Soetikno R, Carlisle M et al (2005) 18-Fluorodeoxyglucose positron emission tomography has limited sensitivity for colonic adenoma and early stage colon cancer. Gastrointest Endosc 61:395–400
7. Gutman F, Alberini JL, Wartski M et al (2005) Incidental colonic focal lesions detected by FDG PET/CT. AJR Am J Roentgenol 185:495–500

8. Kamel EM, Thumshirn M, Truninger K et al (2004) Significance of incidental ¹⁸F-FDG accumulations in the gastrointestinal tract in PET/CT: correlation with endoscopic and histopathologic results. J Nucl Med 45:1804–1810

9. van Kouwen MC, Nagengast FM, Jansen JB et al (2005) 2-(¹⁸F)-fluoro-2-deoxy-D-glucose positron emission tomography detects clinical relevant adenomas of the colon: a prospective study. J Clin Oncol 23:3713–3717

10. Galandiuk S, Wieand HS, Moertel CG et al (1992) Patterns of recurrence after curative resection of carcinoma of the colon and rectum. Surg Gynecol Obstet 174:27–32

11. Sagar PM, Pemberton JH (1996) Surgical management of locally recurrent rectal cancer. Br J Surg 83:293–304

12. Fong Y, Cohen AM, Fortner JG et al (1997) Liver resection for colorectal metastases. J Clin Oncol 15:938–946

13. Gayowski TJ, Iwatsuki S, Madariaga JR et al (1994) Experience in hepatic resection for metastatic colorectal cancer: analysis of clinical and pathologic risk factors. Surgery 116:703–710; discussion 710–711

14. Scheele J, Stangl R, Altendorf-Hofmann A (1990) Hepatic metastases from colorectal carcinoma: impact of surgical resection on the natural history. Br J Surg 77:1241–1246

15. Fortner JG, Silva JS, Golbey RB et al (1984) Multivariate analysis of a personal series of 247 consecutive patients with liver metastases from colorectal cancer. I. Treatment by hepatic resection. Ann Surg 199:306–316

16. Steele G Jr, Ravikumar TS (1989) Resection of hepatic metastases from colorectal cancer. Biologic perspective. Ann Surg 210:127–138

17. Moss AA (1989) Imaging of colorectal carcinoma. Radiology 170:308–310

18. Leen E, Angerson WJ, Wotherspoon H et al (1995) Detection of colorectal liver metastases: comparison of laparotomy CT, US, and Doppler perfusion index and evaluation of postoperative follow-up results. Radiology 195:113–116

19. Moertel CG, Fleming TR, Macdonald JS et al (1993) An evaluation of the carcinoembryonic antigen (CEA) test for monitoring patients with resected colon cancer. JAMA 270:943–947

20. Balthazar EJ (1991) CT of the gastrointestinal tract: principles and interpretation. AJR Am J Roentgenol 156:23–32

21. Valk PE, Abella-Columna E, Haseman MK et al (1999) Whole-body PET imaging with [¹⁸F]fluorodeoxyglucose in management of recurrent colorectal cancer. Arch Surg 134:503–511; discussion 511–513

22. Yonekura Y, Benua RS, Brill AB et al (1982) Increased accumulation of 2-deoxy-2-[¹⁸F]Fluoro-D-glucose in liver metastases from colon carcinoma. J Nucl Med 23:1133–1137

23. Ogunbiyi OA, Flanagan FL, Dehdashti F et al (1997) Detection of recurrent and metastatic colorectal cancer: comparison of positron emission tomography and computed tomography. Ann Surg Oncol 4:613–620

24. Schiepers C, Penninckx F, De Vadder N et al (1995) Contribution of PET in the diagnosis of recurrent colorectal cancer: comparison with conventional imaging. Eur J Surg Oncol 21:517–522

25. Abdel-Nabi H, Doerr RJ, Lamonica DM et al (1998) Staging of primary colorectal carcinomas with fluorine-18 fluorodeoxyglucose whole-body PET: correlation with histopathologic and CT findings. Radiology 206:755–760

26. Kantorova I, Lipska L, Belohlavek O et al (2003) Routine (¹⁸)F-FDG PET preoperative staging of colorectal cancer: comparison with conventional staging and its impact on treatment decision making. J Nucl Med 44:1784–1788

27. Mukai M, Sadahiro S, Yasuda S et al (2000) Preoperative evaluation by whole-body ¹⁸F-fluorodeoxyglucose positron emission tomography in patients with primary colorectal cancer. Oncol Rep 7:85–87

28. Takeuchi O, Saito N, Koda K, Sarashina H et al (1999) Clinical assessment of positron emission tomography for the diagnosis of local recurrence in colorectal cancer. Br J Surg 86:932–937

29. Ruhlmann J, Paulus P, Kaschten BJ et al (1997) Fluorodeoxyglucose whole-body positron emission tomography in colorectal cancer patients studied in routine daily practice. Dis Colon Rectum 40:1195–1204

30. Rigo P, Paulus P, Kaschten BJ et al (1996) Oncological applications of positron emission tomography with fluorine-18 fluorodeoxyglucose. Eur J Nucl Med 23:1641–1674

31. Falk PM, Gupta NC, Thorson AG et al (1994) Positron emission tomography for preoperative staging of colorectal carcinoma. Dis Colon Rectum 37:153–156

32. Chen YM, Ott DJ, Wolfman NT et al (1987) Recurrent colorectal carcinoma: evaluation with barium enema examination and CT. Radiology 163:307–310

33. Charnsangavej C, Whitley NO (1993) Metastases to the pancreas and peripancreatic lymph nodes from carcinoma of the right side of the colon: CT findings in 12 patients. AJR Am J Roentgenol 160:49–52

34. Granfield CA, Charnsangavej C, Dubrow RA et al (1992) Regional lymph node metastases in carcinoma of the left side of the colon and rectum: CT demonstration. AJR Am J Roentgenol 159:757–761

35. McDaniel KP, Charnsangavej C, DuBrow RA et al (1993) Pathways of nodal metastasis in carcinomas of the cecum, ascending colon, and transverse colon: CT demonstration. AJR Am J Roentgenol 161:61–64

36. Steele G Jr, Bleday R, Mayer RJ et al (1991) A prospective evaluation of hepatic resection for colorectal carcinoma metastases to the liver: Gastrointestinal Tumor Study Group Protocol 6584. J Clin Oncol 9:1105–1112

37. Sugarbaker PH, Gianola FJ, Dwyer A et al (1987) A simplified plan for follow-up of patients with colon and rectal cancer supported by prospective studies of laboratory and radiologic test results. Surgery 102:79–87

38. Nelson RC, Chezmar JL, Sugarbaker PH et al (1989) Hepatic tumors: comparison of CT during arterial portography, delayed CT, and MR imaging for preoperative evaluation. Radiology 172:27–34

39. Peterson MS, Baron RL, Dodd GD 3rd et al (1992) Hepatic parenchymal perfusion defects detected with CTAP: imaging-pathologic correlation. Radiology 185:149–155

40. Small WC, Mehard WB, Langmo LS et al (1993) Preoperative determination of the resectability of hepatic tumors: efficacy of CT during arterial portography. AJR Am J Roentgenol 161:319–322

41. Soyer P, Levesque M, Elias D et al (1992) Detection of liver metastases from colorectal cancer: comparison of intraoperative US and CT during arterial portography. Radiology 183:541–544

42. August DA, Ottow RT, Sugarbaker PH (1984) Clinical perspective of human colorectal cancer metastasis. Cancer Metastasis Rev 3:303–324

43. Fletcher RH (1986) Carcinoembryonic antigen. Ann Intern Med 104:66–73

44. Engaras B (2003) Individual cutoff levels of carcinoembryonic antigen and CA 242 indicate recurrence of colorectal cancer with high sensitivity. Dis Colon Rectum 46:313–321

45. McCall JL, Black RB, Rich CA et al (1994) The value of serum carcinoembryonic antigen in predicting recurrent disease following curative resection of colorectal cancer. Dis Colon Rectum 37:875–881

46. Bipat S, van Leeuwen MS, Comans EF et al (2005) Colorectal liver metastases: CT, MR imaging, and PET for diagnosis–meta-analysis. Radiology 237:123–131

47. Delbeke D, Vitola JV, Sandler MP et al (1997) Staging recurrent metastatic colorectal carcinoma with PET. J Nucl Med 38:1196–1201

48. Hustinx R, Paulus P, Jacquet N et al (1998) Clinical evaluation of whole-body ^{18}F-fluorodeoxyglucose positron emission tomography in the detection of liver metastases. Ann Oncol 9:397–401

49. Kalff V, Hicks RJ, Ware RE et al (2002) The clinical impact of ([18])F-FDG PET in patients with suspected or confirmed recurrence of colorectal cancer: a prospective study. J Nucl Med 43:492–499

50. Kinkel K, Lu Y, Both M et al (2002) Detection of hepatic metastases from cancers of the gastrointestinal tract by using noninvasive imaging methods (US, CT, MR imaging PET): a meta-analysis. Radiology 224:748–56

51. Lai DT, Fulham M, Stephen MS et al (1996) The role of whole-body positron emission tomography with ^{18}F]fluorodeoxyglucose in identifying operable colorectal cancer metastases to the liver. Arch Surg 131:703–707

52. Staib L, Schirrmeister H, Reske SN et al (2000) Is (18)F-fluorodeoxyglucose positron emission tomography in recurrent colorectal cancer a contribution to surgical decision making? Am J Surg 180:1–5

53. Vitola JV, Delbeke D, Sandler MP et al (1996) Positron emission tomography to stage suspected metastatic colorectal carcinoma to the liver. Am J Surg 171:21–26

54. Whiteford MH, Whiteford HM, Yee LF et al (2000) Usefulness of FDG-PET scan in the assessment of suspected metastatic or recurrent adenocarcinoma of the colon and rectum. Dis Colon Rectum 43:759–767; discussion 767–770

55. Beets G, Penninckx F, Schiepers C et al (1994) Clinical value of whole-body positron emission tomography with [18F]fluorodeoxyglucose in recurrent colorectal cancer. Br J Surg 81:1666–1670

56. Flamen P, Stroobants S, Van Cutsem E et al (1999) Additional value of whole-body positron emission tomography with fluorine-18-2-fluoro-2-deoxy-D-glucose in recurrent colorectal cancer. J Clin Oncol 17:894–901

57. Imbriaco M, Akhurst T, Hilton S et al (2000) Whole-body FDG-PET in patients with recurrent colorectal carcinoma. A comparative study with CT. Clin Positron Imaging, 2000. 3:107–114

58. Imdahl A, Reinhardt MJ, Nitzsche EU et al (2000) Impact of ^{18}F-FDG-positron emission tomography for decision making in colorectal cancer recurrences. Langenbecks Arch Surg 385:129–134

59. Ito K, Kato T, Tadokoro M et al (1992) Recurrent rectal cancer and scar: differentiation with PET and MR imaging. Radiology 182:549–552

60. Strauss LG, Clorius JH, Schlag P et al (1989) Recurrence of colorectal tumors: PET evaluation. Radiology 170:329–332

61. Berger KL, Nicholson SA, Dehdashti F et al (2000) FDG PET evaluation of mucinous neoplasms: correlation of FDG uptake with histopathologic features. AJR Am J Roentgenol 174:1005–1008

62. Flanagan FL, Dehdashti F, Ogunbiyi OA et al (1998) Utility of FDG-PET for investigating unexplained plasma CEA elevation in patients with colorectal cancer. Ann Surg 227:319–323

63. Gambhir SS, Czernin J, Schwimmer J et al (2001) A tabulated summary of the FDG PET literature. J Nucl Med 42 [5 Suppl]:1S–93S

64. Huebner RH, Park KC, Shepherd JE et al (2000) A meta-analysis of the literature for whole-body FDG PET detection of recurrent colorectal cancer. J Nucl Med 41:1177–1189

65. Ruers TJ, Langenhoff BS, Neeleman N et al (2002) Value of positron emission tomography with [F-18]fluorodeoxyglucose in patients with colorectal liver metastases: a prospective study. J Clin Oncol 20:388–395

66. Cohade C, Osman M, Leal J, Wahl RL (2003) Direct comparison of ([18])F-FDG PET and PET/CT in patients with colorectal carcinoma. J Nucl Med 44:1797–1803

67. Antoch G, Freudenberg LS, Egelhof T et al (2002) Focal tracer uptake: a potential artifact in contrast-enhanced dual-modality PET/CT scans. J Nucl Med 43:1339–1342

68. Cohade C, Osman M, Nakamoto Y et al (2003) Initial experience with oral contrast in PET/CT: phantom and clinical studies. J Nucl Med 44:412–416

69. Dizendorf E, Hany TF, Buck A et al (2003) Cause and magnitude of the error induced by oral CT contrast

agent in CT-based attenuation correction of PET emission studies. J Nucl Med 44:732–38

70. Goerres GW, Hany TF, Kamel E et al (2002) Head and neck imaging with PET and PET/CT: artefacts from dental metallic implants. Eur J Nucl Med Mol Imaging 29:367–370

71. Nakamoto Y, Osman M, Cohade C et al (2002) PET/CT: comparison of quantitative tracer uptake between germanium and CT transmission attenuation-corrected images. J Nucl Med 43:1137–1143

72. Foster JH, Lundy J (1981) Liver metastases. Curr Probl Surg 18:157–202

73. Holm A, Bradley E, Aldrete JS (1989) Hepatic resection of metastasis from colorectal carcinoma. Morbidity, mortality, and pattern of recurrence. Ann Surg 209:428–434

74. Vitola JV, Delbeke D, Meranze SG et al (1996) Positron emission tomography with F-18-fluorodeoxyglucose to evaluate the results of hepatic chemoembolization. Cancer 78:2216–2222

75. Rosa F, Meimarakis G, Stahl A et al (2004) Colorectal cancer patients before resection of hepatic metastases. Impact of (^{18})F-FDG PET on detecting extrahepatic disease. Nuklearmedizin 43:135–140

76. Venook A (2005) Critical evaluation of current treatments in metastatic colorectal cancer. Oncologist 10:250–261

77. Findlay M, Young H, Cunningham D et al (1996) Noninvasive monitoring of tumor metabolism using fluorodeoxyglucose and positron emission tomography in colorectal cancer liver metastases: correlation with tumor response to fluorouracil. J Clin Oncol 14:700–708

78. Kahn H, Alexander A, Rakinic J et al (1997) Preoperative staging of irradiated rectal cancers using digital rectal examination, computed tomography, endorectal ultrasound, and magnetic resonance imaging does not accurately predict T0, N0 pathology. Dis Colon Rectum 40:140–144

79. Guillem JG, Moore HG, Akhurst T et al (2004) Sequential preoperative fluorodeoxyglucose-positron emission tomography assessment of response to preoperative chemoradiation: a means for determining long-term outcomes of rectal cancer. J Am Coll Surg 199:1–7

80. Amthauer H, Denecke T, Rau B et al (2004) Response prediction by FDG-PET after neoadjuvant radiochemotherapy and combined regional hyperthermia of rectal cancer: correlation with endorectal ultrasound and histopathology. Eur J Nucl Med Mol Imaging 31:811–819

81. Barker DW, Zagoria RJ, Morton KA et al (2005) Evaluation of liver metastases after radiofrequency ablation: utility of ^{18}F-FDG PET and PET/CT. AJR Am J Roentgenol 184:1096–1102

82. Solbiati L, Livraghi T, Goldberg SN et al (2001) Percutaneous radio-frequency ablation of hepatic metastases from colorectal cancer: long-term results in 117 patients. Radiology 221:159–166

83. Limanond P, Zimmerman P, Raman SS et al (2003) Interpretation of CT and MRI after radiofrequency ablation of hepatic malignancies. AJR Am J Roentgenol 181:1635–1640

84. Goldberg SN, Gazelle GS, Mueller PR (2000) Thermal ablation therapy for focal malignancy: a unified approach to underlying principles, techniques, and diagnostic imaging guidance. AJR Am J Roentgenol 174:323–331

85. Lencioni R, Cioni D, Bartolozzi C (2001) Percutaneous radiofrequency thermal ablation of liver malignancies: techniques, indications, imaging findings, and clinical results. Abdom Imaging 26:345–360

86. Langenhoff BS, Oyen WJ, Jager GJ et al (2002) Efficacy of fluorine-18-deoxyglucose positron emission tomography in detecting tumor recurrence after local ablative therapy for liver metastases: a prospective study. J Clin Oncol 20:4453–4458

87. Donckier V, Van Laethem JL, Goldman S et al (2003) [F-18] fluorodeoxyglucose positron emission tomography as a tool for early recognition of incomplete tumor destruction after radiofrequency ablation for liver metastases. J Surg Oncol 84:215–223

88. Antoch G, Vogt FM, Veit P et al (2005) Assessment of liver tissue after radiofrequency ablation: findings with different imaging procedures. J Nucl Med 46:520–525

89. Dancey JE, Shepherd FA, Paul K et al (2000) Treatment of nonresectable hepatocellular carcinoma with intrahepatic ^{90}Y-microspheres. J Nucl Med 41:1673–1681

90. Wong CY, Salem R, Raman S et al (2002) Evaluating ^{90}Y-glass microsphere treatment response of unresectable colorectal liver metastases by [18F]FDG PET: a comparison with CT or MRI. Eur J Nucl Med Mol Imaging 29:815–820

91. Wong CY, Salem R, Qing F et al (2004) Metabolic response after intraarterial ^{90}Y-glass microsphere treatment for colorectal liver metastases: comparison of quantitative and visual analyses by ^{18}F-FDG PET. J Nucl Med 45:1892–1897

92. Bienert M, McCook B, Carr BI et al (2005) Sequential FDG PET/CT in ^{90}Y microsphere treatment of unresectable colorectal liver metastases. Eur J Nucl Med Mol Imaging 32:723

93. Bienert M, McCook B, Carr BI et al (2005) 90Y microsphere treatment of unresectable liver metastases: changes in ^{18}F-FDG uptake and tumour size on PET/CT. Eur J Nucl Med Mol Imaging 32:778–787

94. Delbeke D, Martin WH (2004) PET and PET-CT for evaluation of colorectal carcinoma. Semin Nucl Med 34:209–223

95. Strasberg SM, Dehdashti F, Siegel BA et al (2001) Survival of patients evaluated by FDG-PET before hepatic resection for metastatic colorectal carcinoma: a prospective database study. Ann Surg 233:293–299

96. Meta J, Seltzer M, Schiepers C et al (2001) Impact of ^{18}F-FDG PET on managing patients with colorectal cancer: the referring physician's perspective. J Nucl Med 42:586–590

10 FDG-PET and FDG-PET/CT in Breast Cancer

A. Haug, R. Tiling, and H. L. Sommer

Recent Results in Cancer Research, Vol. 170
© Springer-Verlag Berlin Heidelberg 2008

10.1 Introduction: Epidemiology

Breast cancer is the most frequent malignant disease in women worldwide and the second leading cause of cancer death in Western countries. In Germany, 46,000 women per year suffer from breast cancer. Of these women, 18,000 died from it [1]. In the USA, 211,240 new cases of breast cancer were diagnosed in women in 2004 and 40,410 died from it. The incidence has been increasing from 1940 until the present, to 110 per 100,000 women annually, and is higher in white women then in African-Americans. Statistics indicate that one in nine women will develop breast cancer during her lifetime [2].

In the last decade, there has been progress in understanding risk factors for breast cancer. Female breast cancer is a complex multifactorial disease, the etiology of which involves a strong interplay between environmental and genetic factors. The highest risk factor is age. The relative risk (RR) increases from 1 to 56 from the age of 25 to 74. The incidence rises from 1.9 in the 20–24 age group to 387.2 in the 80–84 age group per 100,000 white women in the USA. The probability is also higher in Western countries (RR 5), if relatives have had breast cancer (RR 1, 4–6), in case of contralateral breast cancer (RR 5), and if breast parenchyma is dense in mammography (RR up to 4.3) [3]. Even though breast cancer is uncommon in women younger than 30 years, women with inherited specific genetic abnormalities such as the BRCA gene have a high risk of developing breast cancer at young ages.

Approximately 60%–80% of invasive breast cancers are ductal carcinomas. These often present as a firm to hard lump. Invasive lobular carcinomas account for approximately 10%–20% and are more difficult to detect due to diffuse infiltration of the surrounding tissue and a multicentric appearance. Five percent are medullary carcinomas; the remaining tumors comprise a variety of histological types. However, most patients initially present with a breast lump. In all patients with a lump, a definite diagnosis should made.

10.2 Conventional Imaging

10.2.1 Mammography

Mammography is indicated in clinically symptomatic women and for screening for breast cancer in asymptomatic women. After clinical examination and palpation, mammography is useful to improve the diagnosis in cases of a breast lump, asymmetry of breast contour, protrusion, or dimpling of the skin. Two or three views of each breast are obtained – mediolateral, oblique, and craniocaudal – during which the breast is compressed between two plates.

Breast cancer often shows distinct, irregular, sometimes crab-like densities and clusters of microcalcifications (Fig. 10.1). Ninety percent of all diagnosed in-situ breast cancers

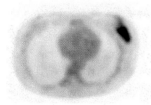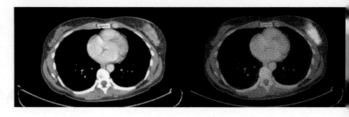

Fig. 10.1. Coronal slices of FDG-PET, CT, and PET/CT showing a large malignant primary breast tumor

and 60% of all invasive cancers show microcalcifications. Lobular carcinomas are harder to detect than ductal carcinomas because microcalcifications are rare (roughly 5%) and the diffuse infiltration of the surrounding tissue with no change in tissue density. Carcinomas can be diagnosed more easily in fatty transformed breasts than in mastopathically changed breasts because of the higher density of the breast tissue and the lower normal tissue-to-tumor contrast. Approximately 10% of carcinomas cannot be detected by mammography even when they are palpable.

Mammography has a high sensitivity of 69%–90% in detecting breast cancer [4–9]. However, approximately 80% of suspicious microcalcifications are benign, resulting in a high number of false-positive diagnoses and a low specificity. Consequentially, only approximately 30% of all women with suspicious mammography who undergo surgery turn out to have breast cancer in histology.

Nevertheless, mammography is at the moment the best modality for screening asymptomatic women for breast cancer and for follow-up after breast cancer. Because screening has now been implemented, mortality in women aged 50 and over has decreased by more than 30% [10]. The age the screening should be started and the frequency remains controversial and differs from country to country.

10.2.2 Sonography

Indications for sonography are a palpable lump in women younger than 30 years, especially when presenting dense breast tissue, or older than 30 with an unsuspicious mammography and to differentiate between solid and cystic

lesions diagnosed in mammography. Signs of malignancy are irregularly shaped hypoechoic masses and ill-defined demarcation against surrounding tissue. Microcalcifications, as the most common sign of malignancy, are not detectable by sonography. The quality of sonography depends greatly on the experience of the physician. For these reasons, it is difficult to discriminate between benign and malignant tumors with the necessary investigator-independent certainty. The sensitivity is high, but because of many false-positive diagnoses specificity is low. Sonography as a single examination for screening is not recommended, but is useful in combination with mammography to increase sensitivity [11].

10.2.3 Magnetic Resonance Imaging

Magnetic resonance imaging (MRI) is a modern breast imaging technique that is gaining popularity. Breast MRI has been shown to have sensitivities between 95% and 100% in detecting early breast cancer [12, 13]. Especially in young women with dense breast tissue, the sensitivity of MRI is higher than mammography [14]. Enhancement of the contrast agent (mostly chelates of gadolinium) and dynamic contrast-enhanced examination of the lesions reflects local tissue changes in blood flow, capillary permeability, and extracellular volume due to angiogenesis, a hallmark of cancer. The reported specificity of MRI ranges between 37% and 97% [15–18]. A high rate of false positive findings results in many unnecessary biopsies and undue anxiety for patients [19]. Mostly benign tumors (e.g., fibroadenoma and severe fibrocystic disease) are responsible for false-positive findings.

The advantages and well-accepted indications of MRI are the detection of multicentric disease, mapping of the extent of tumor in staging newly diagnosed patients, in cancer diagnosis in the case of breast implants, screening of asymptomatic patients with a family predisposition, and the differentiation between scar and recurrence [4].

In conclusion, MRI combines a high sensitivity in detecting breast cancer with exact anatomical information about the extension of the tumor, but low specificity results in a high number of unnecessary biopsies.

10.3 Other Imaging Modalities

10.3.1 Scintimammography

Tc-99m sestamibi has been shown to accumulate in breast cancer cells [20]. Since 1994, many studies with a large number of patients have been reported. Normally, approximately 740 MBq ^{99m}Tc sestamibi is injected into a cubital vein contralateral to the breast with the suspected abnormality. Five minutes subsequent to injection, planar lateral scintimammograms of the breast are acquired. Patients are examined in the prone position with the arms raised. Acquisition time is 10 min for each breast.

The results of the early studies were promising. Sensitivity was between 78% and 95%, with specificity between 73% and 100% [21–27]. However, in most studies a bias due to the condition of a palpable breast mass was present. In a multicenter study including 673 patients with mammographically detected breast lesions, 286 had palpable masses and 387 nonpalpable [28]. In blinded reading, sensitivity decreased from 95% in palpable lesions to 72% in nonpalpable lesions. No cases of lesion detection of less than 5 mm have yet been reported with the use of the currently available detectors. Because of these limitations, 99m-Tc-scintimammography cannot be used as a screening method. On the other hand, scintimammography is not affected by dense breast tissue [29], which is more common among young women, contrary to conventional mammography. So

in nondiagnostic or difficult mammography in premenopausal women, adjunct scintimammography using ^{99m}Tc-sestamibi has been shown to be useful [30].

In patients with inconclusive findings in physical examination and, due to dense breast tissue, equivocal mammography, a mammographic follow-up study can be suggested instead of performing immediate breast biopsy. Since specificity of scintimammography tends to be high in palpable breast lesions independent of breast density, this modality could possibly be used as a surrogate technique. With respect to a comparatively high positive predictive value, positive scintimammographic findings will force immediate breast biopsy. On the other hand, negative scintimammographic findings would strengthen the decision for a noninvasive strategy and waiting another 6 months for follow-up [31]

Another potential indication of scintimammography may be to evaluate the response of locally advanced breast cancer to neoadjuvant chemotherapy. It has already been shown that the decrease of ^{99m}Tc-sestamibi uptake during chemotherapy correlates well with the pathological response of the tumor [32–34]. In the case of complete response in the following course of primary (neoadjuvant) chemotherapy, an early decline of sestamibi uptake was already present after the first or the second cycle. Especially a negative response in scintimammography indicates chemoresistance with a specificity of 100% [34]. Even when there is no place for scintimammography in clinical routine, there are several niches where this test seems to be useful.

10.3.2 Thermography

Thermography has no role in the diagnosis of breast cancer and is now considered obsolete.

10.4 PET: Diagnosis of Primary Tumors

It is generally accepted that early detection of small lesions is essential to reduce both morbidity and mortality of breast cancer [35]. Early detection of breast tumors has improved in the last few decades. Physical examination, mammography, and ultrasound of the breasts are routinely performed in screening and clinical work-up of breast lesions. However, diagnostic limitations still exist. A major problem is the reliable differentiation of malignant and benign breast lesions, resulting in a high number of unnecessary biopsies.

10.4.1 F-18-Fluoro-2-Deoxyglucose

Tumor cells have an increased metabolism of glucose [36], which has also been shown to be true for breast carcinoma cells [37–40]. FDG-PET may improve the ability to discriminate benign from malignant tumors. FDG uptake is dependent on the histological subtype of carcinoma and on different clinical prognostic markers or molecular biomarkers [41]. Ductal carcinomas show a higher uptake than lobular ones [40, 42–44]. Lower differentiated cancers with grade 3 have a significantly higher FDG uptake compared with grade 1 or 2 carcinomas [44]. The correlation between FDG uptake and molecular biomarkers such as mutations and overexpression of the tumor suppressor gene p53 or the immunohistochemical expression of Ki-67 as a marker of tumor cell proliferation remains controversial [45, 43, 44]. A significant correlation between FDG uptake and the mitotic activity index was described by Bos et al., further confirming a relation between proliferation and glucose metabolism [42]. The prognostic factor of FGD uptake remains unclear, since there have been few studies evaluating the correlation. In one study with 70 patients suffering from primary breast cancer, a high uptake was related with a significantly worse relapse-free and overall survival [46].

As in other oncological FDG-PET studies, standardized activities are injected via a cubital vein contralateral to the suspicious lesion site. Patients must be in a fasting state (> 6 h) and should undergo a blood glucose test before examination. Data acquisition and reconstruction do not differ from other standard oncological FDG PET protocols. Imaging is recom-mended in a prone position with both arms at the side or over the head and the breast hanging free to avoid compression and deformation of the breast.

In general, FDG-PET seems not to be useful for screening because of its low spatial resolution and poor sensitivity in small lesions. PET may add additional information if mammography and sonography remain equivocal in tumors larger than 10 mm.

There are several studies analyzing the value of FDG-PET in the diagnosis of primary breast cancer and demonstrating its limitations in tumors smaller than 10 mm. Rosen et al. examined 23 patients with lesions in mammography and/or ultrasound that were highly suggestive of malignancy using a dedicated PET mammography unit. This system consists of two 15×20-cm planar detectors and 3×3×10-mm lutetium gadolinium oxyorthosilicate scintillator elements. The detectors are positioned above and below the compressed breast and are typically separated by 6–9 cm. For each lesion, image-guided core-needle biopsy was performed immediately after PET mammography. PET mammography demonstrated 20 focal abnormalities, 18 of which were malignant and two were benign. Both benign lesions represented areas of fat necrosis. Three of 20 malignant lesions seen at conventional mammography were not demonstrated at PET mammography, while PET mammography diagnosed one additional malignant focus compared to conventional mammography. The overall sensitivity of PET mammography for malignancy, even using a dedicated PET system, was not higher than 86% (95% confidence interval, 65%–95%), with a positive predictive value of 90% (95% CI, 70%–97%). The calculated specificity was 33% (95% CI, 2%–79%), and the negative predictive value was 25% (95% CI, 1%–70%) [47].

In a retrospective study conducted by Hubner et al., the utility F-18-FDG PET in identifying primary breast cancer was evaluated. Thirty-five women with suspected breast cancer were examined [48]. The sensitivity for PET in detecting primary breast cancer was 96%, with a specificity of 91%. Quantitative standard uptake value (SUV) data was colected, but did not improve the accuracy of -18-FDG PET in identifying primary breast ancers. In a retrospective study with 93 women suffering from breast cancer, Rostom t al. showed the ability of FDG-PET in detecting primary breast cancer [49]. PET showed a sensitivity of 90.7%, a specificity of 83.3%, and n accuracy of 89.2% for the primary tumor, with 3.2% false-positive and 7.6% false-negative findings in carcinomas in situ, tumors smaller than 5 mm, or Paget's disease. In addition, 86/93 patients underwent mammography. ET was more accurate than mammography in 9.5% vs 72% (p=0.0003). In order to study the utility of FDG-PET in the evaluation of breast ancer, 28 patients with a total of 35 suspect reast masses underwent PET [50]. FDG-PET iscriminated between eight benign and 27 malignant breast masses, with a sensitivity of 6% and specificity of 100%. Among the magnancies, there was a significant correlation etween normalized FDG uptake and nuclear rade (p=0.006).

Many studies have compared FDG-PET with onventional imaging methods. Most authors ound PET more accurate than the conventional methods. In a study with 25 patients with ocally advanced breast cancer, the feasibility f a gamma camera PET (GCPET) system was valuated compared with mammography and ltrasonography. GCPET detected 24/25 primary breast tumors with a sensitivity of 96% vs onography (22/25, sensitivity 88%) and mammography (15/25, sensitivity 60%). The tumor missed in GCPET turned out to be a grade 1 invasive ductal tumor, only 8 mm in size [51]. Walter et al. [52] compared the diagnostic value f preoperative dynamic enhanced magnetic resonance (MR) mammography and FDG-PET s single diagnostic tool and in combination in suspicious breast lesions. Forty-two breast sions in 40 patients were examined. The MR and PET examinations were evaluated separately and the results were compared with the istological findings. Nineteen malignant and 3 benign breast tumors were proven histogically. MR and PET showed a sensitivity of 9% and 63%, respectively. Specificity was 74% nd 91%, respectively. In combination, both maging methods decreased the unnecessary

biopsies from 55% to 17%. One false-negative result occurred in both modalities in a patient pretreated with chemotherapy. The authors concluded that the combination of MR and PET can help to decrease biopsies of benign lesions. But given the high costs, both modalities should only be used in problematic cases to either rule out or to demonstrate malignancy. Using PET is recommended only if MR mammography findings remain equivocal.

In another study, the ability of PET and MRI was directly compared to determine whether breast lesions were benign or malignant and of the capability of depicting eventual multifocal disease [53]. Thirty-six patients with 40 lesions were included, who were scheduled for surgery because of suggestive mammographic, sonographic, and/or clinical findings. Sensitivity for lesions, sensitivity for patients, specificity for lesions and specificity for patients were 68.0%, 76.2%, 73.3%, and 73.3% for PET and 92.0%, 95.2%, 73.3%, and 73.3% for MRI, respectively. MRI was more sensitive than FDG-PET in disclosing malignant breast tumors and was also more accurate than FDG-PET in the assessment of multifocal disease. The lower sensitivity of FDG-PET than of MRI seems to be due to difficulties in reliable imaging of carcinomas smaller than 10 mm and of lobular carcinomas.

Rieber et al. examined 43 patients with clinically suspected breast cancer with MR mammography (MRM) and PET [54]. The efficacy of these methods in the diagnosis of primary tumor, contralateral carcinomas, bifocal, trifocal, or multifocal disease, as well as noninvasive cancer portions and tumor size was evaluated. Sensitivities for MRM and PET, respectively, were 100% vs 93.0% in the diagnosis of the primary tumor; 100% vs 100% in the diagnosis of contralateral carcinomas; and 95.2% vs 92.5% in the diagnosis of bifocal, trifocal, or multifocal disease. Specificities for MRM and PET, respectively, were 100% vs 97.5% in the diagnosis of contralateral carcinomas and 96.8% vs 90.3% in the diagnosis of bifocal, trifocal, or multifocal disease. Both methods determined noninvasive cancer portions and tumor sizes equally well. The findings of one or both of the methods changed patients' surgical treatment in 12.5%–15% of cases. The authors' conclusion was that preoperative MRM and/or PET can have a positive influence on surgical treatment planning.

Another study compared the diagnostic accuracy of FDG-PET with conventional techniques [55]. Among other factors the differentiation between malignant and benign lesions was evaluated. A total of 117 female patients were prospectively examined using FDG-PET and conventional staging methods such as chest x-ray, ultrasonography of the breast and liver, mammography, and bone scintigraphy. Histopathological analysis of resected specimens served as the reference method. The sensitivity and specificity of PET in detecting malignant breast lesions were 93% and 75%, respectively. PET was twice as sensitive (sensitivity 63%, specificity 95%) with a comparable specificity in detecting multifocal lesions than the combination of mammography and ultrasonography (sensitivity 32%, specificity 93%).

In summary, FDG-PET should not be considered the first-choice modality in the diagnosis of primary breast masses, because of the high diagnostic efficacy of mammography. For screening, its accuracy does not appear comparable with the standard practice of mammography supplemented by ultrasound and core biopsy. The studies with high sensitivity obviously used a strongly preselected patient population, so the results may not be transferable for clinical routine. Overall sensitivity of FDG-PET is too low because of difficulties in detecting small carcinomas, particularly carcinomas in situ and well-differentiated or lobular carcinomas. Given the spatial resolution of the PET system (approximately 5 mm in dedicated scanners), detection of small tumors is affected. Partial volume effects condition a spread of the signal over a larger area than the true volume. Consequently, the radioactive measurement is significantly underestimated. This weakness of FDG-PET is contrary to the intended benefit of screening to detect breast cancer in an early stage to decrease mortality. FDG-PET may help improve the differentiation between benign and malignant changes, which remain equivocal in conventional imaging. Unnecessary biopsies can be avoided this way.

10.4.2 Other PET Tracers

FDG is not the only tracer used to examine tumors in PET. Recently, F-18-fluorothymidine (FLT) was introduced for tumor imaging [56]. The uptake of FLT correlates with the activity of thymidine kinase 1 (TK-1) in cell cultures, which is related to DNA synthesis during the S-phase [57]. The accumulation of FLT in fast proliferating tissue in vivo was demonstrated in several studies [58, 59]. The aim of a study conducted by Smyczek-Gargya et al. [60] with 12 patients with 14 tumors was to assess the value of FLT-PET in the diagnosis of primary breast cancer. Histological diagnosis was obtained from core biopsy. An increased FLT uptake was found in 13/14 tumors. The missed tumor had a diameter of only 5 mm. A FDG-PET scan was performed in six patients for comparison. The SUVmax and SUVmean of FDG were higher than for FLT, although the difference was not significant. The tumor-to-breast tissue ratio of FLT uptake showed no significant difference from the FDG uptake, but the tumor-to-mediastinum ratio of FLT was significantly higher than that of FDG. In younger patients, a nonpathologic band-like retrosternal FLT-uptake may be observed, perhaps attributable to benign tissue such as residual thymus. The authors conclude that because of high image contrast FLT-PET may facilitate the detection of small foci, especially in the mediastinum. In another study ten patients underwent FLT-PET [61]. In eight of ten patients, the primary tumor showed an increased FLT uptake; in two patients no increased uptake was seen. In conclusion, primary breast tumors can be visualized with FLT-PET, but its value in detecting primary breast cancer has to be evaluated in large patient populations and is not recommended for routine clinical use today.

The development of new PET tracers may contribute additional information on tumor biology and prognosis. But all the following tracers are in experimental use and not yet recommended for clinical routine. The estrogen analog 16-alpha-F-18-fluoroestradiol-17-beta (FES) is able to detect noninvasively the estrogen receptor status of breast cancer and measure the effect of antiestrogen therapy [62]. Overexpression of HER-2 receptor in breast cancer correlates with poor patient prognosis, and visualization of HER-2 expression might provide valuable diagnostic information influencing patient management. Preliminary studies on radiolabeled antibodies against the HER-2 receptor have been conducted [63, 64], but its benefit in clinical routine is not yet clear.

Another promising tracer is F-18-fluoromisonidazole (F-18-FMISO), used as a hypoxia marker in soft tissue sarcomas [65]. Its possible role in breast cancer, especially in therapy planning and monitoring, requires further study. I-124-annexin V, which binds to phosphatidylserine (PS) on the surface of apoptotic cells, has shown its ability to measure apoptosis in animal models [66, 67]. Its potential to assess the clinical effect of cancer therapy has to be evaluated in further clinical trials.

10.4.3 FDG-PET/CT

The clinical interpretation of PET images may be difficult due to the lack of anatomical landmarks. This limitation can be overwhelmed by the use of a combined PET/CT scanner. It is thought that the additional morphologic data will increase sensitivity and specificity. There are only a few studies on PET/CT and the primary diagnosis of breast cancer. Fifteen patients with suspected breast cancer were examined preoperative with FDG-PET/CT [68]: 11 of 15 had histological evidence of breast cancer. The accuracy of PET/CT for the diagnosis of primary breast tumor was 93.3% (14/15), with a sensitivity of 90.9% (10/11) and a specificity of 100% (4/4).

10.5 Axillary Lymph Node Staging

Staging of primary breast cancer can be divided into two concerns: locoregional staging (breast and axillary lymph nodes) and staging for distant metastases. Axillary lymph node involvement is one of the most important predictors and helps the clinician to choose the right adjuvant therapy. Currently, the therapeutic strategy is changing: axillary lymph node dissection is no longer performed in most women, sentinel lymph node mapping with technetium-99m marked nanokolloids and/or blue dye has replaced complete axillary lymph node dissection at least in stage pT1. This is mainly to avoid the risk in developing lymphedema (12%) and upper extremity dysfunction or discomfort, which is seen in more than 50% after axillary nodal dissection [69]. Until now, no imaging modality has been accurate enough to replace diagnostic surgical evaluation of lymph node status. Several studies have looked at the use of FDG-PET in noninvasive axillary staging. In the largest study, 308 women with newly diagnosed invasive breast cancer underwent FDG-PET prospectively in a multicenter investigation [70]. PET diagnosis was evaluated by pathologic findings of conventional axillary dissection: 93.2% of the women suffered from breast cancer at stage pT1 or 2. The sensitivity, specificity, and positive and negative predictive value of PET were 61%, 80%, 62%, and 79%, respectively. The false-negative axillae had significantly smaller and fewer tumor-positive lymph nodes in pathology than true-positive axillae. PET was also less sensitive in detecting metastases of lobular rather than ductal carcinoma. Consequently, PET is not routinely recommended for staging the axillary lymph nodes, because it often fails to detect small and few lymph node metastases (Figs. 10.2, 10.3). These findings are supported by the study of Avril et al. [71].

Weir et al. found similar results: in this study 40 women underwent FDG-PET for staging the axilla [72]. PET identified only 5 of 18 patients with axillary lymph node metastases, resulting in a sensitivity of 28% and a specificity of 86%.

Schirrmeister et al. [73] compared the diagnostic value of FDG-PET with conventional imaging modalities (chest x-ray, mammography, ultrasound, bone scintigraphy) in 93 women. The sensitivity and specificity of PET in detecting axillary lymph node metastases

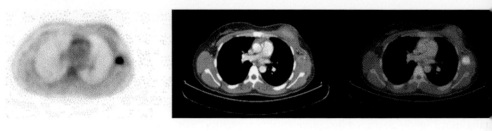

Fig. 10.2. Coronal slices of FDG-PET, CT, and PET/CT presenting an enlarged axillary lymph node with con trast enhancement and increased FDG uptake, which turned out to be a lymph node metastasis

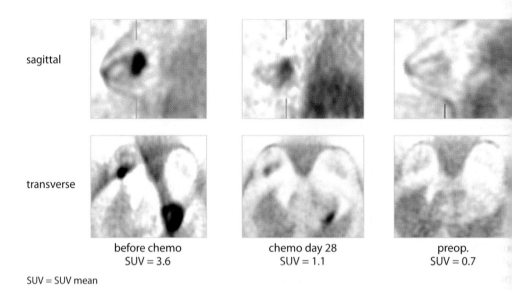

sagittal

transverse

| before chemo | chemo day 28 | preop. |
| SUV = 3.6 | SUV = 1.1 | SUV = 0.7 |

SUV = SUV mean

Fig. 10.3. Clinical complete remission in a patient with locally advanced breast carcinoma. FDG uptal decreased 28 days after the beginning of chemotherapy. In the presurgical studies, PET considered norm; histopathologically, residual invasive tumour with a diameter of 0.3 cm was proven. Retrospectively, faint FD accumulation can be seen in the FDG-PET study

was 79% and 92%, respectively. Sensitivity of the conventional imaging modalities was lower, with an assimilable specificity (41% and 96%).

Greco et al. examined 167 consecutive patients with breast cancers of 50 mm or less preoperatively with FDG-PET [74]. The axillary lymph node status of PET was compared with pathological findings after axillary lymph node dissection. PET detected 68 of 72 patients with axillary lymph node metastases, resulting in a sensitivity of 94.4%. Specificity and accuracy were 86.3% and 89.8%, respectively.

Sensitivity was higher for tumors measurir 21–50 mm (98.0%), specificity for tumors 10 mm or less.

The data indicate that FDG-PET has a hig sensitivity in detecting axillary lymph noc metastases. But because of the importance lymph node involvement in the prognosis ar treatment planning, the diagnostic accurac may be not high enough to replace histopathe logical evaluation after surgical lymph noc dissection. Especially small or micrometast ses are missed frequently because of PET's sp tial resolution.

10.6   Staging

Staging after primary detection of breast cancer consists of routinely performed abdominal sonography, CT, and bone scintigraphy. While conventional imaging methods such as mammography, CT, MRI, or ultrasound can define malignancy only on morphologic criteria, FDG-PET has the potential to detect malignant foci early through its evaluation of glucose metabolism. Another major advantage of PET is its ability to use this method for whole-body staging in a single examination. However, there are only a few studies published in the literature concerning the use of PET as a primary staging procedure. Eubank et al. compared the potential role of FDG-PET in the detection of metastases to the internal mammaria node chain with conventional staging with CT in 73 patients [75]. Sensitivity, specificity, and accuracy for nodal disease was 85%, 90%, and 88%, respectively, by FDG PET, and 54%, 85%, and 83%, respectively, by prospective interpretation of CT. In another study, 28 women with locally advanced breast cancer were examined with FDG-PET [76]. Seven patients presented mediastinal lymph node metastases. As a result, FDG-PET may be useful in staging women with a high risk of presenting (mediastinal) metastases such as women with locally advanced breast cancer.

10.7   Therapy Monitoring

In locally advanced breast cancer, neoadjuvant chemotherapy is used to improve primary tumor resectability, to enable breast-conserving surgery, and to asses the chemosensitivity to the selected chemotherapeutic agents. Complete response to the therapy indicates a better prognosis, whereas the therapeutic regimen should be changed if there is no response to treatment. It is essential to asses the response as early as possible to continue effective therapy or possibly to change therapy. Clinical and conventional imaging information is often inaccurate or slow in detecting a decrease in the size of the tumor [77], because the effect of treatment first influences the metabolism, which is later followed by a decrease in tumor size. Consequently, there is no reliable conventional method of detecting non-responders in the early stage of treatment. FDG-PET measures the metabolism of cells and may be a useful tool to evaluate therapy response earlier and more reliably than conventional imaging modalities.

Another method for therapy monitoring is scintimammography using ^{99m}Tc sestamibi. Tiling et al. conducted a detailed comparison of scintimammography and FDG-PET [33]. He concluded that scintimammography had an assimilable sensitivity in assessing the response to chemotherapy compared to PET. Both methods can predict clinical complete response as early as after the second cycle. However, residual microscopic tumor could not be visualized with both methods.

The potential of FDG-PET to predict the therapeutic outcome very early and with high accuracy was also shown in other studies [78–80]. A decrease in SUV indicates a good response to therapy, whereas unchanged uptake indicates tumor progression. Smith et al. compared PET images before treatment with images after the first and second cycle of chemotherapy in 30 women suffering from locally advanced breast cancer [78]. Findings were compared with histology. Using a 20% threshold of reduction after the first cycle of chemotherapy, they identified pathologic responders with a sensitivity of 90% and a specificity of 74%. A comparable study used a threshold of 55% reduction in uptake after baseline scans in 22 patients [79]. There was a significant difference of tracer uptake in responders and non-responders after the first cycle. They predicted pathologic response with a sensitivity and specificity of 100% and 85%, respectively. The diagnostic accuracy was 88% after the first cycle and 91% after the second cycle. Thus, PET is able to discriminate responders and non-responders early in the course of therapy. On the other hand, single posttreatment PET failed to predict complete pathological response among a group of good clinical responders to neoadjuvant chemotherapy [80]. Of the ten patients enrolled, PET failed to identify residual tumor masses measuring from 2 mm to 20 mm in nine patients. Also, histologically positive axillary lymph nodes were missed in three patients. A possible explanation besides the low spatial resolution of PET could be that carcinomas with high glucose metabolism are more sensitive to chemotherapy and show the greatest differences in FDG uptake after treatment. Perhaps chemoresistant carcinomas a priori have a lower metabolism and are therefore not detectable by PET. Another study showed the value of FDG-PET in the evaluation of antiestrogen therapy [81]. In 11 women with metastatic breast cancer, a PET scan was performed before and after initiation of tamoxifen therapy. Compared to non-responders, responders demonstrated an increased uptake due to the well-known flare reaction. Thus it was possible to discriminate responders and non-responders early. These findings were confirmed by Mortimer et al. in a study with 40 women [82]. FDG uptake after initiation of tamoxifen therapy predicted a subsequent response to therapy consistent with a metabolic flare. They found a significant difference of SUV between responders and non-responders.

10.8 Restaging

Exact restaging of women with breast cancer to detect local recurrence or distant metastases is critical since the survival of women suffering from one of these two entities differs greatly. Women with regional disease have a 5-year survival rate of 80% compared to 25% in women with distant metastatic disease [83]. The follow-up scheme has changed since there

is no treatment available prolonging surviv in patients with recurrent disease detecte early. Until now, only mammography ar clinical examination have been recommende routinely. When the patient becomes sym tomatic or tumor markers are rising, other im aging modalities are used to detect recurrenc Although the knowledge of metastases has r influence on overall survival, there are som benefits in detecting recurrence or metastat disease at an early stage. The right adjuva therapy can be started to avoid complication and to improve quality of life. The therapeut regimen can be modified to the localization the metastases.

10.8.1 Locoregional Recurrence

Local recurrence (Fig. 10.4) appears in ap proximately 5%–9% of women with initial N staging and increases to 20%–28% if axillar lymph nodes are positive. Mammography the modality of choice in suspected local re currence and the only image modality recom mended for yearly screening in the follow-u MRI is often used to differentiate betwee scar and recurrence or when diagnosis complicated because of breast implants. On in mammography equivocal findings, for e ample caused by changes after radiation of th breast or silicone breast implant, can FDG-PE contribute additional information. The mo common sites of locoregional recurrence aft mastectomy, axillary lymph node dissectio and radiation therapy are the chest wall an supraclavicular nodes [84]. FDG-PET has bee shown to be able to detect local recurrence i several studies.

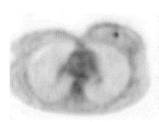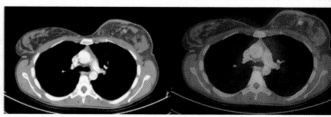

Fig. 10.4. Coronal slices of FDG-PET, CT, and PET/CT showing local recurrence in the left breast

Hathaway et al. compared the value of DG-PET to MRI in ten patients with clinical suspicion of locoregional recurrence [85]. Nine patients suffered from locoregional metastases. While PET identified recurrence in all nine patients, MRI was diagnostic in five and indeterminate in four patients. A similar study compared MRI and FDG-PET in 32 patients with suspected locoregional recurrence (n=19), chest wall recurrence (n=5), and suspected secondary tumor of the contralateral breast (n=8) [86]. PET showed a higher specificity (94% vs 72%) and accuracy (88% vs 84%), but a lower sensitivity (79% vs 100%) than MRI. As an added benefit, additional metastases outside the field of view of MRI were found in PET in five patients. In another study with 62 patients, PET detected more local recurrence than conventional imaging, although the difference was not significant [87]. PET detected ten local recurrences, conventional imaging seven.

Kamel et al. performed FDG-PET in 60 patients with suspected local recurrence [88]. Disease relapse was proven in 40 patients. The overall sensitivity, specificity, and accuracy of PET were 89%, 84%, and 87%, respectively.

In conclusion, FDG-PET can provide useful information in patients with suspected local recurrence, even though mammography remains the first-choice examination. In equivocal findings in mammography, PET can help to detect or rule out local recurrence. PET is also able to detect distant metastases in a single examination. However, the limited number of PET studies precludes any definitive statement on its clinical use in the field of differentiation recurrences.

0.8.2 Distant Metastases

Breast cancer can metastasize to most organs. Most often lymph nodes, lung, liver, and bones are affected. Conventional imaging modalities can be used in addition to FDG-PET. It can scan the whole body in a single examination. Some studies report a high sensitivity and specificity of FDG-PET in detecting metastases at different locations.

Most studies even show the advantage of PET compared to conventional imaging modalities. In a study with 50 patients, FDG-PET showed its advantage compared with chest x-ray, bone scintigraphy, ultrasound of the abdomen, CT, and MRI [89]. The overall sensitivity and specificity of PET were 86% and 90%, respectively. The sensitivity of the conventional imaging modalities was much lower (36%), with a comparable specificity (95%). These findings are supported by the study of Gallowitsch et al. with 62 patients [90]. On a patient basis, sensitivity, specificity, and accuracy for detecting local recurrence or distant metastases were calculated to be 97%, 82%, and 90% compared with 84%, 60%, and 74% with CT. PET findings changed the therapeutic regimen in 13 patients. PET detected significantly more lymph node metastases than conventional imaging. This was confirmed by another study demonstrating the advantage of PET compared to CT in detecting mediastinum and internal mammary node chain metastases [91].

On the other hand, PET seems to be less sensitive than other imaging modalities in detecting bone metastases (Fig. 10.5). Gallowitsch et al. found PET to detect significantly fewer skeleton metastases than bone scintigraphy [87]. Predominantly sclerotic metastases were FDG-negative, but there were also metastases only detected by PET. In another study, bone scintigraphy had a slightly higher sensitivity (88.8% vs 83.3%) and specificity (91.6% vs 89.4%) than FDG-PET [89]. In contrast, other studies show a higher specificity with PET compared with bone scintigraphy, but a similar sensitivity [92, 93]. Preliminary data indicate the superiority of MRI compared to PET/CT in this domain [94]. Forty-one patients suffering from different carcinomas were examined with both modalities. MRI revealed 76 bone metastases, PET/CT only 50. As a result, the value of FDG-PET in skeleton metastases remains controversial.

Frequent problems in evaluating FDG-PET images are false-positive findings, for example resulting from increased uptake of axillary (brown) fat tissue. PET/CT may overcome this particular limitation by adding the necessary anatomical information and thus increasing

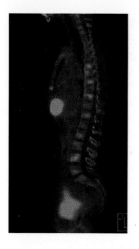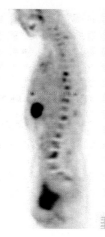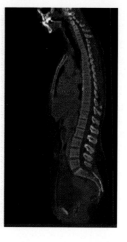

Fig. 10.5. Sagittal slices of PET/CT, FDG-PET, and CT showing a large hepatic metastasis diagnosed in all modalities. PET and PET/CT reveal multiple additional bone metastases of the spine and the sternum

specificity (and sensitivity). In a study with 58 patients, PET/CT staged more women correctly than PET alone (89.7% vs 79.3%), though the difference was not significant [95]. Tatsumi et al. examined another population of 75 patients with known breast cancer using FDG-PET/CT [96]. PET/CT exhibited a significantly better accuracy than CT (p < 0.05). Therefore, integrated PET/CT can improve the accuracy of staging and is a promising new modality. The role of whole-body MRI as another technique covering the whole body has to be evaluated further; preliminary studies show a similar accuracy in staging distant metastases compared to PET/CT [94].

In conclusion, PET and PET/CT are valuable methods for the follow-up of women suffering from breast cancer. It is particularly in cases of clinical suspicion of recurrent disease or rising tumor markers and equivocal findings in conventional imaging modalities that PET can contribute useful information.

10.9   Conclusions

In the diagnosis of primary tumors, FDG-PET is not recommended in routine clinical practice. The sensitivity in small tumors, well-differentiated tumors, and lobular carcinomas is too low to justify its routine use. However, in difficult cases such as equivocal mammo-

graphic and/or MRI findings, dense breast tissue, or posttreatment changes caused by radiation therapy, PET can contribute valuable information in selected patients.

In axillary lymph node staging, FDG-PET cannot replace axillary lymph node dissection or sentinel lymph node mapping because of its low accuracy in small metastases. However, in large primary tumors likely to have lymph node metastases, PET may be useful to choose the right neoadjuvant or adjuvant therapy and can further delineate distant metastases. In tumors of the inner quadrant of the breast, PET imaging may reveal additional metastases of the internal mammaria region lymph nodes.

One major advantage of FDG-PET is its capacity for whole-body staging in a single examination. Though not implemented in a standard follow-up regime, FDG-PET seems to be useful in cases of elevated tumor markers and unsuspicious findings in conventional imaging modalities. Some studies indicate that PET is superior to conventional imaging modalities in suspected recurrent or metastatic breast cancer. If further larger studies confirm these findings conventional imaging may be substituted by FDG-PET, or more likely PET/CT, in the future.

The preliminary results of FDG-PET in monitoring chemotherapy are encouraging but have to be confirmed by larger patient series before it can be recommended routinely.

References

1. Zeeb H, Razum O (2004) Breast cancer among Turkish women in Germany – epidemiology and research agenda. Zentralbl Gynakol 126:77–80
2. Jemal A, Murray T, Ward E, Samuels A, Tiwari RC, Ghafoor A, Feuer EJ, Thun MJ (2005) Cancer statistics, 2005. CA Cancer J Clin 55:10–30
3. Smith RA GR (1996) The epidemiology of breast cancer. Diagnosis of diseases of the breast. 293–316
4. Boetes C, Mus RD, Holland R, Barentsz JO, Strijk SP, Wobbes T, Hendriks JH, Ruys SH (1995) Breast tumors: comparative accuracy of MR imaging relative to mammography and US for demonstrating extent. Radiology 197:743–747
5. Kacl GM, Liu P, Debatin JF, Garzoli E, Caduff RF, Krestin GP (1998) Detection of breast cancer with conventional mammography and contrast-enhanced MR imaging. Eur Radiol 8:194–200
6. Holland R, Hendriks JH, Mravunac M (1983) Mammographically occult breast cancer. A pathologic and radiologic study. Cancer 52:1810–1819
7. Bone B, Pentek Z, Perbeck L, Veress B (1997) Diagnostic accuracy of mammography and contrast-enhanced MR imaging in 238 histologically verified breast lesions. Acta Radiol 38:489–496
8. Rankin SC (2000) MRI of the breast. Br J Radiol 73:806–818
9. Saarenmaa I, Salminen T, Geiger U, Holli K, Isola J, Karkkainen A, Pakkanen J, Piironen A, Salo A, Hakama M (1999) The visibility of cancer on earlier mammograms in a population-based screening programme. Eur J Cancer 35:1118–1122
10. Kopans DB (1997) An overview of the breast cancer screening controversy. J Natl Cancer Inst Monogr (22):1–3
11. Irwig L, Houssami N, van Vliet C (2004) New technologies in screening for breast cancer: a systematic review of their accuracy. Br J Cancer 90:2118–2122
12. Harms SE (1999) Technical report of the international working group on breast MRI J Magn Reson Imaging 10:979
13. Orel SG, Schnall MD, LiVolsi VA, Troupin RH (1994) Suspicious breast lesions: MR imaging with radiologic-pathologic correlation. Radiology 190:485–493
14. Kuhl CK, Schmutzler RK, Leutner CC, Kempe A, Wardelmann E, Hocke A, Maringa M, Pfeifer U, Krebs D, Schild HH (2000) Breast MR imaging screening in 192 women proved or suspected to be carriers of a breast cancer susceptibility gene: preliminary results. Radiology 215:267–279
15. Kaiser WA, Zeitler E (1989) MR imaging of the breast: fast imaging sequences with and without Gd-DTPA Preliminary observations. Radiology 170:681–686
16. Kaiser WA (1992) MRM promises earlier breast cancer diagnosis. Diagn Imaging (San Franc) 14:88–93
17. Boetes C, Barentsz JO, Mus RD, van der Sluis RF, van Erning LJ, Hendriks JH, Holland R, Ruys SH (1994) MR characterization of suspicious breast lesions with a gadolinium-enhanced TurboFLASH subtraction technique. Radiology 193:777–781
18. Gilles R, Guinebretiere JM, Shapeero LG, Lesnik A, Contesso G, Sarrazin D, Masselot J, Vanel D (1993) Assessment of breast cancer recurrence with contrast-enhanced subtraction MR imaging: preliminary results in 26 patients. Radiology 188:473–478
19. Orel SG, Schnall MD (2001) MR imaging of the breast for the detection, diagnosis, and staging of breast cancer. Radiology 220:13–30
20. Aktolun C, Bayhan H, Kir M (1992) Clinical experience with Tc-99m MIBI imaging in patients with malignant tumors. Preliminary results and comparison with Tl-201. Clin Nucl Med 17:171–176
21. Burak Z, Argon M, Memis A, Erdem S, Balkan Z, Duman Y, Ustun EE, Erhan Y, Ozkilic H (1994) Evaluation of palpable breast masses with 99Tcm-MIBI: a comparative study with mammography and ultrasonography. Nucl Med Commun 15:604–612
22. Khalkhali I, Mena I, Jouanne E, Diggles L, Venegas R, Block J, Alle K, Klein S (1994) Prone scintimammography in patients with suspicion of carcinoma of the breast. J Am Coll Surg 178:491–497
23. Taillefer R, Robidoux A, Lambert R, Turpin S, Laperriere J (1995) Technetium-99m-sestamibi prone scintimammography to detect primary breast cancer and axillary lymph node involvement. J Nucl Med 36:1758–1765
24. Kao CH, Wang SJ, Liu TJ (1994) The use of technetium-99m methoxyisobutylisonitrile breast scintigraphy to evaluate palpable breast masses. Eur J Nucl Med 21:432–436
25. Buscombe JR, Cwikla JB, Thakrar DS, Hilson AJ (1997) Uptake of Tc-99m MIBI related to tumour size and type. Anticancer Res 17:1693–1694
26. Scopinaro F, Schillaci O, Ussof W, Nordling K, Capoferro R, De Vincentis G, Danieli R, Ierardi M, Picardi V, Tavolaro R, Colella AC (1997) A three center study on the diagnostic accuracy of ^{99m}Tc-MIBI scintimammography. Anticancer Res 17:1631–1634
27. Tiling R, Khalkhali I, Sommer H, Moser R, Meyer G, Willemsen F, Pfluger T, Tatsch K, Hahn K (1997) Role of technetium-99m sestamibi scintimammography and contrast-enhanced magnetic resonance imaging for the evaluation of indeterminate mammograms. Eur J Nucl Med 24:1221–1229
28. Waxman AD (1997) The role of (^{99m})Tc methoxyisobutylisonitrile in imaging breast cancer. Semin Nucl Med 27:40–54
29. Khalkhali I, Baum JK, Villanueva-Meyer J, Edell SL, Hanelin LG, Lugo CE, Taillefer R, Freeman LM, Neal CE, Scheff AM, Connolly JL, Schnitt SJ, Houlihan MJ, Sampalis JS, Haber SB (2002) (^{99m})Tc sestamibi breast imaging for the examination of patients with dense and fatty breasts: multicenter study. Radiology 222:149–155
30. Lumachi F, Ferretti G, Povolato M, Marzola MC, Zucchetta P, Geatti O, Bui F, Brandes AA (2001) Usefulness of ^{99m}Tc-sestamibi scintimammography in suspected

breast cancer and in axillary lymph node metastases detection. Eur J Surg Oncol 27:256–259

31. Tiling R, Kessler M, Untch M, Sommer H, Linke R, Hahn K (2005) Initial evaluation of breast cancer using Tc-99m sestamibi scintimammography. Eur J Radiol 53:206–212

32. Mankoff DA, Dunnwald LK, Gralow JR, Ellis GK, Drucker MJ, Livingston RB (1999) Monitoring the response of patients with locally advanced breast carcinoma to neoadjuvant chemotherapy using [technetium ^{99m}]-sestamibi scintimammography. Cancer 85:2410–2423

33. Tiling R, Linke R, Untch M, Richter A, Fieber S, Brinkbaumer K, Tatsch K, Hahn K (2001) 18F-FDG PET and ^{99m}Tc-sestamibi scintimammography for monitoring breast cancer response to neoadjuvant chemotherapy: a comparative study. Eur J Nucl Med 28:711–720

34. Cayre A, Cachin F, Maublant J, Mestas D, Feillel V, Ferriere JP, Kwiatkowski F, Chevillard S, Finat-Duclos F, Verrelle P, Penault-Llorca F (2002) Single static view ^{99m}Tc-sestamibi scintimammography predicts response to neoadjuvant chemotherapy and is related to MDR expression. Int J Oncol20:1049–1055

35. Wald N, Chamberlain J, Hackshaw (1994) A consensus conference on breast cancer screening. Paris, February 4–5, 1993. Report of the Evaluation Committee. Oncology 51:380–389

36. Warburg O () The metabolism of tumors. Smith RR 1931:129–169

37. Adler LP, Crowe JP, al-Kaisi NK, Sunshine JL (1993) Evaluation of breast masses and axillary lymph nodes with [F-18] 2-deoxy-2-fluoro-D-glucose PET. Radiology 187:743–750

38. Wahl RL, Cody RL, Hutchins GD, Mudgett EE (1991) Primary and metastatic breast carcinoma: initial clinical evaluation with PET with the radiolabeled glucose analogue 2-[F-18]-fluoro-2-deoxy-D-glucose. Radiology 179:765–770

39. Nieweg OE, Kim EE, Wong WH, Broussard WF, Singletary SE, Hortobagyi GN, Tilbury RS (1993) Positron emission tomography with fluorine-18-deoxyglucose in the detection and staging of breast cancer. Cancer 71:3920–3925

40. Avril N, Menzel M, Dose J, Schelling M, Weber W, Janicke F, Nathrath W, Schwaiger M (2001) Glucose metabolism of breast cancer assessed by ^{18}F-FDG PET: histologic and immunohistochemical tissue analysis. J Nucl Med 42:9–16

41. Buck AK, Schirrmeister H, Mattfeldt T, Reske SN (2004) Biological characterisation of breast cancer by means of PET. Eur J Nucl Med Mol Imaging 31 [Suppl 1]:S80–S87

42. Bos R, van Der Hoeven JJ, van Der Wall E, van Der Groep P, van Diest PJ, Comans EF, Joshi U, Semenza GL, Hoekstra OS, Lammertsma AA, Molthoff CF (2002) Biologic correlates of (^{18})fluorodeoxyglucose uptake in human breast cancer measured by positron emission tomography. J Clin Oncol 20:379–387

43. Buck A, Schirrmeister H, Kuhn T, Shen C, Kalker Kotzerke J, Dankerl A, Glatting G, Reske S, Mattfeldt (2002) FDG uptake in breast cancer: correlation wi biological and clinical prognostic parameters. Eur Nucl Med Mol Imaging 29:1317–1323

44. Crippa F, Seregni E, Agresti R, Chiesa C, Pascali Bogni A, Decise D, De Sanctis V, Greco M, Daidor MG, Bombardieri E (1998) Association betwee [18F]fluorodeoxyglucose uptake and postoperativ histopathology, hormone receptor status, thymidir labelling index and p53 in primary breast cance a preliminary observation. Eur J Nucl Med 25:142§ 1434

45. Avril N, Menzel M, Dose J, Schelling M, Weber V Janicke F, Nathrath W, Schwaiger M (2001) Glucos metabolism of breast cancer assessed by ^{18}F-FD PET: histologic and immunohistochemical tissu analysis. J Nucl Med 42:9–16

46. Oshida M, Uno K, Suzuki M, Nagashima T, Hashimo H, Yagata H, Shishikura T, Imazeki K, Nakajima (1998) Predicting the prognoses of breast carcinom patients with positron emission tomography using ; deoxy-2-fluoro[^{18}F]-D-glucose. Cancer 82:2227–223

47. Rosen EL, Turkington TG, Soo MS, Baker JA, Cole man RE (2005) Detection of primary breast carc noma with a dedicated, large-field-of-view FDG PE mammography device: initial experience. Radiolog 234:527–534

48. Hubner KF, Smith GT, Thie JA, Bell JL, Nelson H Hanna WT (2000) The potential of F-18-FDG PET i breast cancer. Detection of primary lesions, axillar lymph node metastases, or distant metastases. Cli Positron Imaging 3:197–205

49. Rostom AY, Powe J, Kandil A, Ezzat A, Bakheet : el-Khwsky F, el-Hussainy G, Sorbris R, Sjoklint ∢ (1999) Positron emission tomography in breas cancer: a clinicopathological correlation of result Br J Radiol 72:1064–1068

50. Adler LP, Crowe JP, al-Kaisi NK, Sunshine JL (1993 Evaluation of breast masses and axillary lymp nodes with [F-18] 2-deoxy-2-fluoro-D-glucose PE' Radiology 187:743–750

51. Marshall C, Mustafa S, Wheatley DC, Eremin JE, E Sheemy M, Jibril JA, Eremin O, Griffiths PA (2004 A comparison of ^{18}F-FDG gamma camera PET, mam mography and ultrasonography in demonstratin primary disease in locally advanced breast cance Nucl Med Commun 25:721–725

52. Walter C, Scheidhauer K, Scharl A, Goering UJ, The issen P, Kugel H, Krahe T, Pietrzyk U (2003) Clinica and diagnostic value of preoperative MR mammog raphy and FDG-PET in suspicious breast lesions. Eu Radiol 13:1651–1656

53. Heinisch M, Gallowitsch HJ, Mikosch P, Kresnik Kumnig G, Gomez I, Lind P, Umschaden HW, Gasse J, Forsthuber EP (2003) Comparison of FDG-PET an dynamic contrast-enhanced MRI in the evaluation o suggestive breast lesions. Breast 12:17–22

54. Rieber A, Schirrmeister H, Gabelmann A, Nuessle K

Reske S, Kreienberg R, Brambs HJ, Kuehn T (2002) Pre-operative staging of invasive breast cancer with MR mammography and/or PET: boon or bunk? Br J Radiol 75:789–798

5. Schirrmeister H, Kuhn T, Guhlmann A, Santjohanser C, Horster T, Nussle K, Koretz K, Glatting G, Rieber A, Kreienberg R, Buck AC, Reske SN (2001) Fluorine-18 2-deoxy-2-fluoro-D-glucose PET in the preoperative staging of breast cancer: comparison with the standard staging procedures. Eur J Nucl Med 28:351–358

6. Shields AF, Grierson JR, Dohmen BM, Machulla HJ, Stayanoff JC, Lawhorn-Crews JM, Obradovich JE, Muzik O, Mangner TJ (1998) Imaging proliferation in vivo with [F-18]FLT and positron emission tomography. Nat Med 4:1334–1336

7. Rasey JS, Grierson JR, Wiens LW, Kolb PD, Schwartz JL (2002) Validation of FLT uptake as a measure of thymidine kinase-1 activity in A549 carcinoma cells. J Nucl Med 43:1210–1217

8. Buck AK, Schirrmeister H, Hetzel M, Von Der Heide M, Halter G, Glatting G, Mattfeldt T, Liewald F, Reske SN, Neumaier B (2002) 3-deoxy-3-[(18)F]fluorothymidine-positron emission tomography for noninvasive assessment of proliferation in pulmonary nodules. Cancer Res 62:3331–3334

9. Vesselle H, Grierson J, Muzi M, Pugsley JM, Schmidt RA, Rabinowitz P, Peterson LM, Vallieres E, Wood DE (2002) In vivo validation of 3'deoxy-3'-[(^{18})F]fluorothymidine ([(^{18})F]FLT) as a proliferation imaging tracer in humans: correlation of [(^{18})F]FLT uptake by positron emission tomography with Ki-67 immunohistochemistry and flow cytometry in human lung tumors. Clin Cancer Res 8:3315–3323

0. Smyczek-Gargya B, Fersis N, Dittmann H, Vogel U, Reischl G, Machulla H-J, Wallwiener D, Bares R, Dohmen B (2004) PET with [^{18}F]fluorothymidine for imaging of primary breast cancer: a pilot study. Eur J Nucl Med Mole Imaging 31:720–724

1. Been LB, Elsinga PH, de Vries J, Cobben DCP, Jager PL, Hoekstra HJ, Suurmeijer AJH () Positron emission tomography in patients with breast cancer using ^{18}F-3'-deoxy-3'-fluoro-l-thymidine (^{18}F-FLT)–a pilot study. European Journal of Surgical Oncology In Press, Corrected Proof,

2. Mortimer JE, Dehdashti F, Siegel BA, Trinkaus K, Katzenellenbogen JA, Welch MJ (2001) Metabolic flare: indicator of hormone responsiveness in advanced breast cancer. J Clin Oncol 19:2797–2803

3. Robinson MK, Doss M, Shaller C, Narayanan D, Marks JD, Adler LP, Gonzalez Trotter DE, Adams GP (2005) Quantitative immuno-positron emission tomography imaging of HER2-positive tumor xenografts with an iodine-124 labeled anti-HER2 diabody. Cancer Res 65:1471–1478

4. Steffen A-C, Wikman M, Tolmachev V, Adams GP, Nilsson FY, Stahl S, Carlsson J (2005) In vitro characterization of a bivalent anti-HER-2 antibody with potential for radionuclide-based diagnostics. Cancer Biother Radiopharmaceut 20:239–248

65. Bentzen L, Keiding S, Nordsmark M, Falborg L, Hansen SB, Keller J, Nielsen OS, Overgaard J (2003) Tumour oxygenation assessed by ^{18}F-fluoromisonidazole PET and polarographic needle electrodes in human soft tissue tumours. Radiothe Oncol 67:339–344

66. Keen HG, Dekker BA, Disley L, Hastings D, Lyons S, Reader AJ, Ottewell P, Watson A, Zweit J (2005) Imaging apoptosis in vivo using 124I-annexin V and PET. Nucl Med Biol 32:395–402

67. Yagle KJ, Eary JF, Tait JF, Grierson JR, Link JM, Lewellen B, Gibson DF, Krohn KA (2005) Evaluation of 18F-annexin V as a PET imaging agent in an animal model of apoptosis. J Nucl Med 46:658–666

68. Wang Y, Yu J, Liu J, Tong Z, Sun X, Yang G (2003) PET-CT in the diagnosis of both primary breast cancer and axillary lymph node metastasis: initial experience. I. J Radiat Oncolo Biol Phys 57:362–363

69. Kwan W, Jackson J, Weir LM, Dingee C, McGregor G, Olivotto IA (2002) Chronic arm morbidity after curative breast cancer treatment: prevalence and impact on quality of life. J Clin Oncol 20:4242–4248

70. Wahl RL, Siegel BA, Coleman RE, Gatsonis CG (2004) Prospective multicenter study of axillary nodal staging by positron emission tomography in breast cancer: a report of the staging breast cancer with PET Study Group. J Clin Oncol 22:277–285

71. Avril N, Dose J, Janicke F, Ziegler S, Romer W, Weber W, Herz M, Nathrath W, Graeff H, Schwaiger M (1996) Assessment of axillary lymph node involvement in breast cancer patients with positron emission tomography using radiolabeled 2-(fluorine-18)-fluoro-2-deoxy-D-glucose. J Natl Cancer Inst 88:1204–1209

72. Weir L, Worsley D, Bernstein V (2005) The value of FDG positron emission tomography in the management of patients with breast cancer. Breast J 11:204–209

73. Schirrmeister H, Kuhn T, Guhlmann A, Santjohanser C, Horster T, Nussle K, Koretz K, Glatting G, Rieber A, Kreienberg R, Buck AC, Reske SN (2001) Fluorine-18 2-deoxy-2-fluoro-D-glucose PET in the preoperative staging of breast cancer: comparison with the standard staging procedures. Eur J Nucl Med 28:351–358

74. Greco M, Crippa F, Agresti R, Seregni E, Gerali A, Giovanazzi R, Micheli A, Asero S, Ferraris C, Gennaro M, Bombardieri E, Cascinelli N (2001) Axillary lymph node staging in breast cancer by 2-fluoro-2-deoxy-D-glucose-positron emission tomography: clinical evaluation and alternative management. J Natl Cancer Inst 93:630–635

75. Eubank WB, Mankoff DA, Takasugi J, Vesselle H, Eary JF, Shanley TJ, Gralow JR, Charlop A, Ellis GK, Lindsley KL, Austin-Seymour MM, Funkhouser CP, Livingston RB (2001) ^{18}fluorodeoxyglucose positron emission tomography to detect mediastinal or internal mammary metastases in breast cancer. J Clin Oncol 19:3516–3523

76. Bellon JR, Livingston RB, Eubank WB, Gralow JR, Ellis GK, Dunnwald LK, Mankoff DA (2004) Evaluation of the internal mammary lymph nodes by FDG-

PET in locally advanced breast cancer (LABC). Am J Clin Oncol 27:407–410

77. Helvie MA, Joynt LK, Cody RL, Pierce LJ, Adler DD, Merajver SD (1996) Locally advanced breast carcinoma: accuracy of mammography versus clinical examination in the prediction of residual disease after chemotherapy. Radiology 198:327–332

78. Smith IC, Welch AE, Hutcheon AW, Miller ID, Payne S, Chilcott F, Waikar S, Whitaker T, Ah-See AK, Eremin O, Heys SD, Gilbert FJ, Sharp PF (2000) Positron emission tomography using [(^{18})F]-fluorodeoxy-D-glucose to predict the pathologic response of breast cancer to primary chemotherapy. J Clin Oncol 18:1676–1688

79. Schelling M, Avril N, Nahrig J, Kuhn W, Romer W, Sattler D, Werner M, Dose J, Janicke F, Graeff H, Schwaiger M (2000) Positron emission tomography using [(^{18})F]Fluorodeoxyglucose for monitoring primary chemotherapy in breast cancer. J Clin Oncol 18:1689–1695

80. Burcombe RJ, Makris A, Pittam M, Lowe J, Emmott J, Wong WL (2002) Evaluation of good clinical response to neoadjuvant chemotherapy in primary breast cancer using [^{18}F]-fluorodeoxyglucose positron emission tomography. Eur J Cancer 38:375–379

81. Dehdashti F, Flanagan FL, Mortimer JE, Katzenellenbogen JA, Welch MJ, Siegel BA (1999) Positron emission tomographic assessment of «metabolic flare» to predict response of metastatic breast cancer to antiestrogen therapy. Eur J Nucl Med 26:51–56

82. Mortimer JE, Dehdashti F, Siegel BA, Trinkaus K, Katzenellenbogen JA, Welch MJ (2001) Metabolic flare: indicator of hormone responsiveness in advanced breast cancer. J Clin Oncol 19:2797–2803

83. Ries LAG, Eisner MP, Kosary CL (2004) SEER cancer statistics review, 1975–2001. National Cancer Institute, Bethesda

84. Katz A, Strom EA, Buchholz TA, Thames HD, Smith CD, Jhingran A, Hortobagyi G, Buzdar AU, Theriault R, Singletary SE, McNeese MD (2000) Locoregional recurrence patterns after mastectomy and doxorubicin-based chemotherapy: implications for postoperative irradiation. J Clin Oncol 18:2817–2827

85. Hathaway PB, Mankoff DA, Maravilla KR, Austin-Seymour MM, Ellis GK, Gralow JR, Cortese AA, Hayes CE, Moe RE (1999) Value of combined FDG PET and MR imaging in the evaluation of suspected recurrent local-regional breast cancer: preliminary experience. Radiology 210:807–814

86. Goerres GW, Michel SC, Fehr MK, Kaim AH, Steinert HC, Seifert B, von Schulthess GK, Kubik-Huch RA (2003) Follow-up of women with breast cancer: comparison between MRI and FDG PET. Eur Radiol 13:1635–1644

87. Gallowitsch HJ, Kresnik E, Gasser J, Kumnig G, Igerc I, Mikosch P, Lind P (2003) F-18 fluorodeoxyglucose positron-emission tomography in the diagnosis of

tumor recurrence and metastases in the follow-up of patients with breast carcinoma: a comparison to conventional imaging. Invest Radiol 38:250–256

88. Kamel EM, Wyss MT, Fehr MK, von Schulthess GK, Goerres GW (2003) [^{18}F]-Fluorodeoxyglucose positron emission tomography in patients with suspected recurrence of breast cancer. J Cancer Res Clin Oncol 129:147–153

89. Dose J, Bleckmann C, Bachmann S, Bohuslavizk KH, Berger J, Jenicke L, Habermann CR, Janicke F (2002) Comparison of fluorodeoxyglucose positron emission tomography and "conventional diagnostic procedures" for the detection of distant metastases in breast cancer patients. Nucl Med Commun 23:857–864

90. Gallowitsch HJ, Kresnik E, Gasser J, Kumnig G, Igerc I, Mikosch P, Lind P (2003) F-18 fluorodeoxyglucose positron-emission tomography in the diagnosis of tumor recurrence and metastases in the follow-up of patients with breast carcinoma: a comparison to conventional imaging. Invest Radiol 38:250–256

91. Eubank WB, Mankoff DA, Takasugi J, Vesselle H, Eary JF, Shanley TJ, Gralow JR, Charlop A, Ellis GK, Lindsley KL, Austin-Seymour MM, Funkhouser CP, Livingston RB (2001) ^{18}fluorodeoxyglucose positron emission tomography to detect mediastinal or internal mammary metastases in breast cancer. J Clin Oncol 19:3516–3523

92. Ohta M, Tokuda Y, Suzuki Y, Kubota M, Makuuchi H, Tajima T, Nasu S, Yasuda S, Shohtsu A (2001) Whole-body PET for the evaluation of bony metastases in patients with breast cancer: comparison with 99Tcm MDP bone scintigraphy. Nucl Med Commun 22:875–879

93. Yang SN, Liang JA, Lin FJ, Kao CH, Lin CC, Lee CC (2002) Comparing whole body (^{18})F-2-deoxyglucose positron emission tomography and technetium-99m methylene diphosphonate bone scan to detect bone metastases in patients with breast cancer. J Cancer Res Clin Oncol 128:325–328

94. Schmidt GP, Baur-Melnyk A, Herzog P, Schmid R, Tiling R, Schmidt M, Reiser MF, Schoenberg SO (2005) High-resolution whole-body magnetic resonance image tumor staging with the use of parallel imaging versus dual-modality positron emission tomography-computed tomography: experience on a 32-channel system. Invest Radiol 40:743–753

95. Fueger B, Weber W, Quon A, Crawford T, Allen-Auerbach M, Halpern B, Ratib O, Phelps M, Czernin J (2005) Performance of 2-Deoxy-2-[F-18]fluoro-d-glucose positron emission tomography and integrated PET/CT in restaged breast cancer patients. Mol Imaging Biol 7:369–376

96. Tatsumi M, Cohade C, Mourtzikos KA, Fishman EK, Wahl RL (2005) Initial experience with FDG-PET/CT in the evaluation of breast cancer. Eur J Nucl Med Mol Imaging 33:254–262

11 Gynecologic Tumors

M. J. Reinhardt

Recent Results in Cancer Research, Vol. 170
© Springer-Verlag Berlin Heidelberg 2008

11.1 Introduction

Five years ago, a summary of the literature estimated the average sensitivity and specificity of positron-emission tomography (PET) imaging using 2-18F-fluoro-D-glucose (FDG) across all oncologic applications at 84% and 88%, respectively [1]. The average management change due to the results of FDG-PET imaging was estimated to be 30% [1]. These results make metabolic imaging with FDG-PET an alternative and sometimes complimentary tool to morphologic cross-sectional imaging procedures, such as computed tomography (CT) and magnetic resonance (MR) imaging. In the female reproductive tract, FDG-PET imaging has mainly been applied to primary diagnosis in ovarian and cervical cancer, detection of recurrence in cervical and ovarian cancer, monitoring therapy response in ovarian cancer, and evaluation of individual prognosis in ovarian and cervical cancer. Furthermore, several papers in recent years focused on the diagnostic value of the new dual-modality FDG-PET/CT in ovarian and cervical tumors.

A recent meta-analysis of 25 studies (15 cervical cancer, 10 ovarian cancer) using stringent inclusion criteria reported an overall sensitivity and specificity of FDG-PET for aortic node metastasis of 84% and 95% in cervical cancer patients. These statistical values for detection of pelvic node metastasis were 79% and 99%, which was not significantly better than that for MR imaging with 72% and 96%, respectively.

Pooled sensitivity and specificity of FDG-PET for recurrent cervical cancer were 96% and 81%. Overall sensitivity and specificity for detection of suspected recurrent ovarian cancer were 90% and 86%, which was significantly better than that of conventional imaging with 68% and 58%. Mean sensitivity and specificity of FDG-PET were 54% and 73% when conventional imaging and CA-125 were negative, but raised to 96% and 80% when CA-125 increased and conventional imaging was negative [2].

As a consequence, the authors reported FDG-PET as useful for pretreatment detection of retroperitoneal nodal metastases in cervical cancer and for detection of recurrent cervical cancer as well as for detection of recurrence of ovarian cancer in patients with rising CA-125 and negative conventional imaging studies [2].

The guidelines of the German Cancer Society considered FDG-PET as helpful for diagnosis and detection of metastases of cervical cancer and for diagnosis of recurrent ovarian cancer [3]. Thus, this chapter presents the results of FDG-PET and FDG-PET/CT with respect to the current management of patients with ovarian and cervical cancer.

11.2 Ovarian Cancer

Ovarian cancer accounts for 4% of all cancer diagnoses and 5% of all cancer deaths [4]. The poor prognosis of ovarian cancer at the time of detection makes this tumor the leading cause of death from a gynecologic cancer. Due to the frequently observed advanced stage at diagnosis, the mean 5-year survival rate ranged between 35% and 45%. More than 90% of ovarian carcinomas are epithelial in origin and are diagnosed in postmenopausal women [4]. With currently available tests, routine screening for ovarian cancer cannot be recommended [5]. Ovarian palpation, transvaginal ultrasound, and serum CA-125 determination are not sufficiently accurate for general screening. Ovarian cancer is a surgically staged disease [6]. The International Federation of Gynecology and Obstetrics (FIGO) has defined the most widely accepted staging system for carcinoma of the ovary [7]. Ovarian cancer spreads by direct extension to neighboring organs, by exfoliating cells into the peritoneal cavity that can implant on parietal and visceral peritoneum, and by lymphatic spread to the external iliac and obturator fossa and the common iliac and paraaortic lymph node chains. Epithelial cancers of the ovary have been described as a silent killer because approximately 70% of patients present with disease that has spread outside of the ovary at the time of initial presentation (FIGO stage III and IV) [8]. With aggressive treatment, the stage-related 5-year survival rate in patients with stage I disease reaches 93%, in stage II disease 70%, in stage III disease 37%, and in stage IV disease 25% [9]. The volume of residual tumor tissue following cytoreductive surgery has a significant impact on survival. With residual nodules not greater than 1 cm in the omentum after tumor debulking surgery and subsequent cisplatin-based combination chemotherapy, the 5-year survival rate increased to approximately 35% [10]. The current recommendation for management of patients without evidence of progressive disease at 1 year after diagnosis is to perform second-look laparotomy for restaging and possible secondary cytoreductive surgery [4].

CT has been used to identify the extent of ovarian cancer metastases especially in the upper abdomen [11]. However, CT imaging reflects less than the actual histological findings at the time of surgery. Peritoneal carcinosis is particularly difficult to detect with CT.

FDG-PET has been used to differentiate asymptomatic adnexal masses [12–16]. Inflammatory processes of the ovary presented with increased FDG uptake as well and therefore could not be differentiated from malignant lesions [12]. A direct comparison with MR imaging improved the diagnostic accuracy significantly with respect to areas of unspecific FDG uptake [14]. However, in 85 patients with sonographically suspicious adnexal masses the sensitivity and specificity of FDG-PET for detection of ovarian carcinoma was 50% and 78%, respectively [12]. In a summary of six studies including 286 patients, sensitivity and specificity of FDG-PET for primary diagnosis of ovarian cancer was reported as 66% and 77%, respectively [1]. Therefore, FDG-PET cannot be recommended as a routine procedure in asymptomatic patients with suspicious adnexal masses, the most common clinical setting in which a malignant ovarian tumor has to be excluded. For primary staging, the overall sensitivity of FDG-PET was only 54% [1].

The results of FDG-PET imaging were better for detection of recurrence and restaging than that for primary staging. For this purpose, FDG-PET imaging resulted in sensitivity and specificity of 86% and 90%, while CT reached values of 76% and 75%, respectively [1]. These data were derived from a total of 357 patients studied. Therefore, the third German Interdisciplinary Consensus Conference on indications for FDG-PET in oncology has established the use of FDG-PET for detection and staging of recurrent ovarian cancer as "useful in individual cases" [17]. Change of patient management was estimated to be 17% based on findings in FDG-PET scans [1].

Nonetheless, a study on the predictability of complete clinical response with FDG-PET in comparison to a second-look laparotomy [18] and two studies on the diagnostic accuracy of FDG-PET in comparison to CT for detection of recurrent ovarian cancer [19, 20] showed that the sensitivity of FDG-PET for small-volume disease was low despite several technical improvements. Out of 22 patients with advanced-stage ovarian or peritoneal carcinoma, who had achieved complete clinical and radiological remission and normal CA-125 values, 13 patients (59%) had persistent disease [18]. Only one of nine sites with macroscopic and none of four sites with microscopic disease were detected by FDG-PET [18]. Sensitivity, specificity, and accuracy of FDG-PET, CT, and combined PET and CT in 31 patients with recurrent ovarian cancer who underwent FDG-PET 1 month before second-look surgery were not significantly different, even though best results were obtained after image fusion (58.2%, 99.6%, and 92.4%, respectively) [19]. Detection rates of tumor nodules on CT were reported to be significantly higher than those on FDG-PET, especially when nodule size was between 3 and 7 mm [19]. Sensitivity, specificity, positive predictive value, negative predictive value, and accuracy of FDG-PET in 29 patients with suspected recurrence of ovarian cancer after initial treatment was reported as 84.6%, 100%, 100%, 42.9%, and 86.2%, respectively [20]. The low negative predictive value of FDG-PET was due to a high rate of false-negative findings for microscopic disease. All three studies emphasized the need for significant improvements in PET scanner technology, which allow for a much higher spatial resolution than currently available [18–20].

FDG-PET/CT demonstrated a high sensitivity and positive predictive value of 83.3% and 93.8% for detection of recurrent tumor masses above 1 cm in diameter in 22 patients with advanced ovarian cancer and increasing CA-125 levels after primary therapy [21]. Presurgical primary staging using FDG-PET/CT in 15 patients with FIGO I to FIGO III disease was correct in 87% of them [22].

A recent paper evaluated the prognostic value of FDG-PET in comparison to that of a second-look laparotomy in 30 and 25 patients with advanced ovarian cancer after primary treatment [23]. Recurrence was observed in 37 patients. Neither the progression-free interval nor the disease-free interval showed significant differences between the PET group and the second-look laparotomy group [23]. The authors concluded that FDG-PET may substitute second-look laparotomy in patients with

ovarian cancer and a high-risk for recurrence [23].

Seven studies in recent years focused on the accuracy of FDG-PET/CT for detection of recurrent ovarian cancer [24–28], for detection of persistent ovarian cancer after first-line treatment [29], and for prediction of response to neoadjuvant chemotherapy [30]. Nanni and co-workers prospectively evaluated 41 patients after first-line treatment with FDG-PET/CT in comparison to conventional imaging and CA-125 [24]. Histology, clinical and laboratory follow-up, and repeated conventional imaging techniques served as the standard of reference. Sensitivity, specificity, and accuracy of FDG-PET/CT for detection of early recurrence were 88.2%, 71.4%, and 85.4%, respectively [24]. Pannu and co-workers compared the results of FDG-PET/CT with that of laparotomy in 16 patients with suspected recurrence. The reported sensitivity, specificity, and accuracy were 72.7%, 40%, and 62.5%, respectively. The authors found the sensitivity of FDG-PET/CT moderate for detection of low-volume disease [25]. Hauth and co-workers compared the results of FDG-PET/CT with that of CT in 19 patients with suspected recurrence of ovarian cancer [26]. In this small patient series, FDG-PET/CT correctly identified all 11 patients in whom recurrence was confirmed within 6 months [26]. Bristow and co-workers reported about another small series of 14 patients with rising CA-125 levels but negative conventional imaging results in whom FDG-PET/CT detected retroperitoneal nodal recurrence [27]. After histological analysis of the 143 nodes retrieved, it became evident that PET/CT failed to identify microscopic disease in 59.3% of all pathologically positive nodes [27]. Simcock and co-workers reported the results of FDG-PET/CT in 56 patients undergoing second-look laparotomy [28]. All patients with a CA-125 over 35 IU/ml had a positive PET/CT scan, resulting in a major change of management plan in 58% of patients. FDG-PET/CT further identified a subgroup of women with localized disease or no definite evidence of disease that had improved survival. The authors concluded FDG-PET/CT was useful for identification of patients with improved prognosis [28].

Sironi and co-workers used FDG-PET/CT to demonstrate persistent ovarian carcinoma after first-line treatment of 31 patients prior to second-look laparotomy [29]. Histology revealed a total of 41 tumor sites detected by PET/CT with a sensitivity of 78%, a specificity of 75%, a positive predictive value of 89%, a negative predictive value of 57%, and an accuracy of 77%. The largest tumor size missed with FDG-PET/CT was 5 mm in diameter. The authors concluded that FDG-PET/CT could detect persistent ovarian cancer with a high positive predictive value [29].

Avril and co-workers analyzed the value of FDG-PET/CT to predict the individual patient's outcome after the first and the third cycle of neoadjuvant chemotherapy in 33 patients with FIGO stage III and IV ovarian cancer [30]. At a threshold of a 20% decrease in SUV after the first chemotherapy cycle, there was a significant difference in survival between metabolic responders and nonresponders of 38.3 months vs 23.1 months. A similar difference was observed using a threshold of 55% decrease in SUV after the third cycle of chemotherapy: 38.9 months survival in metabolic responders vs 19.7 months survival in nonresponders. In contrast to the results of FDG-PET/CT, there was no correlation between overall survival and clinical response and CA-125 response and only a weak correlation with histopathologic response. The authors concluded FDG-PET/CT was a promising tool for early prediction of response to chemotherapy [30]. The paper from Avril and co-workers was highlighted with an editorial from Maurie Markman [31]. The major concern of this editorial was that Avril and co-workers claimed a clinical utility of FDG-PET/CT in ovarian cancer that could hardly be justified with the low number of 33 patients studied and it was not clear whether results of FDG-PET/CT influenced patient management or only defined prognosis [31]. Although one must agree that the number of patients has to be increased before current management strategies for patients with ovarian cancer can be changed, it has become evident that FDG-PET/CT has the potential to do exactly this.

11.3 Cervical Cancer

Cancer of the cervix is estimated to be the second most frequently diagnosed cancer in women worldwide, accounting for 6% of all malignancies in women [32]. The American Cancer Society estimated that there were approximately 15,000 new cases of invasive cervical cancer diagnosed in the United States in 1999 [33]. The incidence of cervical cancer is 9 per 100,000 and mortality is 3 per 100,000 [32]. The peak age at diagnosis of invasive cervical cancer is between 45 and 50 years [32]. The age-adjusted mortality of cervical cancer has declined nearly 70% in the last half century, which is at least in part due to the adoption of routine screening programs with pelvic examinations and cervical cytology [34]. However, cancer of the cervix continues to be the leading cause of cancer deaths for women in many second and third world countries [34].

Similar to carcinoma of the ovary, FIGO has defined the most widely accepted staging system [35]. This is a clinical staging system based on careful clinical examination, abdominal and/or endovaginal ultrasound, chest radiography and intravenous urography as well as cystoscopy and proctoscopy in bulky disease. The 5-year survival rate decreases progressively from FIGO stage I through stage IV: 80%–100% in stage IB, 60%–75% in stage II, 30%–60% in stage III, and 10%–20% in stage IVA [32]. Treatment of the earlier stages of cervical cancer can be surgery, radiation therapy or a combined radiochemotherapy with similar results [36]. More advanced stages are favorably treated with a combination of radio- and chemotherapy [36]. Although the survival and pelvic disease control rates of patients with cervical cancer correlate with FIGO stage, the prognosis of disease is also influenced by a number of tumor characteristics that are not included in the staging system [34]. Besides the tumor diameter, the extent of lymphatic spread is the most important predictor of prognosis. Survival rates of patients with FIGO stage IB cervical cancer (tumor confined to the cervix) treated with radical hysterectomy and pelvic lymphadenectomy decrease from 85%–95% for patients with negative nodes to 45%–55% for those with lymph node metastases [37]. Even in stage II cervical cancer (tumor extends beyond the cervix but not onto the pelvic wall), the survival rate is correlated with the number of pelvic lymph nodes involved [38, 39]. Survival rates for patients with positive paraaortic nodes treated with extended-field radiation therapy vary between 10% and 50% depending on the extent of pelvic disease and paraaortic lymph node involvement [34].

Lymphangiography (LAG), CT, and MR imaging are frequently performed to evaluate regional nodes, but the accuracy of these studies is compromised by their failure to depict small metastases, and because patients with bulky necrotic tumors often have enlarged reactive nodes [34]. In a meta-analysis of 38 studies fulfilling stringent inclusion criteria, sensitivity of CT and MR imaging ranged from 0.38 to 0.89 and specificity ranged from 0.78 to 0.99 [40]. FIGO states that findings by LAG, CT, and MR imaging are of value for therapy planning but should not be used to change the clinical stage. Thus, the noninvasive detection of nodal disease remains a difficult task. Identification of a sensitive and specific imaging modality would be a useful adjunct to the clinical evaluation of cervical cancer, as it might improve the individual therapy planning. The delineation of the extent of metastatic disease gained increasing relevance when primary therapy includes irradiation of the pelvic and para-aortic lymph nodes [41].

Between 1999 and 2004, 11 papers with 360 patients focused on the presurgical detection of lymph node metastases [42–51], and one paper further addressed the prognostic value of pretreatment FDG-PET in 101 patients [46].

Sugawara and co-workers [42] compared FDG-PET and CT for detection of lymph node metastases in 17 newly diagnosed and four recurrent cervical cancer patients of stages FIGO IB–IVA. From seven patients with confirmed lymph node metastases, FDG-PET detected six (86%) and CT detected four (57%). No false-positive findings on either FDG-PET or CT were reported [42].

Rose and co-workers [43] studied 32 patients with cervical cancer of stages FIGO IIB–IVA with FDG-PET prior to staging lymphadenec-

tomy. All 10 of 17 patients with lymph node metastases were identified by FDG-PET, while CT identified only five of them. The authors observed a higher sensitivity of FDG-PET for pelvic (1.00) than for paraaortic (0.75) nodes. The positive predictive value was 0.75 for FDG-PET. Only two cases with paraaortic micrometastases were missed on FDG-PET images [43].

Umesaki and co-workers [44] studied nine patients with newly diagnosed and four patients with recurrent cervical cancer. Local recurrence could be reliably detected, as well as metastatic spread when compared with MR imaging.

Reinhardt and co-workers [45] compared FDG-PET and MR imaging results with histological findings of 35 patients with cervical cancer stage FIGO IB and II prior to radical hysterectomy and pelvic and paraaortic lymphadenectomy. On a patient basis, sensitivity and specificity of FDG-PET was 0.91 and 1.00 and for MR imaging it was 0.73 and 0.83, respectively. The positive predictive value was 1.00 for FDG-PET and 0.67 for MR imaging. Similar to the study from Rose and co-workers, only a few micrometastases were missed on FDG-PET images [45].

Grigsby and co-workers [46] compared FDG-PET and CT for lymph node staging in 101 patients of stages FIGO IA–IVB prior to standard irradiation and chemotherapy. CT identified enlarged pelvic lymph nodes in 20%, and enlarged paraaortic nodes in 7% of the patients, while FDG-PET showed focally increased uptake in pelvic nodes in 67%, in paraaortic nodes in 21%, and in supraclavicular nodes in 8% of all patients. Based on the pelvic lymph node status, the 2-year progression-free survival rate was significantly higher for FDG-PET- and CT-negative patients than for CT-negative and FDG-PET-positive or CT- and FDG-PET-positive patients (0.73 vs 0.49 and 0.39; p < 0.001). This difference became even more evident when the paraaortic lymph node status was evaluated. The 2-year progression-free survival was 64% for CT and FDG-PET-negative patients but dropped to 18% or 14%, if FDG-PET was positive and CT was either negative or positive (p < 0.0001). In a multivariate analysis of patient age, tumor stage, tumor histology, lymph node status by CT in the pelvis and paraaortic region, and lymph node status by FDG-PET in the pelvis and paraaortic region, the paraaortic lymph nodes, as determined by FDG-PET, was identified as the most significant independent prognostic factor for progression-free survival [46].

Kerr and co-workers [47] studied ten patients with newly diagnosed and three patients with recurrent cervical cancer with FDG-PET. FDG-PET identified three tumor sites not detected by other imaging techniques, including CT.

Narayan and co-workers [48] compared FDG-PET and MR imaging for presurgical staging of 27 patients with locally advanced cervical cancer. Sensitivity and specificity of FDG-PET in 24 patients in whom pelvic lymph node status was evaluated were 0.83 and 0.92, and the positive predictive value was 0.91. MR imaging identified only 50% of patients with pelvic lymph node metastases, all of which were seen by FDG-PET. However, paraaortic involvement was identified by FDG-PET in only four of seven patients (57%). All histologically confirmed metastatic sites not visualized on FDG-PET images were less than 1 cm in diameter [48].

Kühnel and co-workers [49] analyzed the diagnostic accuracy of FDG-PET for presurgical evaluation of the extent of lymphatic spread in 15 cervical cancer patients. The accuracy of FDG-PET for assessment of pelvic lymph node metastases was 0.73 and 0.86 for paraaortic metastases. Only two cases with micrometastases were missed on FDG-PET images [49].

Yeh and co-workers [50] evaluated the sensitivity and specificity of FDG-PET for presurgical detection of paraaortic lymph node metastases in 42 patients with locally advanced cervical cancer and negative abdominal MR imaging results. FDG-PET was true positive in 10 of 12 patients with histologically confirmed paraaortic lymph node metastases and false positive in one case. Thus, sensitivity and specificity of FDG-PET for paraaortic lymph node staging in cervical cancer patients was 0.83 and 0.97, respectively [50].

Belhocine and co-workers [51] compared the contribution of FDG-PET and MR imaging

to the management of cervical cancer in 22 patients for presurgical staging and in 38 patients for therapy control. FDG-PET identified nine unsuspected extrapelvic lymph node sites but missed eight micrometastases in the pelvis. In 18% of the patients, FDG-PET significantly influenced the therapeutic procedure. In the follow-up, FDG-PET detected 13 cases of recurrent disease, while morphological imaging methods were false-negative [51].

Lin and co-workers reported a sensitivity, specificity and accuracy of 85.7%, 94.4%, and 92% of FDG-PET for presurgical detection of paraaortic lymph node metastases in 50 patients with negative findings on CT [52].

In 2005 and 2006, five further studies with 231 patients analyzed the usefulness of FDG-PET for primary lymph node staging of cervical cancer patients [53–57].

Roh and co-workers evaluated the diagnostic accuracy of FDG-PET in 54 patients with FIGO stage IB–IVA cervical cancer who were about to undergo lymphadenectomy [53]. The authors reported a low sensitivity of 38% and a low positive predictive value of 56%. Even when only metastases larger than 10 mm in diameter were analyzed, the sensitivity rose to only 65% [53].

Wright and co-workers [54] reported a sensitivity and specificity of FDG-PET for presurgical pelvic lymph node staging in 59 patients with FIGO stage IA–IIA cervical cancer patients of 53% and 90%, and for paraaortic lymph node staging of 25% and 98%, respectively. The size of FDG-PET negative lymph node metastases ranged from 0.3 mm to 20 mm. In a subset of 42 patients with additional CT, the combined sensitivity reached 75% [54].

Park and co-workers compared FDG-PET and MRI in 36 patients with cervical cancer prior to surgery [55]. The accuracy for detecting pelvic lymph nodes was better for FDG-PET than for MRI (78% vs 67%). Only microscopic disease was missed on PET images [55].

Chou and co-workers conducted a prospective study to evaluate the accuracy of FDG-PET for detection of metastatic disease in 60 patients with FIGO IA2 and IIA cervical cancer and no enlarged lymph nodes on MRI [56]. FDG-PET detected only 2 of 11 lymph node metastases

(18%). All PET-negative metastases measured less than 7×6 mm. The authors concluded that FDG-PET was of little value in primary stage IA2 and IIA with MRI-defined lymph node-negative cervical cancer [56].

Choi and co-workers prospectively compared FDG-PET and MRI in 22 patients with stage IB–IVA cervical cancer [57]. Sensitivity, specificity, and accuracy of FDG-PET were 57.6%, 92.6%, and 85.1% and with MRI the values were 30.3%, 92.6%, and 72.7%, respectively. The difference between FDG-PET and MRI was significant for sensitivity, but not for specificity and for accuracy [57].

Since 2000, ten papers with 642 patients have focused on the value of FDG-PET for detection of recurrent cervical cancer [51, 58–66], and one paper addressed the prognostic value of posttreatment FDG-PET in 152 patients [67]. The results of FDG-PET for detection of recurrent cervical cancer are summarized in Table 11.1. Mean sensitivity, specificity, and accuracy of FDG-PET for detection of recurrent disease in 642 patients were 92% (82%–100%), 84% (60%–98%), and 87% (70%–97%), respectively. In all of these studies, metabolic imaging was more accurate than morphological imaging using CT or MRI, which were often included in the follow-up of cervical cancer patients. However, the conventional routine protocols for posttherapy surveillance of cervical cancer patients are not standardized and may vary considerably. The efficiency of several surveillance protocols is often suboptimal, especially in asymptomatic patients [68]. Thus, there is a clinical need to improve the posttherapeutic monitoring of cervical cancer patients. FDG-PET may be the method of choice to improve posttherapeutic surveillance of cervical cancer patients, as has been outlined in a study by Grigsby and co-workers [67]. In this retrospective analysis of 152 consecutive patients with cervical carcinoma who underwent external irradiation and intracavitary brachytherapy, it could be shown that either persistent or new focally increased FDG-uptake after primary treatment was the most significant predictive variable of 5-year overall survival. Patients without any abnormal FDG uptake had a cause-specific 5-year survival of 80%, but patients with persistent abnormal uptake had a cause-specific 5-year survival of only 32%, while all patients with pathologic FDG uptake outside the field of irradiation died within 5 years of their disease [67].

The potential role of FDG-PET/CT in cervical cancer needs further evaluation, with only two studies published to date [69, 70]. One showed an improved diagnosis for both PET and CT in 32 of 75 patients by providing better localization and definition of abnormal FDG uptake but a low sensitivity of only 60% for the

Table 11.1. Value of FDG-PET for detection of recurrent cervical cancers: cumulative data from the literature

Author	Ref. no.	Year	Patients	Sensitivity	Specificity	Accuracy
Park et al.	58	2000	36	1.0	0.94	0.97
Sun et al.	59	2001	20	0.96	0.94	0.95
Nakamoto et al.	60	2002	20	1.0	0.60	0.70
Belhocine et al.	51	2002	38	1.0	0.77	0.92
Havrilesky et al.	61	2003	28	0.86	0.87	0.86
Ryu et al.	62	2003	249	0.90	0.76	0.78
Lai et al.	63	2004	40	0.91	0.98	0.97
Wong et al.	64	2004	35	0.82	0.97	0.92
Yen et al.	65	2004	55	0.89	0.98	0.97
Chung et al.	66	2006	121	0.96	0.84	0.92
Total/mean			642	0.92	0.84	0.87

fused imaging modalities [69]. The other detected 13 of 18 positive lymph nodes that were all larger than 5 mm in diameter in 47 patients with FIGO stage IA and IB, with an overall patient-based sensitivity, specificity, and accuracy of 73%, 97%, and 89%, respectively [70]. These preliminary results of PET/CT were in fact not better than that for FDG-PET alone. However, PET/CT may be helpful to reduce the number of false-positive results of FDG-PET.

In summary, FDG-PET provided with a high sensitivity ranging from 0.75 to 1.00 and a high specificity ranging from 0.92 to 1.00 for pretherapeutic assessment of lymph node metastases in cervical cancer patients, which was significantly better than that reported for CT and MR imaging with sensitivities between 0.38 and 0.89 and specificities between 0.78 and 0.99 [40]. On the basis of the literature presented, FDG-PET should be applied to primary lymph node staging in cervical cancer patients of stages IIB and higher. The value of FDG-PET in stages IA–IIA cervical cancer patients continues to be debated. However, the detection limit of metastatic lymph nodes can be reduced to 5–7 mm in diameter using current high-resolution PET scanners.

FDG-PET may further play a pivotal role in detection of recurrent cervical cancer by providing the clinician with crucial information from diagnosis to prognosis.

References

1. Gambhir SS, Czernin J, Schwimmer J, Silverman DHS, Coleman RE, Phelps ME (2001) A tabulated summary of the FDG PET literature. J Nucl Med 42 [Suppl]:1–93
2. Havrilesky LJ, Kulasingam SL, Matchar DB, Myers ER (2005) FDG-PET for management of cervical and ovarian cancer. Gynecol Oncol 97:183–191
3. Qualitätssicherung in der Onkologie (2002) Kurzgefasste Interdisziplinäre Leitlinien 2002. In: von Deutsche Krebsgesellschaft (ed) Informationszentrum für Standards in der Onkologie (ISTO). W. Zuckschwerdt, Munich
4. Ozols RF, Schwartz PE, Eifel PJ (1997) Ovarian cancer, fallopian tube carcinoma, and peritoneal carcinoma. In: de Vita VT, Hellman S, Rosenberg SA (eds) Cancer: principles & practice of oncology, 5th edn. Lippincott-Raven, Philadelphia, pp 1502–1539
5. National Institutes of Health Consensus Development Conference Statement (1994) Ovarian cancer: screening, treatment, and follow-up. Gynecol Oncol 55 Suppl: S4
6. Yankic R (1993) Cancer in older persons: magnitude of the problem – how do we apply what we know? Cancer 74:1995–1999
7. Schwartz PE (1981) Surgical management of ovarian cancer. Arch Surg 116:99–106
8. Anonymous (1987) Changes in definition of clinical staging for carcinoma of the cervix and ovary: International Federation of Gynecology and Obstetrics. Am J Obstet Gynecol 156:263–264
9. Holschneider CH, Berek JS (2000) Ovarian cancer: epidemiology, biology, and prognostic factors. Sem Surg Oncol 19:3–10
10. Hoskins WJ, Bundy BN, Thigpen JP, Omura GA (1992) The influence of cytoreductive surgery on recurrence-free interval and survival in small volume stage III epithelial ovarian cancer: a Gynecologic Oncology Group study. Gynecol Oncol 47:159–166
11. Nelson BE, Rosenfield AT, Schwartz PE (1993) Preoperative abdominopelvic computed tomographic prediction of optimal cytoreduction in epithelial ovarian carcinoma. J Clin Oncol 111:166–172
12. Römer W, Avril N, Dose J, Ziegler S, Kuhn W, Herz M et al (1997) Metabolic characterisation of ovarian tumors with positron emission tomography and F-18 fluorodeoxyglucose. Röfo 166:62–68
13. Zimny M, Schröder W, Wolters S, Cremerius U, Rath W, Büll U (1997) 18F-fluoro-deoxy-glucose PET in ovarian carcinoma: methodology and preliminary results. Nuklearmedizin 36:228–233
14. Fenchel S, Kotzerke J, Stöhr I, Grab D, Nussle K, Rieber A et al (1999) Preoperative assessment of asymptomatic adnexal tumors by positron emission tomography and F-18 fluorodeoxyglucose. Nuklearmedizin 38:101–107
15. Grab D, Flock F, Stöhr I, Nussle K, Rieber A, Fenchel S et al (2000) Classification of asymptomatic adnexal masses by ultrasound, magnetic resonance imaging, and positron emission tomography. Gynecol Oncol 77:454–459
16. Kubik-Huch RA, Dörffler W, von Schulthess GK, Marincek B, Kochli OR, Seifert B et al (2000) Value of (18F)-FDG positron emission tomography, computed tomography, and magnetic resonance imaging in diagnosing primary and recurrent ovarian carcinoma. Eur Radiol 10:761–767
17. Reske SN, Kotzerke J (2001) FDG-PET for clinical use Results of the 3rd German Interdisciplinary Consensus Conference "Onko-PET III", 21 July and 19 September 2000. Eur J Nucl Med 28:1707–1723
18. Rose PG, Faulhaber P, Miraldi F, Abdul-Karim FW (2001) Positron emission tomography for evaluating a complete clinical response in patients with ovarian cancer or peritoneal carcinoma: correlation with second-look laparotomy. Gynecol Oncol 82:17–21
19. Cho SM, Ha HK, Byun JY, Lee JM, Kim CJ, Nam-Koong SE, Lee JM (2002) Usefulness of FDG PET for assess

ment of early recurrent epithelial ovarian cancer. Am J Roentgenol 179:391–395

20. Takekuma M, Maeda M, Ozawa T, Yasumi K, Torizuka T (2005) Positron emission tomography with ^{18}F-fluoro-2-deoxyglucose for the detection of recurrent ovarian cancer. Int J Clin Oncol 10:177–181

21. Bristow RE, del Carmen MG, Pannu HK, Cohade C, Zahurak ML, Fishman EK, Wahl RL, Montz FJ (2003) Clinically occult recurrent ovarian cancer: patient selection for secondary cytoreductive surgery using combined PET/CT. Gynecol Oncol 90:519–528

22. Yoshida Y, Kurokawa T, Kawahara K, Tsuchida T, Okazawa H, Fujibayashi Y, Yonekura Y, Kotsuji F (2004) Incremental benefits of FDG positron emission tomography over CT alone for the preoperative staging of ovarian cancer. Am J Roentgenol 182:227–233

23. Kim S, Chung JK, Kang SB, Kim MH, Jeong JM, Lee DS, Lee MC (2004) 18F-FDG PET as a substitute for second-look laparotomy in patients with advanced ovarian carcinoma. Eur J Nucl Med Mol Imaging 31:196–201

24. Nanni C, Rubello D, Farsad M, De Iaco P, Sansovini M, Erba P, Rampin L, Mariani G, Fanti S (2005) (18)F-FDG PET/CT in the evaluation of recurrent ovarian cancer: a prospective study on forty-one patients. Eur J Surg Oncol 31:792–797

25. Pannu HK, Cohade C, Bristow RE, Fishman EK, Wahl RL (2004) PET-CT detection of abdominal recurrence of ovarian cancer: radiologic-surgical correlation. Abdom Imaging 29:398–403

26. Hauth EA, Antoch G, Stattaus J, Kuehl H, Veit P, Bockisch A, Kimmig R, Forsting M (2005) Evaluation of integrated whole-body PET/CT in the detection of recurrent ovarian cancer. Eur J Radiol 56:263–268

27. Bristow RE, Giuntoli RL 2nd, Pannu HK, Schulick RD, Fishman EK, Wahl RL (2005) Combined PET/CT for detecting recurrent ovarian cancer limited to retro-peritoneal lymph nodes. Gynecol Oncol 99:294–300

28. Simcock B, Neesham D, Quinn M, Drummond E, Milner A, Hicks RJ (2006) The impact of PET/CT in the management of recurrent ovarian cancer. Gynecol Oncol 103:271–276

29. Sironi S, Messa C, Mangili G, Zangheri B, Aletti G, Garavaglia E, Vigano R, Picchio M, Taccagni G, Maschio AD, Fazio F (2004) Integrated FDG PET/CT in patients with persistent ovarian cancer: correlation with histologic findings. Radiology 233:433–440

30. Avril N, Sassen S, Schmalfeldt B, Naehrig J, Rutke S, Weber WA, Werner M, Graeff H, Schwaiger M, Kuhn W (2005) Prediction of response to neoadjuvant chemotherapy by sequential F-18-fluorodeoxyglucose positron emission tomography in patients with advanced-stage ovarian cancer. J Clin Oncol 23:7445–7453

31. Markman M (2005) Use of positron emission tomography scans in ovarian cancer: a diagnostic technique in search of an indication. J Clin Oncol 23:7385–7387

32. Hempling RE (1996) Cervical cancer. In: Piver MS (ed) Handbook of gynecologic oncology, 2nd edn. Little, Brown, Boston1, pp 103–130

33. Wingo PA, Tong T, Bolden S (1999) Cancer statistics 1999. CA Cancer J Clin 49:8–31

34. Eifel PJ, Berek JS, Thighpen JT (1997) Cancer of the cervix, vagina and vulva. In: de Vita VT, Hellman S, Rosenberg SA (eds) Cancer: Principles & Practice of Oncology, 5th edn. Lippincott-Raven, Philadelphia, pp 1433–1478

35. International Federation of Gynecology and Obstetrics (1995) FIGO staging of gynecologic cancers: cervical and vulva. Int J Gynecol Cancer 5:319–324

36. Beck L, Smit BJ, Roth SL (1999) Gynäkologische Tumoren. Zervixkarzinom. In: Schmitt G (ed) Onkologie systematisch. UNI-MED Verlag, Bremen, pp 121–125

37. Delgado G, Bundy B, Zaino R, Sevin B, Creasman WT, Major F (1990) Prospective surgical-pathological study of disease-free interval in patients with stage IB squamous cell carcinoma of the cervix: a Gynecology Oncology Group study. Gynecol Oncol 38:352–357

38. Kamura T, Tsukamoto N, Tsuruchi N, Saito T, Matsuyama T, Akazawa K et al (1992) Multivariate analysis of the histopathologic prognostic factors of cervical cancer in patients undergoing radical hysterectomy. Cancer 69:181–186

39. Inoue T, Morita K (1990) The prognostic significance of number of positive nodes in cervical carcinoma stages IB, IIA, and IIB. Cancer 65:1923–1927

40. Scheidler J, Hricak H, Yu KK, Subak L, Segal MR (1997) Radiological evaluation of lymph-node metastases in patients with cervical cancer. JAMA 278:1091–1101

41. Keys HM, Bundy BN, Stehman FB, Muderspach LI, Chafe WE, Suggs CL 3rd et al (1999) Cisplatin, radiation, and adjuvant hysterectomy for bulky stage IB cervical carcinoma. N Engl J Med 340:1154–1161

42. Sugawara Y, Eisbruch A, Kosuda S, Recker BE, Kison PV, Wahl RL (1999) Evaluation of FDG-PET in patients with cervical cancer. J Nucl Med 40:1125–1131

43. Rose PG, Adler LP, Rodriguez M, Faulhaber PF, Abdul-Karim FW, Miraldi F (1999) Positron emission tomography for evaluating para-aortic nodal metastasis in locally advanced cervical cancer before surgical staging: a surgicopathologic study. J Clin Oncol 17:41–45

44. Umesaki N, Tanaka T, Miyama M, Kawabe J, Okamura T, Koyama K et al (2000) The role of ^{18}F-fluoro-2-deoxy-D-glucose positron emission tomography (^{18}F-FDG-PET) in the diagnosis of recurrence and lymph node metastasis of cervical cancer. Oncol Rep 7:1261–1264

45. Reinhardt MJ, Ehritt-Braun C, Vogelgesang D, Ihling C, Högerle S, Mix M, Moser E, Krause TM (2001) Metastatic lymph nodes in patients with cervical cancer: detection with MR imaging and FDG PET. Radiology 218:776–782

46. Grigsby PW, Siegel BA, Dehdashti F (2001) lymph node staging by positron emission tomography in patients with carcinoma of the cervix. J Clin Oncol 17:3745–3749

47. Kerr IG, Manji MF, Powe J, Bakheet S, Al Suhaibani H, Subhi J (2001) Positron emission tomography for the evaluation of metastases in patients with carcinoma

of the cervix: a retrospective review. Gynecol Oncol 81:477–480

48. Narayan K, Hicks RJ, Jobling T, Bernshaw D, McKenzie AF (2001) A comparison of MRI and PET scanning in surgically staged loco-regionally advanced cervical cancer: potential impact on treatment. Int J Gynecol Can 11:263–271

49. Kühnel G, Horn LC, Fischer U, Hesse S, Seese A, Georgi P, Kluge R (2001) ^{18}F-FDG positron-emission-tomography in cervical carcinoma: preliminary findings. Zbl Gynäkol 123:229–235

50. Yeh LS, Hung YC, Shen YY, Kao CH, Lin CC, Lee CC (2002) Detecting para-aortic nodal metastasis by positron emission tomography of ^{18}F-fluorodeoxyglucose in advanced cervical cancer with negative magnetic resonance imaging findings. Oncol Rep 9:1289–1292

51. Belhocine T, Thille A, Fridman V, Albert A, Seidel L, Nickers P, Kridelka F, Rigo P (2002) Contribution of whole-body [18]FDG PET imaging in the management of cervical cancer. Gynecol Oncol 87:90–97

52. Lin WC, Hung YC, Yeh LS, Kao CH, Yen RF, Shen YY (2003) Usefulness of ([18])F-fluoro-deoxyglucose positron emission tomography to detect para-aortic lymph nodal metastasis in advanced cervical cancer with negative computed tomography findings. Gynecol Oncol 89:73–76

53. Roh JW, Seo SS, Lee S, Kang KW, Kim SK, Sim JS, Kim JY, Hong EK, Cho DS, Lee JS, Park SY (2005) Role of positron emission tomography in pretreatment lymph node staging of uterine cervical cancer: a prospective surgicopathologic correlation study. Eur J Cancer 41:2086–2092

54. Wright JD, Dehdashti F, Herzog TJ, Mutch DG, Huettner PC, Rader JS, Gibb RK, Powell MA, Gao F, Siegel BA, Grigsby PW (2005) Preoperative lymph node staging of early-stage cervical carcinoma by [18F]-fluoro-2-deoxy-D-glucose-positron emission tomography. Cancer 104:2484–2491

55. Park W, Park YJ, Huh SJ, Kim BG, Bae DS, Lee J, Kim BH, Choi JY, Ahn YC, Lim do H (2005) The usefulness of MRI and PET imaging for the detection of parametrial involvement and lymph node metastasis in patients with cervical cancer. Jpn J Clin Oncol 35:260–264

56. Chou HH, Chang TC, Yen TC, Ng KK, Hsueh S, Ma SY, Chang CJ, Huang HJ, Chao A, Wu TI, Jung SM, Wu YC, Lin CT, Huang KG, Lai CH (2006) Low value of [18F]-fluoro-2-deoxy-D-glucose positron emission tomography in primary staging of early-stage cervical cancer before radical hysterectomy. J Clin Oncol 24:123–128

57. Choi HJ, Roh JW, Seo SS, Lee S, Kim JY, Kim SK, Kang KW, Lee JS, Jeong JY, Park SY (2006) Comparison of the accuracy of magnetic resonance imaging and positron emission tomography/computed tomography in the presurgical detection of lymph node metastases in patients with uterine cervical carcinoma: a prospective study. Cancer 106:914–922

58. Park DH, Kim KH, Park SY, Lee BH, Choi CW, Chin SY (2000) Diagnosis of recurrent uterine cervical cancer: computed tomography versus positron emission tomography. Korean J Radiol 1:51–55

59. Sun SS, Chen TC, Yen RF, Shen YY, Changlai SP, Kao A (2001) Value of whole body ^{18}F-fluoro-2-deoxyglucose positron emission tomography in the evaluation of recurrent cervical cancer. Antican Res 21:2957–2961

60. Nakamoto Y, Eisbruch A, Achtyes ED, Sugawara Y, Reynolds KR, Johnston CM, Wahl RL (2002) Prognostic value of positron emission tomography using F-18-fluorodeoxy-glucose in patients with cervical cancer undergoing radiotherapy. Gynecol Oncol 84:289–295

61. Havrilesky LJ, Wong TZ, Secord AA, Berchuck A, Clarke-Pearson DL, Jones EL (2003) The role of PET scanning in the detection of recurrent cervical cancer. Gynecol Oncol 90:186–190

62. Ryu SY, Kim MH, Choi SC, Choi CW, Lee KH (2003) Detection of early recurrence with ^{18}F-FDG PET in patients with cervical cancer. J Nucl Med 44:347–352

63. Lai CH, Huang KG, See LC, Yen TC, Tsai CS, Chang TC, Chou HH, Ng KK, Hsueh S, Hong JH (2004) Restaging of recurrent cervical carcinoma with dual-phase [18F]fluoro-2-deoxy-D-glucose positron emission tomography. Cancer 100:544–552

64. Wong TZ, Jones EL, Coleman RE (2004) Positron emission tomography with 2-deoxy-2-[([18])F]fluoro-D-glucose for evaluating local and distant disease in patients with cervical cancer. Mol Imaging Biol 6:55–62

65. Yen TC, See LC, Chang TC, Huang KG, Ng KK, Tang SG, Chang YC, Hsueh S, Tsai CS, Hong JH, Lin CT, Chao A, Ma SY, Lin WJ, Fu YK, Fan CC, Lai CH (2004) Defining the priority of using ^{18}F-FDG PET for recurrent cervical cancer. J Nucl Med 45:1632–1639

66. Chung HH, Kim SK, Kim TH, Lee S, Kang KW, Kim JY, Park SY (2006) Clinical impact of FDG-PET imaging in post-therapy surveillance of uterine cervical cancer: from diagnosis to prognosis. Gynecol Oncol 103:165–170

67. Grigsby PW, Siegel BA, Dehdashti F, Rader J, Zoberi I (2004) Posttherapy [18F] fluorodeoxy-glucose positron emission tomography in carcinoma of the cervix: response and outcome. J Clin Oncol 22:2167–2171

68. Olaitan A, Murdoch J, Anderson R, James J, Graham J, Barley V (2001) A critical evaluation of current protocols for the follow-up of women treated for gynecological malignancies: a pilot study. Int J Gynecol Cancer 11:349–353

69. Amit A, Beck D, Lowenstein L, Lavie O, Bar Shalom R, Kedar Z, Israel O (2006) The role of hybrid PET/CT in the evaluation of patients with cervical cancer. Gynecol Oncol 100:65–69

70. Sironi S, Buda A, Picchio M, Perego P, Moreni R, Pellegrino A, Colombo M, Mangioni C, Messa C, Fazio F (2006) Lymph node metastasis in patients with clinical early-stage cervical cancer: detection with integrated FDG PET/CT. Radiology 238:272–279

12 Cutaneous Melanoma

M. J. Reinhardt

Recent Results in Cancer Research, Vol. 170
© Springer-Verlag Berlin Heidelberg 2008

12.1 Introduction

The incidence of malignant melanoma is increasing dramatically in people with light-colored skin in all parts of the world [1]. In 2004, an estimated 55,000 Americans were diagnosed with cutaneous melanoma, and 7,900 died from the disease [2]. Melanoma prognosis is linked to the stage at diagnosis. Fortunately, most new patients are diagnosed early in the clinical course of disease, when it can be cured with excision of the primary tumor and sentinel lymphadenectomy. Histologic confirmation of diagnosis and microstaging with an accurate tumor thickness are essential before embarking on treatment [3, 4]. Invasive primary melanomas to a depth of 2.0 mm or less without ulceration and negative nodal metastases are essentially curable, whereas melanomas of increasing depth become progressively less curable [4, 5]. Thus, the relationship between tumor thickness and 10-year survival rates is pivotal [5]. Once a melanoma has acquired the ability to invade tissues, to continue to proliferate, and to escape immune recognition, metastatic spread is possible. Thus, accurate staging is essential to implement appropriate management and to improve prognosis. Substantial progress has been made in identifying the most significant clinical and histological criteria that predict melanoma metastasis and survival [4]. In 2001, the American Joint Committee on Cancer (AJCC) introduced a revised staging system for malignant melanoma based on the

analysis of prognostic factors in 17,600 melanoma patients with complete clinical, pathologic, and follow-up information [4, 5]. Clinical staging includes microstaging of the primary melanoma and clinical/radiological evaluation for metastases. In addition to clinical staging, pathologic staging includes pathologic information about the regional lymph nodes after selective sentinel or complete lymphadenectomy. Melanoma patients without evidence for regional or distant metastases are assigned to two stages: stage I refers to early-stage patients at low risk and stage II refers to patients with intermediate risk for metastases and mortality [5]. Patients with regional metastases, i.e., regional lymph nodes, cutaneous satellites and in-transit metastases belong to stage III melanoma, and patients with distant metastases, i.e., distant metastases to skin, subcutaneous tissues, or distant lymph nodes, metastases to the lungs and to other organs are considered as stage IV melanoma [5]. The mean 10-year survival rates for stage I were 79%–88%, for stage IIA and IIB they were 51%–64%, for stage IIC (primary tumor larger than 4.0 mm in depth without local and distant metastases) it was 32%, for stage IIIA they were 57%–63%, for stage IIIB and IIIC they were 15%–48%, and for stage IV 3%–16% depending on the number of nodal metastases and/or the site of distant metastases [5].

Cutaneous melanoma and its metastases usually present with a high uptake of the glucose analog 2-[F-18]-fluoro-2-deoxy-D-glucose (FDG) [6, 7]. This high FDG uptake suggests the frequent use of functional imaging with whole-body positron emission tomography (PET) [8, 9]. Unfortunately, FDG-PET has shown a limited sensitivity for initial regional staging, especially in AJCC stage I and II disease because sentinel node biopsy is much more sensitive in detecting microscopic lymph node metastases [10, 11]. However, FDG-PET performance significantly improved for regional staging of AJCC stage III and stage IV disease with a positive predictive value of up to 90%, and for detection and differentiation of distant metastases [9, 11]. Thus, the Centers for Medicare and Medicaid Services (CMS) decided in July 2001 to cover FDG-PET studies for diagnosis, staging, and restaging of malignant melanoma with the exception of evaluation of regional nodes (http://www.cms.hhs.gov/manuals/downloads/Pub06_PART_50.pdf).

The latest development in the field of diagnostic imaging is the combination of functional and morphological cross-sectional imaging using FDG-PET and computed tomography (CT). The new dual-modality FDG-PET/CT is assumed to provide superior performance in overall TNM staging of various oncologic diseases and to be significantly more accurate than CT alone and/or PET alone [12, 13]. This chapter presents the results of FDG-PET and FDG-PET/CT with respect to the current management of patients with malignant melanoma.

12.2 Diagnostic Accuracy of FDG-PET in Cutaneous Melanoma

A meta-analysis in 2001 analyzed the diagnostic accuracy of FDG-PET reported in eight prospective and in three retrospective studies with 517 melanoma patients until 1999 considering the level of evidence as recommended by the Centre for Evidence Based Medicine of the National Health Service Research and Development (http://cebm.jr2.ox.ac.uk/docs/levels/html) [11]. The pooled sensitivity and specificity of FDG-PET for detection of mela-

noma metastases were 79% and 86%, respectively [11]. The pooled diagnostic odds ratio of 33.1 suggested a high diagnostic accuracy for PET, which was higher for systemic staging than for regional staging (36.4 vs 19.5) [11]. Another meta-analysis investigating FDG-PET for detection of recurrent melanoma reported an overall sensitivity and specificity of 92% and 90%, respectively [14]. This study also suggested a change in patient management directed by FDG-PET in 22% of all cases [14].

A significant problem of FDG-PET was the low sensitivity for detection of lymph node metastases in stage I and stage II disease [15–18]. Several studies compared the results of sentinel node biopsy with that of whole-body FDG-PET for primary staging of melanoma [15–18]. All studies but one included AJCC stage I and II patients and observed FDG-PET to be an insensitive indicator of occult regional lymph node metastases [16–18]. The better results of FDG-PET in the other study may be a result of higher tumor masses, because 60% of patients in this study were AJCC stage III [15]. Thus, the average sensitivity of FDG-PET for subclinical nodal disease in stage I and II melanoma was 14%–17%, whereas sentinel node biopsy reached 86%–94% in sensitivity [15–18]. As a consequence, FDG-PET was not recommended for staging regional lymph nodes in melanoma patients with AJCC stage I and stage II disease [11].

The results of FDG-PET in AJCC stage III and stage IV disease were quite different to that obtained in stage I and stage II disease. The higher tumor burden in these higher stages was more likely to be detected by means of FDG-PET [16]. In a prospective study of 106 PET scans in 95 melanoma patients with AJCC stage III regional disease, a sensitivity of 87% and a positive predictive value (PPV) of 90% were observed when pertinent clinical information was used to reduce the number of false-positive PET findings [19]. More importantly, it was shown that unexpected findings on PET imaging resulted in a change in management in 15% of patients, including the detection of distant metastases [19]. A prospective study compared performance of PET for detection of distant metastases to that of conventional imaging including CT and/or MRI in 18 patients with AJCC stage IV melanoma scheduled for metastasectomy [20]. The authors reported a comparable sensitivity for FDG-PET and conventional imaging of 79% and 76% and the same PPV of 86%, which could be increased to 88% sensitivity and 91% PPV with side-by-side reading of PET and CT [20]. The detection rate of FDG-PET for nodal metastases was size-dependent: in a series of 114 histologically proven lymph node metastases, FDG-PET detected only 23% of lymph node metastases up to 5 mm in diameter, but 83% of lymph node metastases between 6 and 10 mm in diameter, whereas lymph-node metastases larger than 10 mm were always seen [21]. In this study, only lymph nodes with more than 50% metastatic involvement were detected, with a high sensitivity of 93% [21].

In general, FDG-PET appeared to be more accurate for detection of distant metastases than for the detection of regional metastatic nodes [11]. Mijnhout and co-workers reported a diagnostic odds ratio of 36.4 for systemic staging but only 19.5 for regional staging [11]. Several studies reported the overall sensitivity of FDG-PET for detection of visceral metastases as 80%–100% [22–26]. Whereas metastases to the bones and the liver could be detected with a very high accuracy, the detection rate of pulmonary metastases with FDG-PET did not exceed 70% due to blurring caused mainly by respiratory movement [10, 22]. For detection of pulmonary metastases, the complementary use of CT was recommended [27]. Paquet and co-workers suggested that FDG-PET and CT should be regarded as complementary rather than competing imaging modalities for staging of melanoma patients [25].

It has further been assumed that FDG-PET should be considered as the first-line imaging procedure for recurrent disease because it had a higher sensitivity and specificity than CT in three series including 84, 104, and 156 melanoma patients, respectively [26, 28, 29]. These three studies reported sensitivities for FDG-PET and CT of 74%–85% and 58%–81%, respectively, and the specificities for PET and CT were 86%–97% and 45%–87%, respectively [26, 28, 29]. Despite all these promising data, a sys-

tematic review of the PET literature until 1999 concluded that guidelines for the effective use of FDG-PET in melanoma patients could not be developed because most of the available studies reached only a low level of evidence [11].

12.3 Diagnostic Accuracy of FDG-PET/CT in Cutaneous Melanoma

A more recent study from Reinhardt and co-workers reported a significant increase in sensitivity and accuracy for M-stage assessment of 250 consecutive melanoma patients following image fusion with PET/CT in comparison to FDG-PET alone and CT alone [30]. The sensitivity and accuracy increased from 73.4% and 83.5% for CT to 89.0% and 93.2% for FDG-PET and to 98.8% and 98.0% for PET/CT, respectively. PET/CT was further significantly more specific and accurate than CT alone but not than PET alone for N-stage assessment (100% and 98.4% vs 87.2% and 86.3% and vs 97.6% and 96.0%, respectively). Thus, the most significant advantage of combined PET/CT imaging in comparison to the single modalities was an improved detection and differentiation of distant metastases, especially of visceral metastases [30]. An example for improved detection and differentiation of distant nodal metastases by means of PET/CT is shown in Figure 12.1. Specificity of PET significantly improved following image fusion with CT from 90% to 97% for distant lymph node metastases and from 88% to 95% for visceral metastases. An example of improved specificity by means of fused imaging with PET/CT is shown in Figure 12.2. Furthermore, the accurate anatomical correlation of areas of increased FDG-uptake led to a significant reduction of false-positive and false-negative findings [30]. A similar observation was made for PET/CT imaging of tumors other than cutaneous melanoma [13]. It may be assumed that the complementary information from CT imaging to FDG-PET imaging can hardly be overestimated.

In the study from Reinhardt et al., FDG-PET alone provided the same high sensitivity

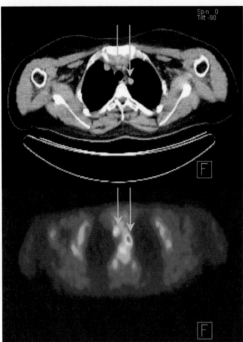
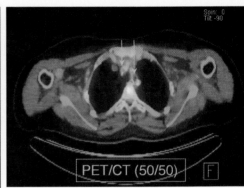

Fig. 12.1a,b. Female patient, 28 years old, nodular melanoma 0.8 mm deep on the left neck, primary staging. CT: two lymph nodes in the mediastinum (1.0–1.2 cm ∅). PET: two foci in the mediastinum (SUV 4.0 and 5.7). Conclusion: PET/CT enabled assignment of hypermetabolic foci to morphologically unsuspicious lymph nodes

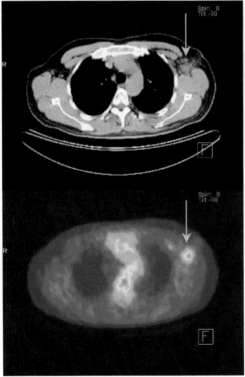
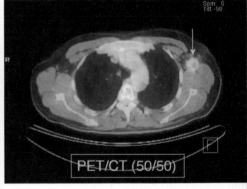

Fig. 12.2a,b. Male patient, 48 years old, superficial spreading melanoma 2.3 mm deep on the left back, staging after primary surgery. CT: hematoma in the left axilla. PET: hypermetabolic focus in the left axilla (SUV 2.9). Conclusion: PET/CT enabled assignment of hypermetabolic focus to a benign hematoma, confirmed during follow-up

as PET/CT for detection of distant lymph node metastases and metastases to all other organs but the lungs [30]. Pulmonary metastases could be detected with a sensitivity of 100% compared to 93.8% by CT (not significant) and to 65.6% by FDG-PET (p < 0.0005) [30].

The usefulness of combined PET/CT imaging for assessment of pulmonary metastases from different malignancies including melanoma was recently evaluated in a series of 92 patients with 438 metastases to the lungs of different primary tumors including malignant melanoma [31]. FDG-PET performed as a part of PET/CT imaging detected only 39.7% of all lung metastases [31]. In this study, only pulmonary metastases greater than 10 mm in diameter were detected by FDG-PET with a high sensitivity of 93.5%, but sensitivity fell rapidly below that nodule size [31].

A few years ago, a clear volume dependency of FDG-PET for detection of lymph node metastases was reported with a reliable detection of tumor deposits of approximately 80 mm3 volume and more [32]. This amount of tumor is most likely to occur in melanoma patients with AJCC stages III and IV. Because axial and transaxial spatial resolution of the current generation PET in PET/CT scanners is approximately 6–7 mm according to National Electrical Manufactures Association standards, the detection limit of lymph-node metastases may be further reduced to that size [33]. However, the use of PET/CT for smaller metastases must await further technological refinements.

Whether the use of intravenous contrast medium for CT imaging performed as a part of a PET/CT study would increase the detection rate of nodal disease, particularly in AJCC stage I and stage II melanoma patients, has not been studied so far [30]. Nonetheless, it has been shown that contrast-enhanced CT performed in addition to a PET/CT study with oral contrast only was of limited value in Hodgkin's and non-Hodgkin's lymphoma patients [34].

From the referring physician's perspective, the use of FDG-PET resulted in a change of intermodality management in 29% and in a change of intramodality management in 18% of melanoma patients, i.e., an overall treatment change in 47% of all cases [35]. A recent retro-spective analysis reported an impact of FDG-PET on the clinical decision-making process in 34% of 126 melanoma patients with stage III or IV disease [36]. This study used a rigorous approach to impact on clinical management such that the FDG-PET results were not considered to have affected decision making if they confirmed the CT or clinical impression of multiple metastases or of no active disease [36]. FDG-PET/CT resulted in an overall treatment change in 48.4% of melanoma patients [30]. The frequency of intermodality management change following FDG-PET/CT imaging was 40.4%, which was higher than that reported of FDG-PET alone [30, 35, 36].

The most interesting question for the near future would be whether whole-body MRI could replace FDG-PET/CT for that purpose. Preliminary results in 25 patients with AJCC stage III and stage IV melanoma suggested a higher sensitivity and specificity of FDG-PET/CT compared to whole-body MRI for detection of metastatic disease (94% and 83% vs 79% and 43%, respectively) [36]. In this abstract, 96% of 48 metastatic lymph node sites were detected with PET/CT and 89% were detected with MRI [36].

As a consequence, the superior diagnostic performance of FDG-PET/CT for N- and M-staging of melanoma patients suggests its use for whole-body tumor staging, especially for detection or exclusion of distant metastases.

References

1. Thompson JF, Scolyer RA, Kefford RF (2005) Cutaneous melanoma. Lancet 365:687–701
2. Jemal A, Tiwari RC, Murray T et al (2004) American Cancer Society. Cancer statistics, 2004. Ca: a Cancer Journal for Clinicians 54:8–29
3. Breslow A (1970) Thickness, cross-sectional areas and depth of invasion in the prognosis of cutaneous melanoma. Ann Surg 172:902–908
4. Balch CM, Soong SJ, Gershenwald JE et al (2001) Prognostic factors analysis of 17,600 melanoma patients: validation of the American Joint Committee on Cancer melanoma staging system. J Clin Oncol 19:3622–3634
5. Balch CM, Buzaid AC, Soong SJ et al (2001) Final version of the American Joint Committee on Cancer

staging system for cutaneous melanoma. J Clin Oncol 19:3635–3648

6. Kern KA (1991) [^{14}C]deoxyglucose uptake and imaging in malignant melanoma. J Surg Res 50:643–647

7. Wahl RL, Hutchins GD, Buchsbaum DJ et al (1991) ^{18}F-2-deoxy-2-fluoro-D-glucose uptake into human tumor xenografts. Feasibility studies for cancer imaging with positron-emission tomography. Cancer 67:1544–1550

8. Gambhir SS, Czernin J, Schwimmer J et al (2001) A tabulated summary of the FDG PET literature. J Nucl Med 42 Suppl:1S–93S

9. Friedman KP, Wahl RL (2004) Clinical use of positron emission tomography in the management of cutaneous melanoma. Sem Nucl Med 34:242–253

10. Prichard RS, Hill AD, Skehan SJ, O'Higgins NJ (2002) Positron emission tomography for staging and management of malignant melanoma. Br J Surg 89:389–396

11. Mijnhout GS, Hoekstra OS, van Tulder MW et al (2001) Systematic review of the diagnostic accuracy of (^{18})F-fluorodeoxyglucose positron emission tomography in melanoma patients. Cancer 91:1530–1542

12. Antoch G, Vogt FM, Freudenberg LS et al (2003) Whole-body dual-modality PET/CT and whole-body MRI for tumor staging in oncology. JAMA 290:3199–3206

13. Antoch G, Saoudi N, Kuehl H et al (2004) Accuracy of whole-body dual-modality fluorine-18-2-fluoro-2-deoxy-D-glucose positron emission tomography and computed tomography (FDG-PET/CT) for tumor staging in solid tumors: comparison with CT and PET. J Clin Oncol 22:4357–4368

14. Schwimmer J, Essner R, Patel A et al (2000) A review of the literature for whole-body FDG-PET in the management of patients with melanoma. Q J Nucl Med 4:153–167

15. Macfarlane DJ, Sondak V, Johnson T, Wahl RL (1998) Prospective evaluation of 2-[^{18}F]-2-deoxy-D-glucose positron emission tomography in staging of regional lymph nodes in patients with cutaneous malignant melanoma. J Clin Oncol 16:1770–1776

16. Wagner JD, Schauwecker D, Davidson D et al (1999) Prospective study of fluorodeoxyglucose-positron emission tomography imaging of lymph node basins in melanoma patients undergoing sentinel node biopsy. J Clin Oncol 17:1508–1515

17. Belhocine T, Pierard G, De Labrassinne M et al (2002) Staging of regional nodes in AJCC stage I and II melanoma: ^{18}FDG PET imaging versus sentinel node detection. Oncologist 7:271–278

18. Havenga K, Cobben DC, Oyen WJ et al (2003) Fluorodeoxyglucose-positron emission tomography and sentinel lymph node biopsy in staging primary cutaneous melanoma. Eur J Surg Oncol 29:662–664

19. Tyler DS, Onaitis M, Kherani A et al (2000) Positron emission tomography scanning in malignant melanoma. Cancer 89:1019–1025

20. Finkelstein SE, Carrasquillo JA, Hoffman JM et al (2004) A prospective analysis of positron emission tomography and conventional imaging for detection of stage IV metastatic melanoma in patients undergoing metastasectomy. Ann Surg Oncol 11:731–738

21. Crippa F, Leutner M, Belli F et al (2000) Which kind of lymph node metastases can FDG PET detect? A clinical study in melanoma. J Nucl Med 41:1491–1494

22. Rinne D, Baum RP, Hör G, Kaufmann R (1998) Primary staging and follow-up of high risk melanoma patients with whole-body ^{18}F-fluorodeoxyglucose positron emission tomography: results of a prospective study of 100 patients. Cancer 82:1664–1671

23. Holder WD Jr, White RL Jr, Zuger JH, Easton EJ Jr, Greene FL (1998) Effectiveness of positron emission tomography for the detection of melanoma metastases. Ann Surg 227:764–769

24. Eigtved A, Andersson AP, Dahlstrom K et al (2000) Use of fluorine-18 fluorodeoxyglucose positron emission tomography in the detection of silent metastases from malignant melanoma. Eur J Nucl Med 27:70–75

25. Paquet P, Henry F, Belhocine T et al (2000) An appraisal of ^{18}fluorodeoxyglucose positron emission tomography for melanoma staging. Dermatology 200:167–169

26. Swetter SM, Carroll LA, Johnson DL, Segall GM (2002) Positron emission tomography is superior to computed tomography for metastatic detection in melanoma patients. Ann Surg Oncol 9:646–653

27. Krug B, Dietlein M, Groth W et al (2000) Fluor-18-fluorodeoxyglucose positron emission tomography (FDG-PET) in malignant melanoma. Diagnostic comparison with conventional imaging methods. Acta Radiol 41:446–452

28. Stas M, Stroobants S, Dupont P et al (2002) ^{18}FDG PET scan in the staging of recurrent melanoma: additional value and therapeutic impact. Melanoma Res 12:479–490

29. Fuster D, Chiang S, Johnson G et al (2004) Is ^{18}F-FDG PET more accurate than standard diagnostic procedures in the detection of suspected recurrent melanoma? J Nucl Med 45:1323–1327

30. Reinhardt MJ, Joe AY, Jaeger U et al (2006) Diagnostic performance of whole body dual modality ^{18}F-FDG PET/CT imaging for N- and M-staging of malignant melanoma: experience with 250 consecutive patients. J Clin Oncol 24:1178–1187

31. Reinhardt MJ, Wiethoelter N, Matthies A et al (2006) PET recognition of pulmonary metastases on PET/CT imaging: impact of attenuation-corrected and non-attenuation corrected PET images. Eur J Nucl Med Mol Imaging 33:134–139

32. Wagner JD, Schauwecker DS, Davidson D et al (2001) FDG-PET sensitivity for melanoma lymph node metastases is dependent on tumor volume. J Surg Oncol 77:237–242

33. Beyer T, Townsend DW, Brun T et al (2000) A combined PET/CT scanner for clinical oncology. J Nucl Med 41:1369–1379

34. Schaefer NG, Hany TF, Taverna C et al (2004) Non-Hodgkin lymphoma and Hodgkin's disease: coregistered FDG PET and CT at staging and restaging – do we need contrast-enhanced CT? Radiology 232:823–829

35. Wong C, Silverman DH, Seltzer M et al (2002) The impact of 2-deoxy-2[^{18}F] fluoro-D-glucose whole body positron emission tomography for managing patients with melanoma: the referring physician's perspective. Mol Imaging Biol 4:185–190

36. Harris MT, Berlangieri SU, Cebon JS, Davis ID, Scott AM (2005) Impact of 2-deoxy-2[^{18}F] fluoro-D-glucose positron emission tomography on the management of patients with advanced melanoma. Mol Imaging Biol 7:304–308

37. Eschmann SM, Pfannenberg AC, Plathow C et al (2006) Vergleich von FDG-Ganzkörper-PET/CT und Ganzkörper-MRT in der Ausbreitungsdiagnostik bei Patienten mit fortgeschrittenem Melanom. Nuklearmedizin 45:A7

13 Value of PET and PET/CT in the Diagnostics of Prostate and Penile Cancer

B. Scher, M. Seitz, W. Albinger, M. Reiser, B. Schlenker, Ch. Stief, U. Mueller-Lisse, and S. Dresel

Recent Results in Cancer Research, Vol. 170
© Springer-Verlag Berlin Heidelberg 2008

13.1 Value of PET and PET/CT in the Diagnostics of Prostate Cancer

13.1.1 Introduction

Prostate cancer accounts for the most frequent cancer in the elderly man and is one of the most common causes of cancer-related death in Europe and the USA (Sarma and Schottenfeld 2002). An annual urological screening is generally recommended for male patients aged 45 years or older. A 50-year-old man with a 25-year life expectancy has a 42% risk of developing microscopic prostate cancer, a 9.5% risk of developing clinically evident prostate cancer, and a 3% risk of dying from this malignancy (Scardino 1989). The vast majority of prostate carcinomas originate in the peripheral portion (70%–80%) of the prostate gland and are frequently multifocal in appearance. Conventional diagnostic work-up of patients with suspected prostate cancer consists of digital rectal examination (DRE), assessment of the serum prostate specific antigen (PSA), and transrectal ultrasound (TRUS). The use of PSA as a screening method combined with the increasing public awareness of prostate cancer as a malignant entity with high prevalence, has resulted in an increased detection rate. Therefore, PSA screening complemented by DRE are considered valuable first-line methods for selecting patients at risk of having prostate cancer.

Once suspicion of prostate cancer arises, histologic evaluation is mandatory. However, it is known that the accuracy of transrectal biopsy may yield unsatisfactory results. In this respect, Wefer et al. found that the accuracy of biopsy depends on the location of the primary carcinoma and is comparatively low when the malignant process is located in the prostate apex (Wefer et al. 2000). Therefore, in case of rising PSA levels but repeated negative biopsies, patients find themselves in a diagnostic dilemma. Presumably, imaging procedures with high diagnostic accuracy in the detection of prostate cancer lesions would be of value in these patients.

13.1.2 Radiologic Imaging Modalities

Because prostate cancer varies widely with regard to the rate of growth, its aggressiveness, and the tendency to metastasize, and because benign hyperplasia of the prostate (BPH) also has a high incidence, proper diagnostic work-up of patients with suspected prostate cancer is of high relevance. Transrectal ultrasound (TRUS) as a ubiquitous imaging modality has to be considered the front-line diagnostic imaging procedure in patients with suspected prostate cancer or patients with suspected local recurrence of prostate cancer. Generally, TRUS is performed by the urologist and offers as a real-time procedure the possibility of guiding biopsies in addition to providing morphologic information of the prostate gland. Not surprisingly, TRUS is the most commonly used imaging procedure. However, the diagnostic efficacy of this imaging technique has its limitations, with sensitivities in detecting prostate cancer in the range of 17%–57% and specificities in the range of 40%–63%. Regarding the detection of extracapsular extension and seminal vesicle invasion, the accuracy of TRUS ranges from 58% to 86% (Cornud et al. 1997; Halpern et al. 2000; Heuck et al. 2003; Wijkstra et al. 2004; Wilkinson and Hamdy 2001). Interestingly, recent multicenter studies conducted on large groups of 386 and 558 patients showed no clinically relevant superiority of TRUS when compared to DRE (Liebross et al. 1999; Smith et al. 1997).

Conventional radiologic imaging modalities such as computed tomography (CT) and magnetic resonance imaging (MRI) have been in use for imaging prostate cancer. While CT has a broader availability, MRI provides superior soft-tissue contrast and is therefore generally favored. MRI has high accuracy in distinguishing tissues of different chemical composition. This is particularly the case when T2-weighted sequences are used. Therefore, T2-weighted sequences are most frequently utilized in the search for prostate cancer foci. When located in the peripheral zone, prostate cancer can frequently be demarcated by revealing lower signal intensity than normal surrounding tissue (Engelbrecht et al. 2002; Heuck et al. 2003; Mueller-Lisse et al. 2005). However, the detection of prostate cancer in the central portion of the prostate gland is much more difficult, because here the surrounding parenchyma also displays a low signal in T2-weighted sequences. As has been shown in a meta-analysis, an important factor in increasing the diagnostic efficacy of MRI is the use of an endorectal coil (Engelbrecht et al. 2002). This approach, however, contributes to a complex and time-consuming patient preparation and an increase in examination costs. In contrast to T2-weighted images, T1-weighted sequences are better suited for revealing intraprostatic hemorrhage or detecting metastatic spread to lymph nodes or osseous lesions in the pelvis. In addition, the use of gadolinium-enhanced contrast media may help to visualize prostate cancer foci in T1-weighted images.

An intrinsic shortcoming of imaging modalities primarily relying on morphologic criteria, is the limited ability to differentiate between benign and malignant changes with high diagnostic assertiveness. A reason for this is that visible anatomic changes are not always present in early tumor stages. As is the case for several other malignant entities, it is known that prostate cancer cells exhibit certain metabolic changes. Proton magnetic resonance spectroscopy (MRS) is capable of assessing metabolic changes typical for prostate cancer by providing information on the citrate, creatine, and choline metabolism. As prostate cancer exhibits an increased citrate utilization for energy generation, citrate concentration in tumor tissue is lower than in normal tissue. On the other hand, choline, as a cell membrane phospholipid, has a higher concentration in prostate cancer tissue, reflecting an increased proliferation rate. By means of certain MRS spectra, representing the relative concentration of choline, creatine, and citrate in predefined volume elements inside the prostate gland, it is possible to detect prostate cancer foci by using this metabolic information (Costello et al. 1999; Heerschap et al. 1997; Kurhanewicz et al. 1996a; Mueller-Lisse et al. 2001a). However this novel diagnostic approach is limited to the evaluation of the peripheral zone of the prostate, but not the central and transitional zones. Another limitation of this procedure must be considered: the problems discriminating malignant foci from benign prostatic diseases such as BPH (Kurhanewicz et al. 1996b) Furthermore, previously performed therapeutic procedures, such as hormone therapy or intraprostatic bleeding due to recent biopsy can lead to a significant reduction in the ability to detect prostate cancer by means of both MR and MRS (Qayyum et al. 2004).

A methodical advantage of MRI combined with MRS is the capability to visualize extracapsular tumor growth because of its excellent soft tissue contrast. According to preliminary publications, particularly with the use of endorectal coils, MRI provides sensitivities and specificities in the range of 80%–90% in the evaluation of extracapsular tumor growth (Engelbrecht et al. 2002; Heuck et al. 2003)

Furthermore, recent studies show that MRI complemented by MRS is capable of identifying prostate cancer foci in patients with elevated PSA but previously negative biopsy Amsellem-Ouazana et al. 2005; Beyersdorff et al. 2002; Yuen et al. 2004). Other fields of investigation are the potential usefulness of MRI/MRS for treatment planning and localization of local recurrence or metastatic spread (Coakley et al. 2004; DiBiase et al. 2002; Huisman et al. 2005; Kurhanewicz et al. 1996b; Menard et al. 2001; Mueller-Lisse et al. 2001a, 2001b; Parivar et al. 1996).

3.1.3 Positron Emission Tomography

The complementary use of imaging procedures that provide functional information such as single photon emission computed tomography (SPECT), positron emission tomography (PET), and MRS helps to differentiate benign from malignant processes. In the mid-1990s, SPECT utilizing the monoclonal antibody capromab pendetide (Prostascint (R)), which targets the prostate-specific membrane antigen, was investigated in several studies (Hinkle et al. 1998; Sodee et al. 2000). While this procedure has shown some promising results regarding certain indications, it could not be transferred into routine clinical use. An intrinsic shortcoming of SPECT is its inferior overall image quality in comparison to PET.

In much the same way as MRS, PET allows noninvasive assessment of metabolic processes in normal and diseased tissue. PET as functional procedure has been shown to be in principle suitable for the detection of malignant processes with high diagnostic accuracy by providing information on tumor metabolism. Among the many radiotracers in use, the most common is the glucose analog ^{18}F-fluorodeoxyglucose (^{18}F-FDG). Accumulation of ^{18}F-FDG correlates with proliferate activity and can be therefore used to visualize malignant tissue (Okada et al. 1992). Unfortunately, even though ^{18}F-FDG uptake of prostate cancer correlates with the Gleason score, PSA level and PSA velocity (Agus et al. 1998; Effert et al. 1996; Oyama et al. 2002; Seltzer et al. 1999),

this radiotracer has limited suitability for the diagnosis of prostate cancer. Prostate carcinomas show rather discrete ^{18}F-FDG uptake in comparison to other, more aggressively proliferating malignant entities (Hara et al. 1998; Heicappell et al. 1999; Inaba 1992; Oyama et al. 1999). The low rate of glucose metabolism typical for prostate cancer can be primarily attributed to the generally slow growth rate of this malignant tumor. In only a few cases did ^{18}F-FDG reveal sufficiently high sensitivity for the detection of prostate cancer lesions. This is particularly true for prostate carcinomas with high histologic grade, high clinical stage, or in malignancies accompanied by high PSA levels (Seltzer et al. 1999). However, a sensitivity in the detection of prostate cancer in the range of 60%–70%, as reported in previous studies, does not warrant its routine clinical use (Seltzer et al. 1999). At present, there are several innovative PET radiotracers which seem to be promising for the detection of prostate cancer.

13.1.4 PET Radiotracers for Imaging Prostate Cancer

13.1.4.1 ^{11}C-Choline

One of the most widely investigated substances among the variety of novel PET radiotracers available to image prostate cancer is radiolabeled choline. MRS has demonstrated that a characteristic of prostate cancer is an increased choline uptake (Ackerstaff et al. 2001). Hara et al. (1998) showed that prostate cancer tissue is characterized by an increased amount of intracellular choline metabolism to meet the high demand for phosphatidylcholine, an elementary cell membrane component. Choline is a substrate for the synthesis of phosphatidylcholine and is integrated at the end of its metabolic pathway into cell membrane phospholipids. High proliferative activity of malignant cell membrane components leads to a significantly increased intracellular uptake of ^{11}C-choline in prostate cancer tissue. As a consequence, increased accumulation of ^{11}C-choline indicates the integration of this radiotracer into the cell membrane. Therefore, ^{11}C-choline uptake reflects the proliferate activity of cell membrane components (Hara et al. 1997). In 1997, Hara et al. successfully visualized brain tumors by utilizing ^{11}C-choline PET (Hara et al. 1997). Subsequently, they used this radiotracer to image a variety of malignant entities. In 1998, Hara et al. used ^{11}C-choline for the visualization of prostate carcinomas with PET. By investigating a group of ten prostate cancer patients, they revealed that ^{11}C-choline uptake of malignant prostatic tissue was generally intense and significantly higher than the uptake of ^{18}F-FDG (Hara et al. 1998). In this pilot study, ^{11}C-choline PET was successfully utilized for the detection of the primary malignancy as well as for the localization of bone and lymph node metastases. They also found that ^{11}C-choline PET had a higher sensitivity in detecting bone metastases than bone scintigraphy. Interestingly, in a consecutive study Breeuwsma et al. found that the in vivo uptake of ^{11}C-choline in prostate cancer tissue does not correlate with the amount of proliferating cells (Breeuwsma et al. 2005). With regard to the diagnosis of prostate cancer, ^{11}C-choline has to be considered superior to ^{18}F-FDG. A further advantage of ^{11}C-choline is its comparatively low urinary excretion compared to ^{18}F-FDG, providing improved evaluation of pelvic structures.

13.1.4.2 ^{18}F-Choline

[18]F-labeled tracers are in general more convenient for routine diagnostic procedures because of the comparatively great half-decay time, which is 110 min. In contrast, the half-decay time of ^{11}C is approximately 20 min. In 2000, Coleman et al. (2000) evaluated in a pilot study the use of ^{18}F-labeled choline (^{18}F-choline) and found encouraging results for the evaluation of metastatic prostate cancer. DeGrado et al. (2001) confirmed these findings and reported, that ^{18}F-labeled choline may be useful for the detection and localization of prostate cancer. Hara et al. (2002) demonstrated that ^{18}F-choline, equivalent to normal choline, is incorporated into tumor cells by an active transport mechanism. Following that, it is phosphorylated intracellularly, and integrated into phospholipids. In addition, no significant differences between ^{18}F-choline and ^{11}C-choline regarding the pattern of tracer uptake in malignant lesions were found. A shortcoming of ^{18}F-labeled choline analogs is the high urinary bladder activity when compared to ^{11}C choline.

13.1.4.3 ^{11}C-Acetate

In cardiac diagnostics, ^{11}C-acetate has been utilized as a radiotracer for visualizing the myocardial oxidative metabolism. ^{11}C-acetate was first introduced for cancer imaging by Shreve et. al in the mid-1990s (Shreve et al 1995; Shreve and Gross 1997). The exact pathway of acetate metabolism in cancerous tissue is still unclear; however, there is consensus that accelerated lipid synthesis plays a principle role (Swinnen et al. 2003; Yoshimoto et al. 2001). Therefore, similarly to choline, ^{11}C-acetate has to be considered an indicator for the highly increased lipid metabolism rate due to the accelerated cell membrane synthesis in malignant tissue. In a study investigating 513 patients ^{11}C-acetate was utilized for imaging different malignant diseases (Liu 2000). The findings of this publication imply that ^{11}C-acetate may be useful for the visualization of other tumor entities besides prostate cancer. Oyama et al. found ^{11}C-acetate to be more accurate than ^{18}F-FDG in the detection of prostate cancer (Oyama et al. 2002). Although an overlap of ^{11}C-acetate uptake between benign prostatic diseases such as BPH and prostate cancer may occur, recent studies hint that ^{11}C-acetate is a valuable PET tracer for imaging prostate cancer and its metastases (Oyama et al. 2002, 2003). While ^{11}C-choline has the advantage of a better understood metabolic pathway, this radiotracer may exhibit urinary excretion in up to 30% of cases. While bladder activity of ^{11}C-choline is significantly lower than that of ^{18}F-FDG and most often too low to profoundly interfere with the visualization of pelvic structures, ^{11}C-acetate completely lacks urinary excretion. Urinary accumulation of ^{11}C-choline may be the result of incomplete tubular reabsorption or enhanced excretion of oxidative metabolites of the radiotracer. Kotzerke et al. conducted a ntraindividual comparison of ^{11}C-acetate and ^{1}C-choline (Kotzerke et al. 2003) for the visu-lization of metastasized prostate cancer. The attern of tracer uptake was found to be nearly dentical for both radiotracers and it was con-luded that both radiotracers are equivalently iseful for detecting prostate cancer lesions. 3oth radiotracers demonstrated a sensitivity f 100% in the detection of prostate cancer in his small patient sample.

3.1.4.4 Other Potentially Useful PET Tracers for Imaging Prostate Cancer

everal other PET radiotracers have been devel--ped for imaging prostate cancer, among them ^{3}F-fluorodihydrotestosterone. This radiotracer s a radiolabeled analog of dihydrotestosterone, he primary ligand of the androgen receptor. 'he majority of prostate cancer lesions showed acreased uptake of ^{18}F-fluorodihydrotestoster-ne in a pilot study (Larson et al. 2004). Another 'ET radiotracer in use for imaging prostate can-er is ^{11}C-methionine. Its uptake pattern basi-ally reflects regional protein synthesis and it s therefore related to cellular proliferation ac-ivity. Toth et al. demonstrated in a group of 0 patients that ^{11}C-methionine PET is a use-al method to ensure a high detection rate of rostate cancer in patients with increased PSA evels but repeated negative biopsies (Toth et al. 005). Further investigation is needed to assess ie value of the above-mentioned PET tracers, 'hich are not related to lipid synthesis, for im-ging prostate cancer.

3.1.5 Value of PET in the Primary Staging of Prostate Cancer

enerally, Choline metabolism in paren-hymatous organs is comparatively high. herefore, even the normal prostate gland 1ows a significant amount of choline metabo-sm. In consequence, the uptake of PET trac-rs related to lipid synthesis is relatively high 1 the normal prostate gland. In addition, the 1ajority of patients presenting with suspicion f prostate cancer also reveal accompanying enign changes of the prostate, such as BPH

and chronic prostatitis. This may result in a further increase in ^{11}C-choline or ^{11}C-acetate uptake. Therefore, a possible limitation of ^{11}C-choline or ^{11}C-acetate PET may lie in an over-lap between tracer uptake of benign prostatic changes and prostate cancer.

In a recent study carried out by Yoshida et al. (2005) prostate cancer lesions could be visualized as a focal tracer accumulation within the prostate in five of six patients. It was noted that BPH and primary prostate cancer revealed an overlap regarding the stan-dardized uptake value (SUV). However, there were differences in the pattern of tracer up-take between benign and malignant prostatic changes in terms of homogeneous vs focal ac-cumulation. Interestingly, no correlation be-tween ^{11}C-choline uptake, PSA level or tumor stage was found. Yoshida et al. concluded that ^{11}C-choline PET may be of limited value in the detection of prostate cancer, because BPH also exhibits increased choline metabolism (Yoshida et al. 2005). In addition, in some of the patients included in the study, nonspecific accumulation of ^{11}C-choline in the small in-testine was found, which made it difficult to assess lymph node status. On the other hand, in a study covering 25 consecutive patients with histopathologically proven prostate can-cer (de Jong et al. 2002), the SUV of primary malignancies ranged from 2.4 to 9.5, with a mean SUV of 5.0. In contrast, the SUV of the prostate gland in five patients with BPH but without malignancy ranged from 1.3 to 3.2, with a mean SUV of 2.3. The difference in SUV between BPH and prostate cancer was found to be significant in this study. In the detection of the primary malignancy sensitivity was 96%, specificity was 100%, PPV was 100%, and NPV was 83%. Lymph node metastases could be verified in five cases and ^{11}C-choline PET was read as true-positive in four of these five cases. The single false-negative PET finding could be attributed to a lymph node micrometastasis. The tracer-independent inability to detect micrometastases due to its limited spatial resolution is a known shortcoming of PET. In addition, PET interpreted a lymph node with inflammatory changes and increased choline metabolism as a false-positive result.

In a subsequent study, de Jong et al. (2003b) analyzed the diagnostic efficacy of ^{11}C-choline PET in preoperative staging of pelvic lymph nodes in 67 prostate cancer patients. In addition to ^{11}C-choline PET, MRI and CT were performed. Fifteen patients revealed histopathologically proven lymph node metastases and 12 of 15 were correctly classified by ^{11}C-choline PET. PET was false-negative in three patients with lymph node micrometastases. The authors also noted that unspecific bowel activity sometimes hampered the interpretation of foci seen in the pelvic or abdominal region. In 52 cases without metastatic spread to the lymphatic system, ^{11}C-choline PET was read as true-negative in 50 patients. In two patients false-positive findings occurred due to inflammatory lymph node changes in one case and because of recurrent inguinal hernia mimicking a nodal metastasis in the other. In this study, sensitivity, specificity, and accuracy in diagnosing lymph node metastases have been reported to be 80%, 96%, and 93%, respectively. In contrast, sensitivity, specificity, and accuracy of radiologic cross-sectional imaging modalities were found to be 47%, 98%, and 86%, respectively. De Jong et al. concluded that ^{11}C-choline PET is an appropriate tool for the preoperative staging of pelvic lymph nodes in patients with histologically proven prostate cancer (de Jong et al. 2003b).

With regard to ^{11}C-acetate for imaging prostate cancer, Oyama et al. (2002) found in 22 biopsy proven prostate cancer patients that ^{11}C-acetate uptake in cancerous tissue was significantly increased in all cases (sensitivity 100%). In contrast, sensitivity of ^{18}F-FDG PET was 83% in this selected patient population. As the findings of Yoshida et al. using ^{11}C-choline, ^{11}C-acetate uptake did not correlate with the Gleason score or PSA level. While ^{11}C-acetate exhibits no renal excretion at all (Shreve et al. 1995), ^{11}C-choline, even though predominantly excreted with the bile, can show a variable amount of renal elimination. However, in a series of publications, the impact of bladder activity of ^{11}C-choline was found not to be a major issue in image interpretation (de Jong et al. 2002; Hara et al. 1998; Sutinen et al. 2004; Yoshida et al. 2005). Kotzerke et al. found no

difference in the diagnostic efficacy comparing ^{11}C-acetate and ^{11}C-choline (Kotzerke et al. 2003).

With regard to logistics, ^{18}F-labeled cholin may eventually be favored over ^{11}C-cholin for routine clinical use. Price et al. found ^{18}F fluorocholine to be a suitable radiotracer fo imaging prostate cancer and demonstrate that androgen-dependent as well as androgen independent prostate cancer cells metaboliz more ^{18}F-fluorocholine in vitro than ^{18}F-FD (Price et al. 2002). Kwee et al. found that ^{18}F fluorocholine is potentially useful for the T staging of prostate cancer and for localizin cancer foci within the prostate gland (Kwee e al. 2005). In comparison to ^{11}C-choline, on particular shortcoming of ^{18}F-choline is it extremely high bladder activity as early a 6 min after intravenous injection, making i difficult to discriminate malignant foci in th proximity of the urinary bladder (DeGrado e al. 2001).

13.1.5.1 Presentation of Our Study Results

The value and limitations of ^{11}C-choline PE for imaging prostate cancer seem insufficientl clarified in the literature today, notably in th contradictory reports on the ability to differ entiate between BPH/prostatitis and prostat cancer. In a recent study, Farsad et al. corre lated the ^{11}C-choline uptake of prostate cance foci with a histopathologic step-section analy sis (Farsad et al. 2005) of the resected prostat gland. Sensitivity of ^{11}C-choline PET/CT on per lesion basis was found to be comparativel poor at 66%. However, on a per patient bas PET/CT would have yielded a detection ra of 35 out of 36 true-positive findings. In cor sequence, per patient-based sensitivity, whic has to be considered the primary factor r garding therapeutic consequences, would hav been 97%. However, no healthy subjects we included in this study; therefore data regardir the per patient-based specificity could not b provided. Therefore, we see still a need for fu ther investigation of the value of ^{11}C-cholir PET or PET/CT in a clinical setting. To defir clear indications for this novel diagnostic ap proach, data regarding patient-based sensiti ty and specificity is mandatory. The aim of his prospective study was to investigate the diagnostic efficacy of PET and PET/CT using ^{11}C-choline in patients with suspected prostate cancer in a large sample of patients.

Forty-three patients with a clinical high level of suspicion of prostate carcinoma underwent ^{11}C-choline PET or PET/CT scanning; 24 of these patients were examined on a combined PET/CT scanner and the remaining 19 patients were examined on a dedicated full-ring PET scanner. Regarding the primary cancer, a reference standard based on histopathological examination of specimens obtained at biopsy or during surgery was established.

PET scans where performed with a standard whole-body staging clinical protocol; patients fasted the day of examination in order to reduce biliary excretion of choline into the bowel. We administered 500 MBq of ^{11}C-choline intravenously with the patient already positioned on the PET or PET/CT scanner. Immediately after administration of the total activity, a low-dose CT scan covering the area from the base of the skull to the proximal thighs was carried out for attenuation correction. Thereafter, emission measurement was performed in caudocranial orientation. After finishing PET acquisition, a contrast-enhanced diagnostic CT of the abdomen and pelvis was conducted.

Data from both scanners was reconstructed iteratively with and without attenuation correction and reoriented in axial, sagittal, and coronal planes. With all PET/CT studies, all CT data underwent multiplanar reconstruction. SUV measurement was performed using manually defined polymorphic ROIs tightly surrounding the focus of increased ^{11}C-choline uptake seen on attenuation-corrected PET images. Studies were interpreted prospectively by readers blinded to any clinical information as well as blinded to the results of other diagnostic procedures. Attenuation-corrected and noncorrected PET images were interpreted in consensus by two experienced nuclear medicine physicians. The classification of a respective lesion was based primarily on a qualitative image analysis taking into account the visual pattern of tracer uptake. The maximum SUV (SUV_{max}) of a suspected lesion was used as guidance only. When patients underwent a PET/CT examination, the diagnostic contrast-enhanced CT was exclusively used for anatomic allocation of foci seen in PET. All lesions classified as malignant by PET maintained a malignant status, if the pathologic tracer uptake has been verified to be located inside the prostate gland or if the corresponding CT revealed any other morphologic correlate, for example a lymph node. Abnormalities seen in CT without a pathologic correlate in the respective PET scan were classified as nonmalignant.

Primary Malignancies

In 19 of 43 patients, prostate cancer could be ruled out on the basis of the reference standard. In six of these cases, BPH was present and in eight cases chronic prostatitis could be verified histopathologically. In two cases acute prostatitis was present. In only 5 of the 19 patients without malignancy, neither BPH nor prostatitis was present. ^{11}C-choline PET or PET/CT was true-negative in 12 of 19 cases. In these 12 patients, tracer uptake was rather homogeneous and SUV_{max} levels ranged from 1.4 to a maximum level of 4.0 in a patient with chronic prostatitis. In seven of 19 cases, PET was interpreted as false-positive. SUV_{max} levels ranged from 3.3 to 4.7. Acute prostatitis was found in one of these cases and chronic prostatitis was present in another three. BPH could be verified in two of these cases. The false-positive cases revealed an inhomogeneous pattern of ^{11}C-choline uptake, possibly due to inflammatory changes and BPH.

In 24 of 43 cases, prostate cancer could be verified. Gleason scores of the 24 patients with proven prostate cancer ranged from 2+2 to 4+3 and the mean PSA level was 39.5 ± 71.1 ng/ml (range, 2.4–266.0). Twenty-one of the 24 primary cancers exhibited increased ^{11}C-choline uptake with a pattern of tracer uptake inside the prostate that was focal or inhomogeneous (Figs. 13.1, 13.2). The mean SUV_{max} of the primary malignancies was 4.3 ± 1.9, ranging from 2.2 to 9.8. The SUV_{max} of prostate glands in patients without malignancy was 3.3 ± 1.9, ranging from 1.4 to 4.7. The SUV_{max} of primary can-

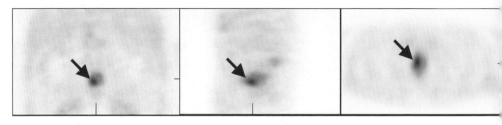

Fig. 13.1. Coronal, sagittal, and axial PET images of a patient (65 years old) with histopathologically proven cancer in the right lobe of the prostate gland. ^{11}C-choline PET shows corresponding focal tracer uptake

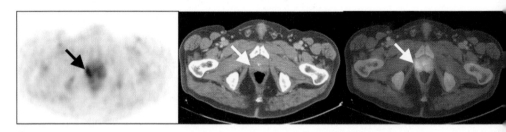

Fig. 13.2. PET (*left*), CT (*middle*), and fused PET/CT (*right*) images of a patient (69 years old) with histopathologically proven prostate cancer on the right side with corresponding focal tracer accumulation (*arrows*)

cers was significantly higher than the SUV_{max} of prostate glands without malignant changes. Twenty-one cases were true-positive by ^{11}C-choline PET or PET/CT, while three cases were interpreted as false-negative. The three primary malignancies missed by PET exhibited SUV_{max} levels ranging from 2.2 to 2.9. The pattern of tracer uptake had no focal or inhomogeneous character. Histopathologic work-up revealed a Gleason score ranging from 2+3 to 3+3 in those cases. T-stage was T2 in one case and T3 in another case and could not be assessed in one patient without surgery. These patients had neither lymph node nor distant metastases.

ROC analysis of the assessed SUV_{max} levels of the prostate gland suggests a cut-off value of 3.3 for differentiation between benign and malignant processes. This approach would yield a sensitivity of 75% with a specificity of 58% in the detection of the primary malignancy. On the basis of a predominantly visual image analysis, however, ^{11}C-choline PET and PET/CT showed a sensitivity and specificity of 88% and 63%, respectively, in the detection of the primary malignancy.

Metastases

In 15 of the 24 patients with proven prostate cancer, metastatic spread could be ruled out on the basis of histopathologic examination of resection specimens obtained in surgery or by a follow-up period of at least 6 months. Follow-up included digital-rectal palpation, assessment of PSA levels, and transrectal ultrasonography. Fourteen patients received a MRI of the pelvis received in addition to the PET scan. In case of suspected metastatic spread to the bone, bone scintigraphy or ^{18}F-PET were conducted. In nine patients, metastatic spread could be verified histopathologically or by follow-up. On the basis of the underlying reference standard, four patients had lymph node metastases and another five patients suffered from osseous metastases. Metastases exhibited focal accumulation of ^{11}C-choline typical for malignant lesions (Figs. 13.3–13.5). On a per-patient basis, lymph node metastases were interpreted as true-positive by PET in three of four cases and in one case a histopathologically confirmed lymph node micrometastasis located in the left obturatoris region was

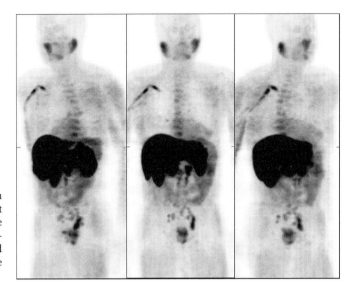

Fig. 13.3. Coronal projection images of a prostate cancer patient (51 years of age) with multiple pathologic ^{11}C-choline foci located bilaterally in the parailiac and paraaortal region due to multiple lymph node metastases

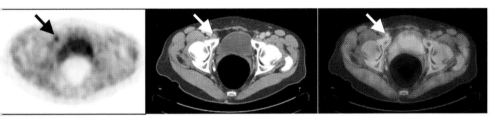

Fig. 13.4. PET (*left*), CT (*middle*), and fused PET/CT (*right*) images of a patient (71 years of age) with histopathologically proven prostate cancer. PET shows focal tracer accumulation in an iliac lymph node on the right side (*arrows*). This lesion turned out to be a lymph node metastasis

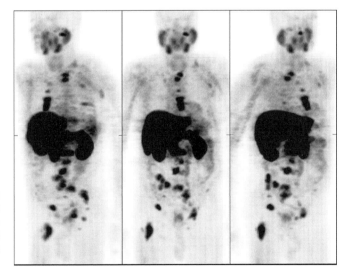

Fig. 13.5. Patient (58 years old) with histopathologically proven prostate cancer. Coronal projection images of ^{11}C-choline PET. ^{11}C-choline PET shows multiple bone metastases

missed. With regard to bone metastases, PET provided true-positive results for four of five patients and missed an osseous metastasis located in the spine. This lesion was positive in bone scintigraphy. On a per patient basis, PET demonstrated a sensitivity in the detection of metastatic lesions of 77% and produced no false positive findings.

Interpretation of Preliminary Study Results

Based on our results, we see an indication for ^{11}C-choline PET and PET/CT for the detection of the primary malignancy as well as for the visualization of local and distant metastases. PET, as a whole body procedure, may be of value particularly with regard to the search for distant metastases. Skip lesions are not uncommon for this tumor entity. The detection of distant metastatic spread would imply a change in the therapeutic regimen in the majority of cases. Contrary to the findings of Yoshida et al., we believe that ^{11}C-choline PET can also be used successfully to detect the primary cancer with sufficiently high diagnostic assertiveness. We found a significantly higher SUV_{max} of prostate carcinomas when compared to the SUV_{max} of prostate glands without malignancy. De Jong et al. corroborate our findings and also report significantly higher ^{11}C-choline uptake in prostate cancer (mean SUV_{max} = 5.0) than in the benign prostate (mean SUV_{max} = 2.3) (de Jong et al. 2002). Using the SUV_{max} primarily as guidance, our results of a predominantly visual image analysis provided high sensitivity. Only three of 24 primary malignancies were interpreted as false-negative by ^{11}C-choline PET. Specificity, however, was hampered by eight false-positive findings, a comparatively high number. Acute prostatitis was verified histopathologically in two of the included patients without malignancy. The pattern of tracer uptake was markedly inhomogeneous in one of these cases and SUV_{max} was 4.6 and PET was interpreted as false-positive. In four other cases with chronic prostatitis, the pattern of tracer uptake was to a greater or lesser extent inhomogeneous and PET was interpreted as

false-positive. We therefore can conclude tha particularly acute but also chronic prostatiti mimicking prostate cancer may be a limita tion of this diagnostic procedure. But BPH may also exhibit a markedly inhomogeneou pattern of tracer uptake and showed SUV_{max} levels as high as 3.7 in our patient group. Onl two of the seven cases that were interpreted a false-positive by PET revealed neither prosta titis nor BPH.

ROC analysis was carried out to assess a ideal SUV_{max} threshold value to differentiat benign from malignant intraprostatic pro cesses. In our patient group, a cut-off value c 3.3 above which the SUV_{max} is considered to b malignant would yield the best compromis between sensitivity and specificity. This ap proach would result in a sensitivity of 75% wit a specificity of 58%. However, these values d not warrant the definition of a clear SUV_{max} cut-off value providing a valid differentiatio between malignant and benign processes. I contrast, a primarily qualitative image inter pretation taking into account the actual pat tern of tracer uptake and using the SUV_{max} primarily as guidance yielded better results The moderate specificity may be explained b an overlap of the ^{11}C-choline uptake in benig and malignant prostatic changes.

We found significant urinary bladder activ ity in 14 out of 43 of the patients included i the study, which sometimes interfered with th visualization of the prostate gland and pelvi structures. Interestingly, readers found blad der activity as well as unspecific intestinal ac tivity to be an issue only in some of the stand alone PET studies but not PET/CT. Althoug it was beyond the scope of this study to com pare stand-alone PET and PET/CT, a combine PET/CT system may eventually be favore and may even be mandatory when using ^{18}F labeled choline. This may be substantiated b the fact that radiolabeled choline provides gen erally poorer anatomic information than doe ^{18}F-FDG. Also, from a clinical point of view combined PET/CT scanners may be favored i certain scenarios, for example for planning bi opsy or surgery.

13.1.6 PET and PET/CT in Detecting Local Recurrence After Definitive Therapy

The definite value of PET or PET/CT in identifying local recurrence of prostate cancer after therapy has yet to be determined. Preliminary reports in the literature are available with regard to PET tracers related to lipid synthesis. In a study carried out by Kotzerke et al., 31 patients with PSA recurrence after definitive therapy were investigated with ^{11}C-acetate PET (Kotzerke et al. 2002). Thirteen patients had negative biopsy and revealed no evidence of manifest disease in a follow-up period of 6 months, including TRUS. No pathologic ^{11}C-acetate accumulation was found in the region of the prostate bed in these patients. Sixteen patients revealed local recurrence verified at biopsy and in two further patients local recurrence was clinically verified. ^{11}C-acetate PET detected true-positive local recurrence in 15 of these 18 patients. PSA levels of the three patients classified false-negative by PET were found to be 1.3, 4.4, and 12.6 ng/ml, respectively. In a subgroup of patients with PSA recurrence of less than 2.0 ng/ml, five patients revealed pathologic tracer uptake in the prostate bed. Local recurrence could be verified in four of these patients at biopsy. Another study investigated the diagnostic efficacy of ^{11}C-acetate PET after radical prostatectomy and radiation therapy (Oyama et al. 2003). In general, sensitivity of PET in detecting recurrent prostate cancer was encouraging. However, the sensitivity was highly dependent on the PSA level and was markedly reduced in cases with low PSA. Fricke et al. (2003) reported a sensitivity of 70% and a specificity of 100% for the detection of local recurrence in a study covering 25 patients examined with ^{11}C-acetate PET. The comparatively low sensitivity found may be explained by the fact that 14 patients underwent anti-androgen therapy. A positive correlation between PSA levels and SUV ($r = 0.864$, $p < 0.005$) was found in this study. Furthermore, sensitivity in the detection of lymph node and bone metastases was 75% and 50%, respectively.

With regard to the PET tracer ^{11}C-choline, Yoshida et al. performed PET scans in eight patients with PSA recurrence after definitive therapy. Clinical follow-up was used as the standard of reference. PET was found to be of value in detecting recurrent prostate cancer in this study (Yoshida et al. 2005). In another study on 36 patients, De Jong et al. (2003a) revealed that 13 had PSA failure after radical prostatectomy. ^{11}C-choline PET revealed pathologic tracer accumulation in 5 of these 13 cases. However, local recurrence could be verified in only 3 of 13 patients. On the basis of histopathological examination after lymphadenectomy, lymph node metastases could be verified in four patients. ^{11}C-choline PET detected metastatic spread in all four patients. In a large group of 100 patients investigated using ^{11}C-choline PET, Picchio et al. found concordant results between PET imaging and conventional imaging (MRI, CT, bone scintigraphy) in 86 patients (Picchio et al. 2003). Six of the remaining 14 patients had pathologic tracer uptake in ^{11}C-choline PET but were negative in conventional imaging modalities. Two patients with suspected local recurrence demonstrated decreasing PSA levels after antihormonal therapy. The elevated PSA levels could not be attributed to local recurrence or distant metastases during follow-up in these patients. ^{11}C-choline PET raised suspicion of lymph node metastases in three patients and metastatic spread to the bone in another patient. However, on the basis of the underlying reference standard, ^{11}C-choline PET was interpreted as false-positive in these four cases. Eight cases without pathologic PET findings revealed local recurrence on the basis of biopsy and were consequently classified false-negative. Conventional imaging modalities were also false-negative in these patients. In this study, no correlation of serum PSA with the SUV was found in patients with positive PET findings. In a recent study carried out by Kotzerke et al., PET failed to detect two of four local recurrences with low PSA values (0.3 ng/ml and 3.4 ng/ml) (Kotzerke et al. 2003). In addition, PET missed one of three lymph node metastases but all bone metastases were true-positive.

The preliminary studies carried out thus far suggest that PET imaging using ^{11}C-choline or ^{11}C-acetate may be of value in identifying recurrent disease after definitive treatment. This seems to be especially true for cases with significantly elevated serum PSA levels. However, in cases with comparatively low serum PSA (< 5 ng/ml), the rate of false-negative findings seems to be high. In some patients, local radiation therapy may be based on the identification of local recurrence and the exclusion of distant metastases by PET.

13.1.7 Outlook

Modern metabolic imaging procedures such as PET and MRI/MRS will have their indications in patients with a high risk of prostate cancer due to persistently elevated serum PSA. This could also be true in cases with repeated negative biopsies of the prostate gland, as it is known that false-negative biopsy findings can occur. At present, PET is the only diagnostic procedure at hand providing functional information of the primary prostate cancer as well as its metastases. MRI complemented by MRS as a competing procedure provides similar results in the detection rate of the primary malignancy (Amsellem-Ouazana et al. 2005; van Dorsten et al. 2004; Yu et al. 1999). However, in contrast to PET, MRS does not provide functional information beyond that of the prostate gland. The detection of metastatic spread or local recurrence with MRI is again primarily based on morphologic criteria, such as the size of a respective lymph node. It may therefore be speculated that ^{11}C-choline PET and PET/CT, as a whole-body functional imaging modality, should have a methodical advantages over MRI/MRS with regard to the search for metastatic spread or local recurrence. An intrinsic advantage of MRI when used with dedicated endorectal coils is its superior anatomic information, particularly regarding soft tissue contrast. Therefore, it is frequently possible to detect tumor growth exceeding the prostate capsule by means of MRI. Tumor spread beyond the prostate capsule would in many cases imply changing the therapeutic regimen. In contrast, even with the use of modern PET/CT scanners exact evaluation of involvement of the prostate capsule cannot be provided, because CT simply does not provide as detailed

anatomic information of the prostate gland as does MRI. Nevertheless, in a first comparison of 11C-choline PET vs MRI combined with MRS, PET had a slight advantage in the detection rate of the primary prostate cancer (Yamaguchi et al. 2005).

In summary, we can conclude that according to the data available in the literature and our own study results, ^{11}C-choline PET and PET/CT has high sensitivity in the detection of the primary prostate cancer. However, false-positive findings may occur because of an overlap of ^{11}C-choline uptake between benign prostatic processes such as BPH or prostatitis and prostate cancer. A valid differentiation between benign and malignant prostatic changes is feasible in the majority of cases by taking into account the actual pattern of tracer uptake. The use of combined PET/CT scanners may be especially useful in scenarios where exact anatomic allocation of PET foci is of high relevance, such as planning of biopsy or surgery.

With regard to the evaluation of recurrent prostate cancer, PET and PET/CT may also play an important role in the future diagnostic workup of these patients. PET using ^{11}C-choline or ^{11}C-acetate is an improvement over a therapeutic regime based solely on the assessment of the PSA level and morphologic imaging procedures. Metastatic spread demonstrated by PET would frequently imply hormonal therapy instead of local radiation therapy. Therefore PET could be of value in selecting an adequate, stage-appropriate therapy. However, further systematic studies on larger patient cohorts are needed to corroborate the potential value of PET and PET/CT in therapy planning.

13.2 ^{18}F-FDG PET/CT for Staging Penile Cancer

13.2.1 Introduction

Penile cancer is a rare tumor entity in industrial countries. In Europe and the United States, penile carcinomas, measured as a percentage of all type of malignant diseases in males, amount to only 0.4%–0.6% and these tumors are responsible for less than 1%–2% of all deaths (Derakhshani et al. 1999; Misra et al. 2004). Conversely, the incidence of penile carcinomas is considerably higher in developing countries such as Puerto Rico or Uganda. In these regions, penile cancer represents up to 10%–22% of all malignancies in males (Derakhshani et al. 1999). Decisive prognostic factors are tumor grade and stage as well as the presence of lymph node metastases (Chen et al. 2004; Misra et al. 2004).

Approximately 97% of penile cancers are squamous cell carcinomas (Ravizzini et al. 2001). The majority of the primary malignancies are located at the glans of the penis or at the preputium (Algaba et al. 2002). Solsona et al. demonstrated in a group of 103 patients that the likelihood of the presence or absence of occult lymph node metastases is associated with tumor grade and stage (Solsona et al. 2001). Distant metastases occur in only 1%–10% of cases and are generally associated with regional lymph node involvement (Misra et al. 2004). Curative surgical resection of the primary malignancy with a safety margin of 2 cm or partial amputation of the penis generally provides a good chance for cure (Syed et al. 2003). Another therapeutic option is laser ablation of the primary penile cancer in early disease stages. Bilateral radical lymphadenectomy is indicated in patients with suspected lymph node spread. However, there are some centers that perform prophylactic bilateral lymphadenectomy at stage T2 or above, although this approach is accompanied by a high morbidity rate. In advanced stages, radiation therapy will be used as well as chemotherapy in cases with systemic tumor manifestation. Despite surgical therapy and lymphadenectomy, tumor progression will take place in roughly 40% of cases (Syed et al. 2003). Prognosis of penile cancer depends on tumor stage, histologic grade, and involvement of regional lymph nodes (Chen et al. 2004; Singh and Khaitan 2003).

13.2.2 Conventional Imaging Modalities

Diagnosis of penile cancer is generally established on the basis of histopathological examination of tissue samples taken at biopsy of the suspected area (Algaba et al. 2002; Micali et al. 2004). When the presence of penile carcinoma is verified, clinical palpation will be performed as a first-line diagnostic method for N-staging. Complementary, morphologic imaging techniques such as US, CT, and MRI will be carried out (Micali et al. 2004). Ultrasound, as a ubiquitously available front-line imaging modality is considered unreliable with regard to N-staging (Algaba et al. 2002). CT and MRI, mainly relying on a system of classification based on morphological criteria, also have proven insufficiently robust in evaluating patients for possible regional lymph node involvement (Derakhshani et al. 1999). In this respect, Lont et al. reported a relatively high risk of false-positive findings in CT and MRI with regard to N-staging (Lont et al. 2003). One reason for this may be the fact that lymph nodes often exhibit reactive changes caused by the underlying malignant disease in the penis (Chen et al. 2004). In addition, even under physiological conditions, the diameter of lymph nodes in the inguinal region can exceed 2 cm in the absence of malignancy. Algaba et al. report that 20%–96% of penile cancer patients have palpable lymph nodes at the time of first diagnosis, although actual lymphogenic metastasis is present in only 17%–45% of these patients (Algaba et al. 2002).

13.2.3 Sentinel Lymph Node Biopsy and Prophylactic Lymphadenectomy

N-staging is established in some centers on the basis of sentinel lymph node biopsy (SLNB), which is an invasive option for assessing lymphogenic metastasis, after peritumoral injection of nanocolloid particles that are labeled with Tc-99m. For some tumor entities such as mammary cancer, this procedure is known to have high accuracy (Barone et al. 2005). However, Tanis et al. reported a comparatively low overall sensitivity of SLNB at 78% in penile cancer patients (Tanis et al. 2002). In addition, because of the highly variable lymphatic drainage in this region of the body, skip lesions can occur and bilateral infiltration of regional lymph nodes is not uncommon for this tumor entity (Algaba et al. 2002). Because of the frequency and the high prognostic consequence of the presence of inguinal lymph node metastases and because of the unsatisfactory diagnostic accuracy of currently available imaging techniques, general prophylactic lymphadenectomy has been suggested by some authors, even without clinical suspicion of metastatic spread (Chen et al. 2004). In contrast, other centers recommend this procedure only in G3 tumors at stage T2 and above (Mobilio and Ficarra 2001). A reason for this is the fact that lymphadenectomy is accompanied by a high morbidity rate of 30%–50% (Algaba et al. 2002). It may be speculated that noninvasive imaging procedures, robust enough to provide high diagnostic assertiveness in assessing N-stage, could in some cases reduce the utilization of prophylactic lymphadenectomy.

13.2.4 PET and PET/CT

With regard to several malignant diseases, PET has been shown to be of value in differentiating benign and malignant processes. Also, as a whole-body procedure, PET provides high diagnostic accuracy in the search for metastatic spread (Reske and Kotzerke 2001). However, stand-alone PET provides limited anatomical information, making it sometimes difficult to allocate pathologic tracer uptake to a certain anatomic region. Therefore, combined PET/CT systems, by providing exact image fusion between functional PET images and detailed morphologic CT information, may be preferable in certain scenarios (Ell and von Schulthess 2002; Pelosi et al. 2004; Schoder et al. 2003; Stahl et al. 2004). In this respect, Schoder et al. assume a 10%–20% change in therapeutical management on the basis of PET/CT in certain tumor entities (Schoder et al. 2004). This innovative imaging modality, using the radiopharmaceutical ^{18}F-fluorodeoxyglucose (^{18}F-FDG-PET/CT) could prove useful in the noninvasive imaging of penile cancer.

Regarding penile cancer imaging with PET or PET/CT, the principle question that has to be answered is, whether penile carcinomas and metastases originating from penile cancer exhibit high enough ^{18}F-FDG uptake to be differentiated from the surrounding tissue with sufficiently high diagnostic certainty. It is known that squamous cell type cancers often exhibit high glucose metabolism in relation to normal tissue and thus be amenable to diagnosis by PET (Laubenbacher et al. 1995). Therefore, in theory penile cancers should be amenable to PET imaging under utilization of ^{18}F-FDG. Until recently, only three case reports existed in the international literature, suggesting that FDG-PET can be used to image penile cancer. In a publication that focused primarily on a novel polychemotherapy approach in a patient with penile cancer, Joerger et al. report that a metastatic lymph node discovered incidentally at follow-up showed increased ^{18}F-FDG uptake (Joerger et al. 2004). In another case report, Ravizzini et al. described a lesion with positive ^{18}F-FDG uptake in a patient with penile cancer (Ravizzini et al. 2001). Finally, Langen et al. demonstrated that a coincidentally discovered metastatic inguinal lymph node of a penile cancer patient exhibited increased ^{18}F-FDG uptake (Langen et al. 2001). In none of these case reports was the diagnostic value of ^{18}F-FDG PET in the diagnosis of penile carcinoma the primary focus.

In a pilot study investigating 13 patients with suspected penile cancer, we demonstrated for the first time that the primary penile cancer as well as lymph node metastases originating from penile cancer exhibit typically increased FDG uptake for malignancy (Scher et al. 2005). Based on these findings, we can conclude that FDG-PET and PET/CT are in principle suitable for staging penile cancer patients. In the following, a consecutive update of the aforementioned study, with a larger patient group, will be provided.

13.2.5 Presentation of Our Study Results

The objective of this clinical study was to investigate the diagnostic value of ^{18}F-FDGPET/CT in the N-staging of patients with suspected penile cancer or history of penile cancer with a large sample of patients. Twenty patients were included into the study. In 15 patients, penile cancer was suspected on the basis of clinical examination. The five remaining patients presented for follow-up after surgery for penile cancer. One of these patients was examined twice by ^{18}F-FDG PET/CT because recurrence of regional lymph node metastases secondary to radical bilateral lymphadenectomy was suspected during clinical follow-up. The reference standard is based on histopathological correlation obtained at biopsy or surgery. The surgical procedures consisted of excision of the primary malignancy, partial penile amputation, and radical bilateral lymphadenectomy. In five patients with histopathologically confirmed penile cancer, lymphadenectomy was not carried out because of tumor stage and grade. After surgical treatment of the primary penile cancer, these patients were validated by a follow-up period of at least 6 months. MRI of the pelvis, ultrasonography of the inguinal region, and clinical inspection and palpation were conducted during this interval. In addition, PET/CT follow-up was performed in two patients.

^{18}F-FDG PET/CT was carried out for whole-body staging in all patients on a dual-slice PET/CT system (Philips Gemini, Philips, Hamburg, Germany). We administered 200 MBq of ^{18}F-FDG intravenously. A low-dose CT scan was started 60 min after administering the total tracer for attenuation correction. Emission scanning was performed in caudocranial orientation and then a diagnostic contrast-enhanced CT of the thorax, abdomen, and pelvis was performed. PET data was reconstructed iteratively with and without attenuation correction. PET and CT data underwent multiplanar reconstructions. Using the attenuation-corrected PET image, manually defined ROIs were placed throughout all axial planes in which a suspected lesion could be delineated, including the focus of increased glucose metabolism.

The results presented are primarily based on the information provided by PET, while CT was mainly used for exact anatomic localization. All studies were evaluated by readers blinded to any clinical information and to results of other imaging procedures. However, readers were aware of the patient's underlying disease. Primarily,

PET examinations were interpreted without access to the respective CT scan. Classifying a lesion as benign or malignant was based predominantly on a visual image analysis. SUV_{max} values were used as guidance. A SUV_{max} cut-off value for differentiation between benign and malignant processes has not been used. After evaluation of the plain PET images, fused PET/CT scans were interpreted in consensus with a radiologist. All lesions classified as malignant by PET maintained a malignant status when a morphologic correlate could be found in the corresponding CT scan, for example a lymph node. Any abnormalities seen in CT without corresponding pathologic tracer accumulation in the respective PET image was interpreted as nonmalignant.

13.2.5.1 Preliminary Study Results

Five patients presented verified penile carcinoma after surgery and 15 patients presented with clinical suspicion of penile cancer prior to treatment. In 11 of these 15 patients, penile cancer was verified. All primary carcinomas were of the squamous cell type, located at the glans penis. Nine of the 11 primary malignancies exhibited focally increased tracer accumulation in the ^{18}F-FDG PET/CT scan (Fig. 13.6). In the remaining two cases, T1G2 tumors with maximum diameters below 1 cm were not detectable by PET/CT. During surgery, the maximum diameter of the primary malignancies was assessed to range from less than 0.5 cm to 3.5 cm. The mean SUV_{max} of the 11 primary malignancies was 5.6 ± 3.5, ranging from 1.9 to 12.1. In two of the 20 patients included in the study, histological work-up revealed carcinoma in situ. The tumor did not penetrate the basilar membrane and PET/CT showed no focal uptake of the radiotracer. In one patient, PET/CT showed discretely increased glucose utilization at the region of the glans penis with a SUV_{max} of 1.3. Histopathological examination, however, revealed inflammatory changes due to Wegener's disease at the penile glans. Another patient suffered from partial necrosis at the penile glans due to peripheral arterial occlusive disease attributable to diabetes mellitus. This lesion was incorrectly suspected

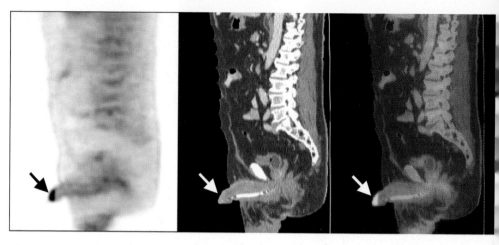

Fig. 13.6. PET (*left*), CT (*middle*), and fused PET/CT (*right*) images of a patient (67 years old) with G2 penile cancer at the glans penis (*arrows*). The maximum diameter of the lesion was approximately 2.5 cm. ^{18}F-FDG uptake is intense

of being penile cancer on clinical inspection. PET/CT, however, showed no increased glucose utilization at the site of necrosis.

Lymph node metastases could be verified in 8 of 20 patients, localized bilaterally in three patients. A total of 21 lymph node metastases were verified by histopathology in these eight patients; 18 of 21 lymph node metastases were rated true-positive using ^{18}F-FDG PET/CT. The majority of the metastatic lesions showed pathologically increased glucose utilization (Figs. 13.7, 13.8). The mean SUVmax of the 20 lymph node metastases was 4.3 ± 2.0, ranging from 0.9 to 7.6. All three lesions missed by PET corresponded to lymph node micrometastases. Six lymph node metastases exhibited a SUV_{max} lower than 3.0. In three of these cases, lesions turned out to be micrometastases. In another two cases, lymph node metastases had maximum diameters as assessed by CT of less than 1 cm. The size dependency of the SUV_{max} is a known effect of SUV quantification in smaller lesions due to partial volume effects caused by the limited spatial resolution of PET. All of the foci interpreted as lymph node metastases by PET corresponded to lymph nodes in the respective CT image. In four cases, lymph nodes were less than 1 cm in diameter. The diameter of the three lymph node metastases missed by PET/CT was 0.6, 0.9, and 1.8 cm.

In 12 of 20 patients, lymph node metastases were neither suspected on the basis of clinical examination nor from diagnostic imaging modalities. With regard to the primary lesion (CIS, Wegener's disease, and partial necrosis) lymph node metastases could be ruled out in 4 of 12 cases. In another three cases, radical bilateral lymphadenectomy was carried out and histopathological work-up showed no signs of malignancy. The remaining five patients were validated by a follow-up period of at least 6 months. PET/CT was true-negative in 11 cases and returned a single false-positive finding in one patient. This patient had penile cancer at stage 2 and grade 2. Focal tracer accumulation with a SUV_{max} of 2.2 could be delineated in the right inguinal region with a corresponding lymph node measuring 1.2 cm in diameter in the respective CT scan. In a follow-up PET/CT examination after excision of the primary malignancy, PET was negative and CT showed no increase in size. The lymph node was therefore rated as nonmalignant on the basis of the reference standard. The discrete tracer uptake in the first PET/CT scan was possibly due to reactive changes secondary to the primary penile cancer.

In summary, ^{18}F-FDG PET/CT was interpreted as true-positive in 18 of 21 lymph node metastases and returned three false-negative

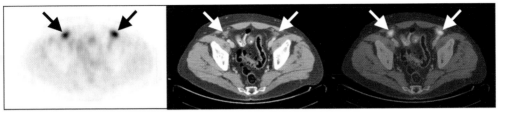

Fig. 13.7. PET (*left*), CT (*middle*), and PET/CT (*right*) images of 63-year-old man with bilateral inguinal lymph node metastases originating from T2G2 penile cancer

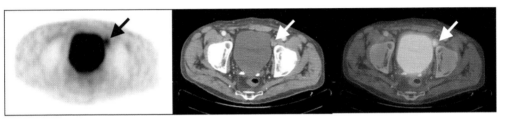

Fig. 13.8. PET (*left*), CT (*middle*), and PET/CT (*right*) images of a penile cancer patient (75 years of age). ^{18}F-FDG PET shows focal tracer uptake in the proximity of the urinary bladder (*arrows*). CT reveals a corresponding lymph node. Based on exact image fusion, this lesion was correctly classified as a lymph node metastasis by PET/CT

findings, corresponding to micrometastases. The sensitivity of PET/CT in the detection of lymph node metastases was 86% on a per lesion basis. On a per patient basis, sensitivity was 75%, with a specificity of 92%.

13.2.5.2 Interpretation of Study Results

An intrinsic advantage of PET/CT is the ability to assess the malignancy of lymph nodes based on functional information, and independently of morphologic criteria, as is the case with stand alone CT and MRI. As the primary penile cancer is generally verified at biopsy and distant metastases are rare, the main indication of ^{18}F-FDG PET/CT in penile cancer patients has to be considered the prognostically crucial search for lymph node metastases. Per lesion-based sensitivity of PET/CT in the detection of lymph node metastases was 86% and only one false-positive finding occurred. Patient-based specificity was 92%. PET/CT missed three lesions, which turned out to be lymph node micrometastases. Because two of the missed micrometastases were the single metastatic

lesions in two patients, both patients would have been incorrectly classified at stage N0 by PET/CT. It may be speculated that because of the limited number of eight patients with metastatic spread to lymph nodes, the 75% per patient-based sensitivity found was comparatively low. More investigations on larger patient groups are needed, to further corroborate the value of PET/CT in the N-staging of penile cancer patients.

Even small lesions can be detected reliably by PET/CT due to the usually intense pattern of tracer uptake of this tumor entity. However, partial volume effects of lesions below 1 cm Must be taken into account during PET interpretation. Because partial volume effects can also occur in lesions significantly exceeding 1 cm in diameter, we recommend using SUV_{max} values only for guidance. False-positive findings can also occur, because often inguinal lymph nodes undergo reactive changes due to the primary malignancy. This could lead to increased glucose utilization of the respective lymph node, as was the case in the single false-positive PET/CT finding of an incorrectly classified inguinal lymph node in our patient sample. Although in general metastatic processes exhibit a higher ^{18}F-FDG uptake than do reactive changes, the possibility of false-positive findings has to be taken into consideration during routine image interpretation, particularly with regard to inguinal lymph nodes.

13.2.6 Outlook

Based on the limited data available in the literature and the results presented of our own study, we can conclude that squamous cell penile cancer is in principle amenable to PET or PET/CT imaging. ^{18}F-FDG PET/CT showed promising preliminary results in staging and re-staging penile cancer patients and may prove a valuable diagnostic tool in the near future. PET already is regarded as the gold standard for whole-body staging and the search for metastatic spread in a variety of malignant entities. This could also hold true for imaging penile cancer.

The inability to detect micrometastases using PET or PET/CT is a known limitation independent of the underlying malignant disease. Although the scanner-specific resolution of modern PET systems is less than 1 cm in lesions with intense tracer accumulation, the detection of micrometastases is generally unsuccessful. Therefore, it may be speculated that using SLNB along with PET/CT may reduce the risk of unrecognized micrometastasis. A combination of both procedures may provide a sufficiently high level of diagnostic certainty to dispense with general lymphadenectomy in cases with low-grade disease and low T-stage. This would have a positive effect on the morbidity rate associated with invasive diagnostic procedures.

With respect to combined PET/CT systems, the additional information provided by CT allows exact anatomic localization of foci seen in PET. Detailed anatomic information provided by CT and the possibility of exact image fusion might prove especially useful in certain scenarios, such as planning for surgery. Implementation of PET and PET/CT into future staging algorithms may lead to an increase in diagnostic efficacy regarding planning of therapy and follow-up.

References

Ackerstaff E, Pflug BR, Nelson JB, Bhujwalla ZM (2001) Detection of increased choline compounds with proton nuclear magnetic resonance spectroscopy subsequent to malignant transformation of human prostatic epithelial cells. Cancer Res 9:3599–3603

Agus DB, Golde DW, Sgouros G, Ballangrud A, Cordon-Cardo C, Scher HI (1998) Positron emission tomography of a human prostate cancer xenograft: association of changes in deoxyglucose accumulation with other measures of outcome following androgen withdrawal. Cancer Res 14:3009–3014

Algaba F, Horenblas S, Pizzocaro-Luigi Piva G, Solsona E, Windahl T (2002) EAU guidelines on penile cancer. Eur Urol 3:199–203

Amsellem-Ouazana D, Younes P, Conquy S, Peyromaure M, Flam T, Debre B, Zerbib M (2005) Negative prostatic biopsies in patients with a high risk of prostate cancer. Is the combination of endorectal MRI and magnetic resonance spectroscopy imaging (MRSI) a useful tool? A preliminary study. Eur Urol 5:582–586

Barone JE, Tucker JB, Perez JM, Odom SR, Ghevariya V (2005) Evidence-based medicine applied to sentinel lymph node biopsy in patients with breast cancer. Am Surg 1:66–70

Beyersdorff D, Taupitz M, Winkelmann B, Fischer T, Lenk S, Loening SA, Hamm B (2002) Patients with a history of elevated prostate-specific antigen levels and negative transrectal US-guided quadrant or sextant biopsy results: value of MR imaging. Radiology 3:701–706

Breeuwsma AJ, Pruim J, Jongen MM, Suurmeijer AJ, Vaalburg W, Nijman RJ, de Jong IJ (2005) In vivo uptake of [(^{11})C]choline does not correlate with cell proliferation in human prostate cancer. Eur J Nucl Med Mol Imaging 32:668–673

Chen MF, Chen WC, Wu CT, Chuang CK, Ng KF, Chang JT (2004) Contemporary management of penile cancer including surgery and adjuvant radiotherapy: an experience in Taiwan. World J Urol 1:60–66

Coakley FV, Teh HS, Qayyum A, Swanson MG, Lu Y, Roach M 3rd, Pickett B, Shinohara K, Vigneron DB, Kurhanewicz J (2004) Endorectal MR imaging and MR spectroscopic imaging for locally recurrent prostate cancer after external beam radiation therapy: preliminary experience. Radiology 2:441–448

Coleman R, DeGrado T, Wang S, Baldwin S, Orr M, Reiman R, Price D (2000) 9:30–9:45. Preliminary evaluation of F-18 fluorocholine (FCH) as a PET tumor imaging agent. Clin Positron Imaging 4:147

Cornud F, Belin X, Piron D, Chretien Y, Flam T, Casanova JM, Helenon O, Mejean A, Thiounn N, Moreau JF

(1997) Color Doppler-guided prostate biopsies in 591 patients with an elevated serum PSA level: impact on Gleason score for nonpalpable lesions. Urology 5:709–715

Costello LC, Franklin RB, Narayan P (1999) Citrate in the diagnosis of prostate cancer. Prostate 3:237–245

De Jong IJ, Pruim J, Elsinga PH, Vaalburg W, Mensink HJ (2002) Visualization of prostate cancer with ^{11}C-choline positron emission tomography. Eur Urol 1:18–23

De Jong IJ, Pruim J, Elsinga PH, Vaalburg W, Mensink HJ (2003a) ^{11}C-choline positron emission tomography for the evaluation after treatment of localized prostate cancer. Eur Urol 1:32–38; discussion 38–39

De Jong IJ, Pruim J, Elsinga PH, Vaalburg W, Mensink HJ (2003b) Preoperative staging of pelvic lymph nodes in prostate cancer by ^{11}C-choline PET. J Nucl Med 3:331–335

DeGrado TR, Coleman RE, Wang S, Baldwin SW, Orr MD, Robertson CN, Polascik TJ, Price DT (2001) Synthesis and evaluation of ^{18}F-labeled choline as an oncologic tracer for positron emission tomography: initial findings in prostate cancer. Cancer Res 1:110–117

Derakhshani P, Neubauer S, Braun M, Bargmann H, Heidenreich A, Engelmann U (1999) Results and 10-year follow-up in patients with squamous cell carcinoma of the penis. Urologia Internationalis 4:238–244

DiBiase SJ, Hosseinzadeh K, Gullapalli RP, Jacobs SC, Naslund MJ, Sklar GN, Alexander RB, Yu C (2002) Magnetic resonance spectroscopic imaging-guided brachytherapy for localized prostate cancer. Int J Radiat Oncol Biol Phys 2:429–438

Effert PJ, Bares R, Handt S, Wolff JM, Bull U, Jakse G (1996) Metabolic imaging of untreated prostate cancer by positron emission tomography with 18-fluorine-labeled deoxyglucose. J Urol 3:994–998

Ell PJ, von Schulthess GK (2002) PET/CT: a new road map. Eur J Nucl Med Mol Imaging 6:719–720

Engelbrecht MR, Jager GJ, Laheij RJ, Verbeek AL, van Lier HJ, Barentsz JO (2002) Local staging of prostate cancer using magnetic resonance imaging: a meta-analysis. Eur Radiol 9:2294–2302

Farsad M, Schiavina R, Castellucci P, Nanni C, Corti B, Martorana G, Canini R, Grigioni W, Boschi S, Marengo M, Pettinato C, Salizzoni E, Monetti N, Franchi R, Fanti S (2005) Detection and localization of prostate cancer: correlation of ^{11}C-choline PET/CT with histopathologic step-section analysis. J Nucl Med 10:1642–1649

Fricke E, Machtens S, Hofmann M, van den Hoff J, Bergh S, Brunkhorst T, Meyer GJ, Karstens JH, Knapp WH, Boerner AR (2003) Positron emission tomography with ^{11}C-acetate and ^{18}F-FDG in prostate cancer patients. Eur J Nucl Med Mol Imaging 4:607–611

Halpern EJ, Verkh L, Forsberg F, Gomella LG, Mattrey RF, Goldberg BB (2000) Initial experience with contrast-enhanced sonography of the prostate. AJR Am J Roentgenol 6:1575–1580

Hara T, Kosaka N, Shinoura N, Kondo T (1997) PET imaging of brain tumor with [methyl-11C]choline. J Nucl Med 6:842–847

Hara T, Kosaka N, Kishi H (1998) PET imaging of prostate cancer using carbon-11-choline. J Nucl Med 6:990–995

Hara T, Kosaka N, Kishi H (2002) Development of (18)F-fluoroethylcholine for cancer imaging with PET: synthesis, biochemistry, and prostate cancer imaging. J Nucl Med 2:187–199

Heerschap A, Jager GJ, van der Graaf M, Barentsz JO, Ruijs SH (1997) Proton MR spectroscopy of the normal human prostate with an endorectal coil and a double spin-echo pulse sequence. Magn Reson Med 2:204–213

Heicappell R, Muller-Mattheis V, Reinhardt M, Vosberg H, Gerharz CD, Muller-Gartner H, Ackermann R (1999) Staging of pelvic lymph nodes in neoplasms of the bladder and prostate by positron emission tomography with 2-[(18)F]-2-deoxy-D-glucose. Eur Urol 6:582–587

Heuck A, Scheidler J, Sommer B, Graser A, Muller-Lisse UG, Massmann J (2003) MR imaging of prostate cancer. Radiologe 6:464–473

Hinkle GH, Burgers JK, Neal CE, Texter JH, Kahn D, Williams RD, Maguire R, Rogers B, Olsen JO, Badalament RA (1998) Multicenter radioimmunoscintigraphic evaluation of patients with prostate carcinoma using indium-111 capromab pendetide. Cancer 4:739–747

Huisman HJ, Futterer JJ, van Lin EN, Welmers A, Scheenen TW, van Dalen JA, Visser AG, Witjes JA, Barentsz JO (2005) Prostate cancer: precision of integrating functional MR imaging with radiation therapy treatment by using fiducial gold markers. Radiology 1:311–317

Inaba T (1992) Quantitative measurements of prostatic blood flow and blood volume by positron emission tomography. J Urol 5:1457–1460

Joerger M, Warzinek T, Klaeser B, Kluckert JT, Schmid HP, Gillessen S (2004) Major tumor regression after paclitaxel and carboplatin polychemotherapy in a patient with advanced penile cancer. Urology 4:778–780

Kotzerke J, Volkmer BG, Neumaier B, Gschwend JE, Hautmann RE, Reske SN (2002) Carbon-11 acetate positron emission tomography can detect local recurrence of prostate cancer. Eur J Nucl Med Mol Imaging 10:1380–1384

Kotzerke J, Volkmer BG, Glatting G, van den Hoff J, Gschwend JE, Messer P, Reske SN, Neumaier B (2003) Intraindividual comparison of [11C]acetate and [11C]choline PET for detection of metastases of prostate cancer. Nuklearmedizin 1:25–30

Kurhanewicz J, Vigneron DB, Hricak H, Narayan P, Carroll P, Nelson SJ (1996a) Three-dimensional H-1 MR spectroscopic imaging of the in situ human prostate with high (0.24–0.7-cm^3) spatial resolution. Radiology 3:795–805

Kurhanewicz J, Vigneron DB, Hricak H, Parivar F, Nelson SJ, Shinohara K, Carroll PR (1996b) Prostate cancer: metabolic response to cryosurgery as detected with

3D H-1 MR spectroscopic imaging. Radiology 2:489–496

Kwee SA, Coel MN, Lim J, Ko JP (2005) Prostate cancer localization with [18]fluorine fluorocholine positron emission tomography. J Urol 1:252–255

Langen KJ, Borner AR, Muller-Mattheis V, Hamacher K, Herzog H, Ackermann R, Coenen HH (2001) Uptake of cis-4-[^{18}F]fluoro-L-proline in urologic tumors. J Nucl Med 5:752–754

Larson SM, Morris M, Gunther I, Beattie B, Humm JL, Akhurst TA, Finn RD, Erdi Y, Pentlow K, Dyke J, Squire O, Bornmann W, McCarthy T, Welch M, Scher H (2004) Tumor localization of 16beta-^{18}F-fluoro-5alpha-dihydrotestosterone versus ^{18}F-FDG in patients with progressive, metastatic prostate cancer. J Nucl Med 3:366–373

Laubenbacher C, Saumweber D, Wagner-Manslau C, Kau RJ, Herz M, Avril N, Ziegler S, Kruschke C, Arnold W, Schwaiger M (1995) Comparison of fluorine-18-fluorodeoxyglucose PET, MRI and endoscopy for staging head and neck squamous-cell carcinomas. J Nucl Med 10:1747–1757

Liebross RH, Pollack A, Lankford SP, Zagars GK, von Eschenbach AC, Geara FB (1999) Transrectal ultrasound for staging prostate carcinoma prior to radiation therapy: an evaluation based on disease outcome. Cancer 7:1577–1585

Liu RS (2000) 31. Clinical Application of. Clin Positron Imaging 4:185

Lont AP, Besnard AP, Gallee MP, van Tinteren H, Horenblas S (2003) A comparison of physical examination and imaging in determining the extent of primary penile carcinoma. BJU Int 6:493–495

Menard C, Smith IC, Somorjai RL, Leboldus L, Patel R, Littman C, Robertson SJ, Bezabeh T (2001) Magnetic resonance spectroscopy of the malignant prostate gland after radiotherapy: a histopathologic study of diagnostic validity. Int J Radiat Oncol Biol Phys 2:317–323

Micali G, Nasca MR, Innocenzi D, Schwartz RA (2004) Invasive penile carcinoma: a review. Dermatol Surg 2:311–320

Misra S, Chaturvedi A, Misra NC (2004) Penile carcinoma: a challenge for the developing world. Lancet Oncol 4:240–247

Mobilio G, Ficarra V (2001) Genital treatment of penile carcinoma. Curr Opin Urol 3:299–304

Mueller-Lisse UG, Swanson MG, Vigneron DB, Hricak H, Bessette A, Males RG, Wood PJ, Noworolski S, Nelson SJ, Barken I, Carroll PR, Kurhanewicz J (2001a) Time-dependent effects of hormone-deprivation therapy on prostate metabolism as detected by combined magnetic resonance imaging and 3D magnetic resonance spectroscopic imaging. Magn Reson Med 1:49–57

Mueller-Lisse UG, Vigneron DB, Hricak H, Swanson MG, Carroll PR, Bessette A, Scheidler J, Srivastava A, Males RG, Cha I, Kurhanewicz J (2001b) Localized prostate cancer: effect of hormone deprivation therapy measured by using combined three-dimensional 1H MR

spectroscopy and MR imaging: clinicopathologic case-controlled study. Radiology 2:380–390

Mueller-Lisse U, Mueller-Lisse U, Scheidler J, Klein G, Reiser M (2005) Reproducibility of image interpretation in MRI of the prostate: application of the sextant framework by two different radiologists. Eur Radiol 9:1826–1833

Okada J, Yoshikawa K, Itami M, Imaseki K, Uno K, Itami J, Kuyama J, Mikata A, Arimizu N (1992) Positron emission tomography using fluorine-18-fluorodeoxyglucose in malignant lymphoma: a comparison with proliferative activity. J Nucl Med 3:325–329

Oyama N, Akino H, Suzuki Y, Kanamaru H, Sadato N, Yonekura Y, Okada K (1999) The increased accumulation of [^{18}F]fluorodeoxyglucose in untreated prostate cancer. Jpn J Clin Oncol 12:623–629

Oyama N, Akino H, Kanamaru H, Suzuki Y, Muramoto S, Yonekura Y, Sadato N, Yamamoto K, Okada K (2002) ^{11}C-acetate PET imaging of prostate cancer. J Nucl Med 2:181–186

Oyama N, Miller TR, Dehdashti F, Siegel BA, Fischer KC, Michalski JM, Kibel AS, Andriole GL, Picus J, Welch MJ (2003) ^{11}C-acetate PET imaging of prostate cancer: detection of recurrent disease at PSA relapse. J Nucl Med 4:549–555

Parivar F, Hricak H, Shinohara K, Kurhanewicz J, Vigneron DB, Nelson SJ, Carroll PR (1996) Detection of locally recurrent prostate cancer after cryosurgery: evaluation by transrectal ultrasound, magnetic resonance imaging, and three-dimensional proton magnetic resonance spectroscopy. Urology 4:594–599

Pelosi E, Messa C, Sironi S, Picchio M, Landoni C, Bettinardi V, Gianolli L, Del Maschio A, Gilardi MC, Fazio F (2004) Value of integrated PET/CT for lesion localisation in cancer patients: a comparative study. Eur J Nucl Med Mol Imaging 7:932–939

Picchio M, Messa C, Landoni C, Gianolli L, Sironi S, Brioschi M, Matarrese M, Matei DV, De Cobelli F, Del Maschio A, Rocco F, Rigatti P, Fazio F (2003) Value of [^{11}C]choline-positron emission tomography for re-staging prostate cancer: a comparison with [18F]fluorodeoxyglucose-positron emission tomography. J Urol 4:1337–1340

Price DT, Coleman RE, Liao RP, Robertson CN, Polascik TJ, DeGrado TR (2002) Comparison of [^{18}F]fluorocholine and [^{18}F]fluorodeoxyglucose for positron emission tomography of androgen dependent and androgen independent prostate cancer. J Urol 1:273–280

Qayyum A, Coakley FV, Lu Y, Olpin JD, Wu L, Yeh BM, Carroll PR, Kurhanewicz J (2004) Organ-confined prostate cancer: effect of prior transrectal biopsy on endorectal MRI and MR spectroscopic imaging. AJR Am J Roentgenol 4:1079–1083

Ravizzini GC, Wagner M, Borges-Neto S (2001) Positron emission tomography detection of metastatic penile squamous cell carcinoma. J Urol 5:1633–1634

Reske SN, Kotzerke J (2001) FDG-PET for clinical use Results of the 3rd German Interdisciplinary Consensus Conference, "Onko-PET III", 21 July and 19 September 2000. Eur J Nucl Med 11:1707–1723

Sarma AV, Schottenfeld D (2002) Prostate cancer incidence, mortality, and survival trends in the United States: 1981–2001. Semin Urol Oncol 1:3–9

Scardino PT (1989) Early detection of prostate cancer. Urol Clin North Am 4:635–655

Scher B, Seitz M, Reiser M, Hungerhuber E, Hahn K, Tiling R, Herzog P, Reiser M, Schneede P, Dresel S (2005) ^{18}F-FDG PET/CT for staging of penile cancer. J Nucl Med 9:1460–1465

Schoder H, Erdi YE, Larson SM, Yeung HW (2003) PET/CT: a new imaging technology in nuclear medicine. Eur J Nucl Med Mol Imaging 10:1419–1437

Schoder H, Larson SM, Yeung HW (2004) PET/CT in oncology: integration into clinical management of lymphoma, melanoma, and gastrointestinal malignancies. J Nucl Med 72S–81S

Seltzer MA, Barbaric Z, Belldegrun A, Naitoh J, Dorey F, Phelps ME, Gambhir SS, Hoh CK (1999) Comparison of helical computerized tomography, positron emission tomography and monoclonal antibody scans for evaluation of lymph node metastases in patients with prostate specific antigen relapse after treatment for localized prostate cancer. J Urol 4:1322–1328

Shreve PD, Gross MD (1997) Imaging of the pancreas and related diseases with PET carbon-11-acetate. J Nucl Med 8:1305–1310

Shreve P, Chiao PC, Humes HD, Schwaiger M, Gross MD (1995) Carbon-11-acetate PET imaging in renal disease. J Nucl Med 9:1595–1601

Singh I, Khaitan A (2003) Current trends in the management of carcinoma penis–a review. Int Urol Nephrol 2:215–225

Smith JA Jr, Scardino PT, Resnick MI, Hernandez AD, Rose SC, Egger MJ (1997) Transrectal ultrasound versus digital rectal examination for the staging of carcinoma of the prostate: results of a prospective, multi-institutional trial. J Urol 3:902–906

Sodee DB, Malguria N, Faulhaber P, Resnick MI, Albert J, Bakale G (2000) Multicenter ProstaScint imaging findings in 2154 patients with prostate cancer. The ProstaScint Imaging Centers. Urology 6:988–993

Solsona E, Iborra I, Rubio J, Casanova JL, Ricos JV, Calabuig C (2001) Prospective validation of the association of local tumor stage and grade as a predictive factor for occult lymph node micrometastasis in patients with penile carcinoma and clinically negative inguinal lymph nodes. J Urol 5:1506–1509

Stahl A, Wieder H, Wester HJ, Piert M, Lordick F, Ott K, Rummeny E, Schwaiger M, Weber WA (2004) PET/CT molecular imaging in abdominal oncology. Abdom Imaging 29:388–397

Sutinen E, Nurmi M, Roivainen A, Varpula M, Tolvanen T, Lehikoinen P, Minn H (2004) Kinetics of [(^{11})C]choline uptake in prostate cancer: a PET study. Eur J Nucl Med Mol Imaging 3:317–324

Swinnen JV, Van Veldhoven PP, Timmermans L, De Schrijver E, Brusselmans K, Vanderhoydonc F, Van de Sande

T, Heemers H, Heyns W, Verhoeven G (2003) Fatty acid synthase drives the synthesis of phospholipids partitioning into detergent-resistant membrane microdomains. Biochem Biophys Res Commun 4:898–903

Syed S, Eng TY, Thomas CR, Thompson IM, Weiss GR (2003) Current issues in the management of advanced squamous cell carcinoma of the penis. Urol Oncol 6:431–438

Tanis PJ, Lont AP, Meinhardt W, Olmos RA, Nieweg OE, Horenblas S (2002) Dynamic sentinel node biopsy for penile cancer: reliability of a staging technique. J Urol 1:76–80

Toth G, Lengyel Z, Balkay L, Salah MA, Tron L, Toth C (2005) Detection of prostate cancer with ^{11}C-methionine positron emission tomography. J Urol 1:66–69; discussion 69

Van Dorsten FA, van der Graaf M, Engelbrecht MR, van Leenders GJ, Verhofstad A, Rijpkema M, de la Rosette JJ, Barentsz JO, Heerschap A (2004) Combined quantitative dynamic contrast-enhanced MR imaging and (1)H MR spectroscopic imaging of human prostate cancer. J Magn Reson Imaging 2:279–287

Wefer AE, Hricak H, Vigneron DB, Coakley FV, Lu Y, Wefer J, Mueller-Lisse U, Carroll PR, Kurhanewicz J (2000) Sextant localization of prostate cancer: comparison of sextant biopsy, magnetic resonance imaging and magnetic resonance spectroscopic imaging with step section histology. J Urol 2:400–404

Wijkstra H, Wink MH, de la Rosette JJ (2004) Contrast specific imaging in the detection and localization of prostate cancer. World J Urol 5:346–350

Wilkinson BA, Hamdy FC (2001) State-of-the-art staging in prostate cancer. BJU Int 5:423–430

Yamaguchi T, Lee J, Uemura H, Sasaki T, Takahashi N, Oka T, Shizukuishi K, Endou H, Kubota Y, Inoue T (2005) Prostate cancer: a comparative study of (^{11})C-choline PET and MR imaging combined with proton MR spectroscopy. Eur J Nucl Med Mol Imaging 32:742–748

Yoshida S, Nakagomi K, Goto S, Futatsubashi M, Torizuka T (2005) C-choline positron emission tomography in prostate cancer: primary staging and recurrent site staging. Urol Int 3:214–220

Yoshimoto M, Waki A, Yonekura Y, Sadato N, Murata T, Omata N, Takahashi N, Welch MJ, Fujibayashi Y (2001) Characterization of acetate metabolism in tumor cells in relation to cell proliferation: acetate metabolism in tumor cells. Nucl Med Biol 2:117–122

Yu KK, Scheidler J, Hricak H, Vigneron DB, Zaloudek CJ, Males RG, Nelson SJ, Carroll PR, Kurhanewicz J (1999) Prostate cancer: prediction of extracapsular extension with endorectal MR imaging and three-dimensional proton MR spectroscopic imaging. Radiology 2:481–488

Yuen JS, Thng CH, Tan PH, Khin LW, Phee SJ, Xiao D, Lau WK, Ng WS, Cheng CW (2004) Endorectal magnetic resonance imaging and spectroscopy for the detection of tumor foci in men with prior negative transrectal ultrasound prostate biopsy. J Urol 4:1482–1486

14 Pediatric PET: Indications and Value of Multimodal Imaging

Th. Pfluger, K. Hahn, and I. Schmid

Recent Results in Cancer Research, Vol. 170
© Springer-Verlag Berlin Heidelberg 2008

Magnetic resonance imaging (MRI) and positron emission tomography (PET) are diagnostic imaging modalities that allow visualization of morphological as well as functional features of different diseases in childhood. Both modalities are often used separately or even in competition. Some of the most important indications for both PET and MRI lie in the field of pediatric oncology. The malignant diseases in children are leukemia, brain tumors, lymphomas, neuroblastoma, soft tissue sarcomas, Wilms' tumor, and bone sarcomas. Apart from leukemia, correct assessment of tumor expansion with modern imaging techniques, mainly consisting of ultrasonography, computed tomography (CT), magnetic resonance imaging (MRI), and positron emission tomography (PET), is essential for cancer staging, for the choice of the best therapeutic approach, and for restaging after therapy or in recurrence [1, 2].

14.1 Indications for MRI in Children

MRI is an excellent tool for noninvasive evaluation of tumor extent and has become the study of choice for evaluating therapy-induced regression in the size of musculoskeletal sarcomas. It directly demonstrates the lesion in relationship to surrounding normal structures with exquisite anatomical detail [3, 4].

Especially in children, MRI offers several fundamental advantages compared to computed tomography (CT) examinations and other whole-body imaging modalities, such as the absence of radiation exposure, non-use of iodinated, potential nephrotoxic contrast agents, a high intrinsic contrast for soft tissue and bone marrow, and accurate morphological visualization of internal structure, all of which are decisive factors in tumor staging [5–7]. Because of its much higher intrinsic soft tissue contrast compared to CT, MRI has been shown to be advantageous in neuroradiological, musculoskeletal, cardiac, and oncologic diseases [2, 6]. On the other hand, CT plays a major role in the assessment of thoracic lesions and masses because of a lower frequency of movement artifacts.

Since structural abnormalities are detected with high accuracy, MRI generally has a high sensitivity for detecting structural alterations, but a low specificity for further characterization of these abnormalities [8]. Frequently, these structural abnormalities are not reliable indicators of viable tumor tissue, especially after treatment [4].

T2-weighted MRI sequences visualize fluid-equivalent changes with a high sensitivity. This is of special importance in detection of cysts and edema in the diagnosis of inflammatory and tumorous diseases. High signal intensity on T1-weighted MRI sequences allows differentiation of adipose tissue and hemorrhage. Depiction of soft tissue or lesion perfusion can be achieved using paramagnetic contrast agents such as Gd-DTPA.

Modern fast and ultrafast sequences permit monitoring of contrast medium perfusion over time, which improves recognition of lesions. These rapid sequences are especially widespread in contrast-enhanced MR angiography (MRA), which provides high-resolution selective arterial and venous vascular imaging.

A further improvement in the contrast medium effect has been achieved by suppression of the signal from adipose tissue in T1-weighted sequences. These fat-suppressed contrast-enhanced sequences are currently considered state of the art in the work-up of tumors and inflammatory processes.

14.2 Necessary Components for Multimodality Imaging

Three basic components are required for multimodal imaging. First, multiple imaging modalities, often including of one nuclear medical (PET, SPECT) and one radiological (CT, MRI) cross-sectional imaging method, must be available. Second, there must be simple and prompt access to the corresponding images or image data sets. Adequate multimodal imaging requires a clinic-wide computer network, a digital archive of radiological and nuclear medical studies, multimodal image viewing workstations, and appropriate software for image correlation and fusion [9, 10]. These requirements are currently satisfied to only a limited extent in hospital departments of radiology and nuclear medicine and in private practices.

Third and probably most important is the competence of the physician in evaluating these different nuclear medical and radiological data sets. Because each individual modality can yield false-negative findings, a careful and time-consuming separate analysis of each individual modality prior to multimodal processing is essential. In combined multimodal image evaluation, there is a tendency to depend primarily on the findings of PET, which usually identifies pathological processes more rapidly. In doing so, one runs the risk of missing diagnoses that would be seen at MRI because of reliance on false-negative PET scans.

Therefore, a mainly PET-guided analysis of MRI should be avoided.

14.3 Algorithms and Accuracy of Combined Image Analysis and Image Registration

The retrospective registration and superimposition of multimodal image data can be done using different approaches and algorithms, which, in general, can be broken down into feature- and volume-based techniques. The image transformation can be static (displacement and rotation in all three spatial axes) or nonlinear (e.g., additional stretching or compression in order to compensate for respiratory movements) [11].

The classical example of a feature-based method is the surface matching or Pelizzari algorithm, which uses organ surfaces as a property [12]. This technique has two disadvantages: the requirement for a potentially quite extensive segmentation of the organ surface in the different modalities and the fact that image registration is based only on the extracted portions of the image (surface pixels).

Simply stated, volume-based techniques analyze similarities of pixel distribution in the two imaging modalities [11]. The widest current application is the mutual information algorithm in which two-dimensional grayscale histograms of the individual modalities and a combined histogram are analyzed and compared in various image transformations [13, 14]. Advantages of the volume-based techniques include the fully automatic application, their robustness compared to a different field of view, and the higher degree of precision in image registration [11].

A meta-analysis by Hutton and Braun quantified the exactness of software-based cerebral image registration at less than 3 mm [10]. For extracerebral applications, the PET and CT registration of pulmonary focal lesions showed a comparable exactness (average position of center of the lesion) of 6.2 mm for separate modalities [15] and 7.6 mm for combined PET/CT scanners [16].

14.4 Analysis and Presentation of Multimodality Images

The evaluation of multimodal imaging data consists of three stages. The first stage corresponds to the separate analysis of the multimodal data in nuclear medicine and diagnostic radiology with subsequent comparison of the reported findings. In case of discrepancies, the imaging data are re-evaluated separately with comparison of the other imaging modality. This is the currently most widely used method and it has the advantage of minimum requirements in terms of hardware and software, together with restricted logistics, time, and personnel requirements. The very great disadvantage is the lack of an exact anatomic–functional comparison of both methods. This disadvantage can be decisive in the recognition and delineation of physiological changes.

The second stage consists of simultaneous interpretation of the multimodal data sets at the same site. Although this is possible using conventional films, it is more practicable when performed at viewing workstations with PACS access. Although this method enhances the capacity for morphological correlation, because of the associated significant increase in personnel, costs, and time requirements, it is advisable to progress directly to the third stage.

In the third stage analysis of spatially synchronized image data is performed simultaneously at a single workstation (Fig. 14.1). Synchronization may be interactive or partially or fully automatic with help of a fusion algorithm [17]. These conditions provide for optimum spatial correlation of findings. Also useful is a common cursor that points to the corresponding location in both modalities, which are displayed side by side [11]. This exact synchronization of data sets with appropriate software provides the additional capacity for image fusion with superimposition of both sets of imaging data in one image. In addition, a three-dimensional reconstruction of the fused imaging data can be used for therapy planning (Fig. 14.2). When using a fused image, it is important to note that original information from the two individual imaging modalities may be partially lost, meaning that the original images of each modality should also be simultaneously displayed [11] (Fig. 14.3).

Following image analysis comes the presentation of multimodal images to one's clinical colleagues, for whom the display of the fused imaging data sets moves to the foreground. Here, image fusion and three-dimensional reconstruction often represent decisive building blocks for understanding the pathology and for further therapeutic planning (Fig. 14.2).

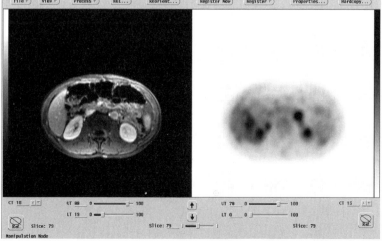

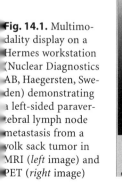

Fig. 14.1. Multimodality display on a Hermes workstation (Nuclear Diagnostics AB, Haegersten, Sweden) demonstrating a left-sided paravertebral lymph node metastasis from a yolk sack tumor in MRI (*left* image) and PET (*right* image)

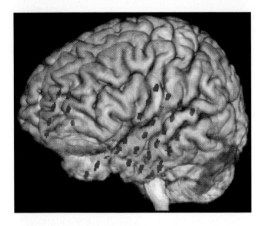

Fig. 14.2. Three-dimensional reconstruction of a registered image data set: cortical surface was rendered from MRI and red dots represent subdural EEG electrodes that were imaged with CT. The functional epileptogenic focus (*orange*) was defined by interictal FDG-PET and ictal ECD-SPECT

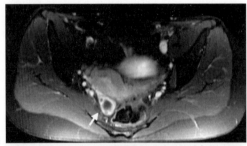

a

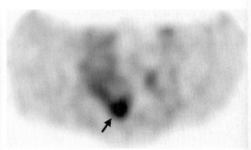

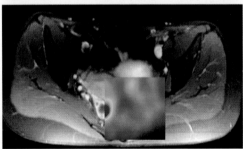

c

Fig. 14.3a–c. Histologically proven nonaffected cystic ovary in a patient with a recurrent yolk sack tumor: T1-weighted, fat-suppressed MR sequence after administration of Gd-DTPA (**a**) depicts a physiological-appearing cystic ovary (*arrow*). Corresponding PET (**b**) revealed a false-positive finding with an increased glucose uptake (*arrow*) suspicious of a recurrent disease. Multimodality display of registered images (**c**) shows exact spatial correlation between the cystic ovary in MRI and increased glucose uptake in PET

14.5 Combination of MRI and PET

In combined imaging, morphological information from MRI is complemented and extended by the functional information supplied by PET on the glucose metabolism of the respective lesions. An important advantage of FDG-PET, especially in staging malignant disease, is the capacity for examining the entire body or whole-body regions, while MRI is usually able to image only fractions of the same area during a single session (Fig. 14.4).

Most publications of clinical applications and usefulness of multimodal diagnostic imaging concern oncological imaging and multimodal diagnosis of epilepsy [7, 18–27].

The major concentration of [F-18]FDG-PET is in oncological diagnostics, where the evaluation of glucose metabolism in the tumor provides information on its viability. For this reason, PET in many cases has a higher specificity, sometimes even a higher sensitivity, than morphological imaging modalities (MRI and CT) [28–33]. Furthermore, a review

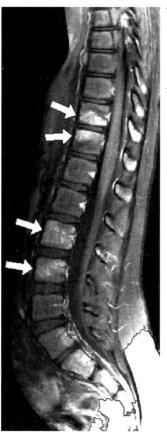

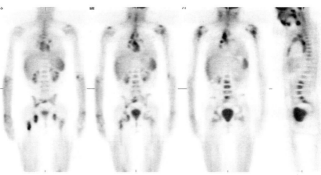

b

Fig. 14.4a,b. Non-Hodgkin lymphoma in a 12-year-old girl with back pain. MRI shows a strong contrast enhancement in vertebral bodies of the thoracic and lumbar spine (*arrows*) (**a**). A clear distinction between inflammatory and tumoral lesions was not possible. PET as a whole body examination tool shows multiple bone and mediastinal lesions with the typical distribution pattern of a malignant lymphoma (**b**)

of the literature shows PET imaging to be suitable for the majority of pediatric malignancies [1, 34–42]. Advances in these two anatomical and functional diagnostic imaging technologies have significantly influenced the staging and treatment approaches for pediatric tumors [8, 38]. The methods provide complementary information and have become essential in modern cancer therapy. Thus, anatomical and functional noninvasive technologies should be viewed as complementary rather than competitive. To identify a change in function without knowing accurately where it is localized, or equivalently, to know there is an anatomical change without understanding the nature of the underlying cause compromises the clinical efficacy of both anatomical and functional imaging techniques [8, 38, 43]. Combination of whole-body PET and state-of-the-art MRI offers accurate registration of metabolic and molecular aspects of a disease with exact correlation to anatomical findings, improving the diagnostic value of PET and MRI in identifying and characterizing malignancies and in tumor staging. PET can be used to detect areas of malignancies, tumor growth, therapeutic response and recurrence. Malignancies with low or normal metabolic activity may show clearly positive or suspicious findings on MRI [6].

In a comparative study demonstrating the potential of combined PET/MRI diagnostics in 42 pediatric examinations, sensitivity and specificity in detecting viable tumor was significantly increased with combined analysis [44]. The main reasons for false-positive PET findings when looking at suspected solitary tumor lesions in children are inflammatory or reactive changes in lymph nodes without tumor infiltration, normal bone marrow after chemotherapy, physiological FDG-uptake of the intestine, the ovary (Fig. 14.3), the ureter, and brown adipose tissue. False-negative findings in FDG-PET primarily occur in bone metastases and tumor-affected lymph nodes resulting from low glucose metabolism or small size (Fig. 14.5). One reason is the limited spatial resolution of PET leading to false-negative findings in very small lesions [45]. Under chemotherapy, active bone metastases may temporarily become PET-negative (Table 14.1) [35].

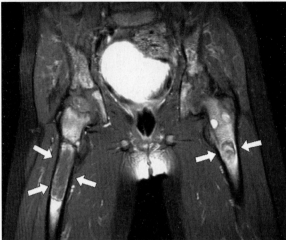

a

Fig. 14.5a,b. Histologically proven metastases of a Ewing sarcoma in the proximal femoral bone on both sides: T1-weighted fat-suppressed MR sequence shows hypointense lesions within the bone (*arrows*) (**a**). Corresponding PET revealed a false-negative finding with no signs of a metastatic spread in both femoral bones (**b**)

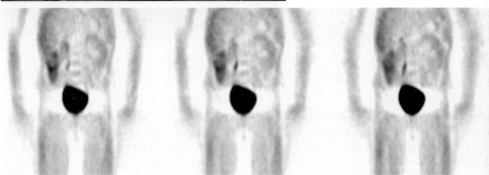

b

Table 14.1. Possible sources for false-positive and false-negative findings in MRI and FDG-PET

False positive: PET	Brown adipose tissue, physiological uptake in the muscles, bowel, ureter, and ovary, inflammatory changes (i.e., in lymph nodes), normal bone marrow after chemotherapy
False positive: MRI	Posttherapeutic changes (i.e., persisting bone marrow edema in treated metastases), enlarged lymph nodes without tumor involvement
False negative: PET	Metastases with a small size and/or low glucose metabolism, tumor lesions under chemotherapy
False negative: MRI	Small lymph node and bone metastases, lesions in the neighborhood of the bowel

In MRI, the main reasons for false-positive findings are enlarged lymph nodes and bone marrow edema without tumor involvement. On the other hand, small bone and lymph node metastases can be responsible for false-negative findings. Tumor lesions adjacent to normal bowel structures quite often cannot be distinguished from the bowel and consequently cannot be detected with MRI (Fig. 14.6). In the diagnosis of lymph nodes, a diameter of more than 1 cm is the leading parameter for the diagnosis of a metastasis. Therefore, lymph node metastases below this size and reactive lymph node enlargement are misinterpreted. Lesion size is not a reliable parameter for metastatic involvement [46]. After successful tumor therapy, bone marrow edema often persists for a long time in MRI and may be responsible for false-positive findings. In

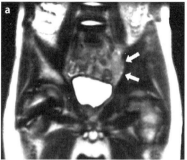
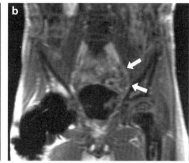
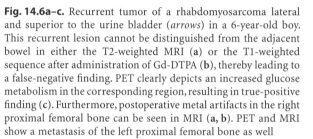
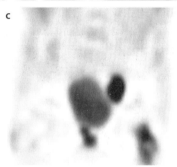

Fig. 14.6a–c. Recurrent tumor of a rhabdomyosarcoma lateral and superior to the urine bladder (*arrows*) in a 6-year-old boy. This recurrent lesion cannot be distinguished from the adjacent bowel in either the T2-weighted MRI (**a**) or the T1-weighted sequence after administration of Gd-DTPA (**b**), thereby leading to a false-negative finding. PET clearly depicts an increased glucose metabolism in the corresponding region, resulting in true-positive finding (**c**). Furthermore, postoperative metal artifacts in the right proximal femoral bone can be seen in MRI (**a, b**). PET and MRI show a metastasis of the left proximal femoral bone as well

summary, MRI is highly sensitive but not very specific (Table 14.1) [35, 45, 47, 48].

When combining FDG-PET and MRI in pediatric oncology, PET as a whole-body imaging tool plays a major role in assessing MRI-positive lesions. The most important benefit of MRI is to distinguish PET-positive tumor lesions from physiologically increased glucose uptake. In addition, MRI is indispensable for surgical and biopsy planning (Fig. 14.7). Combination of PET and MRI improves the respective diagnostic values of PET and MRI in identifying and characterizing tumor tissue [4, 6, 49].

PET is also used in the work-up of inflammatory disease, though far less frequently than for oncological indications. It is the method of choice in the search for a focus of inflammation in a patient with fever of unknown origin and/or unclear sepsis [50–54]. Lesions detected with PET can be further delineated with MRI, which may also be useful for further therapy planning.

[F-18]FDG-PET is also very useful in the presurgical focus localization in the work-up of epilepsy. An exact integration of the findings of morphological, electrophysiological, and nuclear medical examinations is of great importance in planning surgical procedures for the treatment of epilepsy and determining the borders of resection, again underscoring the role of integrative diagnostics [55, 56].

In these patients, functional diagnostic methods include EEG and nuclear medical methods for visualizing cerebral metabolism and perfusion. Frequently, ictal Tc-99m ECD-SPECT is combined interictal FDG-PET, which permits more exact identification of the seizure focus with typical hypometabolism seen on PET [57–60]. Besides conventional EEG leads, subdural electrodes may be implanted prior to the actual surgical procedure for direct measurement of the EEG signal from the cortical surface. These subdural electrodes can also be used for cortical stimulation. This permits delineation of functionally important areas that must be protected during a resective procedure. Knowledge of the exact position of the individual electrode points is important for demarcation of the resection boundaries. Because only CT can visualize these electrode points with sufficient accuracy, integration of CT information into the combined PET-MRI analysis is also necessary [56]. Demarcation of resection boundaries therefore requires integration of all four described modalities: MRI for brain morphology, CT to establish the position of the subdural EEG electrodes, PET for visualization of brain metabolism, and SPECT for visualization of hyperperfusion. This is best achieved with three-dimensional image fusion, which permits exact spatial integration (Fig. 14.2). Here, registration of images is possible within 1.5 mm, which is adequate for clinical application [61]. This method has also been shown to be superior to localization of electrodes using a conventional radiograph [56]. The resulting reconstructed three-dimensional data set provides the neurosurgeon with the information needed for exact preoperative planning, including functional information on the focus of the seizure and important (especially language-related) brain areas, which must be protected during resection.

In conclusion, it is important to emphasize that MRI and PET are not competing modalities. Instead, these two methods in combination can produce a synergy between function and morphology. For planning biopsies and resective surgery, the knowledge of function (i.e.,

tumor viability) provided by PET and of the exact morphology of the tumor provided by MRI is often crucial. In patients with cerebral lesions, the whole spectrum of digital image fusion with direct superimposition of several modalities with subsequent three-dimensional reconstruction should be applied. This provides the surgeon with the tools for exact planning of approach and resection boundaries.

Direct image superimposition is not necessary for extracranial questions because information from individual modalities may be partially lost during fusion. The simultaneous evaluation of both modalities should be emphasized. Synchronized evaluation of corresponding slices from both modalities displayed at a single workstation is very useful. This is the most reliable method of immediately and efficiently correlating pathological and especially unclear findings with the corresponding slice on the other imaging method.

Because of MRI's low specificity in oncological staging and at follow-up monitoring, the addition of PET for evaluating tumor vitality is essential.

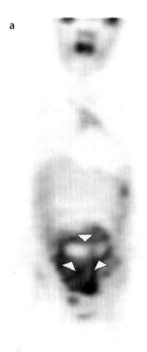

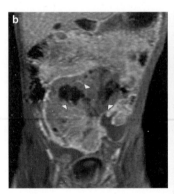

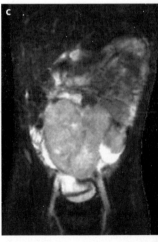

Fig. 14.7a–c. Rhabdomyosarcoma of the lower abdomen in a 6-year-old boy. FDG-PET demonstrates a large area with increased glucose uptake correlating with the primary tumor and a central photopenic defect (*arrowheads*) (**a**). This photopenic defect correlates well with central necrosis visible in the T1-weighted, contrast-enhanced MR sequence (*arrowheads*) (**b**). For operative planning, T2-weighted STIR sequence is necessary for the delineation of tumor borders and course of vessels (**c**)

References

1. Connolly LP, Drubach LA, Ted Treves S (2002) Applications of nuclear medicine in pediatric oncology. Clin Nucl Med 27:117–125

2. Schmidt GP, Baur-Melnyk A, Tiling R, Hahn K, Reiser MF, Schoenberg SO (2004) Comparison of high resolution whole-body MRI using parallel imaging and PET-CT. First experiences with a 32-channel MRI system. Radiologe 44:889–898

3. Bloem JL, van der Woude HJ, Geirnaerdt M, Hogendoorn PC, Taminiau AH, Hermans J (1997) Does magnetic resonance imaging make a difference for patients with musculoskeletal sarcoma? Br J Radiol 70:327–337

4. Bredella MA, Caputo GR, Steinbach LS (2002) Value of FDG positron emission tomography in conjunction with MR imaging for evaluating therapy response in patients with musculoskeletal sarcomas. AJR Am J Roentgenol 179:1145–1150

5. Antoch G, Vogt FM, Bockisch A, Ruehm SG (2004) Whole-body tumor staging: MRI or FDG-PET/CT? Radiologe 44:882–888

6. Gaa J, Rummeny EJ, Seemann MD (2004) Whole-body imaging with PET/MRI. Eur J Med Res 9:309–312

7. Pfluger T, Schmied C, Porn U, Leinsinger G, Vollmar C, Dresel S, Schmid I, Hahn K (2003) Integrated imaging using MRI and 123I metaiodobenzylguanidine scintigraphy to improve sensitivity and specificity in the diagnosis of pediatric neuroblastoma. AJR Am J Roentgenol 181:1115–1124

8. Czernin J (2002) Clinical applications of FDG-PET in oncology. Acta Med Austriaca 29:162–170

9. Alyafei S, Inoue T, Zhang H, Ahmed K, Oriuchi N, Sato N, Suzuki H, Endo K (1999) Image fusion system using PACS for MRI, CT, and PET images. Clin Positron Imaging 2:137–143

10. Hutton BF, Braun M (2003) Software for image registration: algorithms, accuracy, efficacy. Semin Nucl Med 33:180–192

11. Slomka PJ (2004) Software approach to merging molecular with anatomic information. J Nucl Med 45 [Suppl 1]:36S–45S

12. Pelizzari CA, Chen GT, Spelbring DR, Weichselbaum RR, Chen CT (1989) Accurate three-dimensional registration of CT, PET, and/or MR images of the brain. J Comput Assist Tomogr 13:20–26

13. Maes F, Collignon A, Vandermeulen D, Marchal G, Suetens P (1997) Multimodality image registration by maximization of mutual information. IEEE Trans Med Imaging 16:187–198

14. Wells WM 3rd, Viola P, Atsumi H, Nakajima S, Kikinis R (1996) Multi-modal volume registration by maximization of mutual information. Med Image Anal 1:35–51

15. Skalski J, Wahl RL, Meyer CR (2002) Comparison of mutual information-based warping accuracy for fusing body CT and PET by 2 methods: CT mapped onto PET emission scan versus CT mapped onto PET transmission scan. J Nucl Med 43:1184–1187

16. Cohade C, Osman M, Marshall LN, Wahl RN (2003) PET-CT: accuracy of PET and CT spatial registration of lung lesions. Eur J Nucl Med Mol Imaging 30:721–726

17. Stokking R, Zubal IG, Viergever MA (2003) Display of fused images: methods, interpretation, and diagnostic improvements. Semin Nucl Med 33:219–227

18. Aquino SL, Asmuth JC, Alpert NM, Halpern EF, Fischman AJ (2003) Improved radiologic staging of lung cancer with 2-[^{18}F]-fluoro-2-deoxy-D-glucose-positron emission tomography and computed tomography registration. J Comput Assist Tomogr 27:479–484

19. Cohade C, Wahl RL (2003) Applications of positron emission tomography/computed tomography image fusion in clinical positron emission tomography-clinical use, interpretation methods, diagnostic improvements. Semin Nucl Med 33:228–237

20. Coleman RE, Hawk TC, Hamblen SM, Cnmt, Laymon CM, Turkington TG (1999) Detection of recurrent brain tumor. Comparison of MR registered camera-based and dedicated PET images. Clin Positron Imaging 2:57–61

21. Dresel S, Grammerstorff J, Schwenzer K, Brinkbaumer K, Schmid R, Pfluger T, Hahn K (2003) [18F]FDG imaging of head and neck tumours: comparison of hybrid PET and morphological methods. Eur J Nucl Med Mol Imaging 30:995–1003

22. Keidar Z, Israel O, Krausz Y (2003) SPECT/CT in tumor imaging: technical aspects and clinical applications. Semin Nucl Med 33:205–218

23. Murphy M, O'Brien TJ, Morris K, Cook MJ (2001) Multimodality image-guided epilepsy surgery. J Clin Neurosci 8:534–538

24. So EL (2002) Role of neuroimaging in the management of seizure disorders. Mayo Clin Proc 77:1251–1264

25. Tsai CC, Tsai CS, Ng KK, Lai CH, Hsueh S, Kao PF, Chang TC, Hong JH, Yen TC (2003) The impact of image fusion in resolving discrepant findings between FDG-PET and MRI/CT in patients with gynaecological cancers. Eur J Nucl Med Mol Imaging 30:1674–1683

26. Visvikis D, Ell PJ (2003) Impact of technology on the utilisation of positron emission tomography in lymphoma: current and future perspectives. Eur J Nucl Med Mol Imaging 30 [Suppl 1]: S106–S116

27. Zhang W, Simos PG, Ishibashi H, Wheless JW, Castillo EM, Kim HL, Baumgartner JE, Sarkari S, Papanicolaou AC (2003) Multimodality neuroimaging evaluation improves the detection of subtle cortical dysplasia in seizure patients. Neurol Res 25:53–57

28. Anderson H, Price P (2000) What does positron emission tomography offer oncology? Eur J Cancer 36:2028–2035

29. Bar-Shalom R, Valdivia AY, Blaufox MD (2000) PET imaging in oncology. Semin Nucl Med 30:150–185

30. Czech N, Brenner W, Kampen WU, Henze E (2000) Diagnostic value of positron emission tomography (PET) in clinical oncology. Dtsch Med Wochenschr 125:565–567

31. Delbeke D, Martin WH (2001) Positron emission tomography imaging in oncology. Radiol Clin North Am 39:883–917

32. Mankoff DA, Bellon JR (2001) Positron-emission tomographic imaging of cancer: glucose metabolism and beyond. Semin Radiat Oncol 11:16–27

33. Scott AM (2001) Current status of positron emission tomography in oncology. Intern Med J 31:27–36

34. Brisse H, Ollivier L, Edeline V, Pacquement H, Michon J, Glorion C, Neuenschwander S (2004) Imaging of malignant tumours of the long bones in children: monitoring response to neoadjuvant chemotherapy and preoperative assessment. Pediatr Radiol 34:595–605

35. Daldrup-Link HE, Franzius C, Link TM, Laukamp D, Sciuk J, Jurgens H, Schober O, Rummeny EJ (2001) Whole-body MR imaging for detection of bone metastases in children and young adults: comparison with skeletal scintigraphy and FDG PET. AJR Am J Roentgenol 177:229–236

36. Franzius C, Daldrup-Link HE, Wagner-Bohn A, Sciuk J, Heindel WL, Jurgens H, Schober O (2002) FDG-PET for detection of recurrences from malignant primary bone tumors: comparison with conventional imaging. Ann Oncol 13:157–160

37. Hawkins DS, Rajendran JG, Conrad EU 3rd, Bruckner JD, Eary JF (2002) Evaluation of chemotherapy response in pediatric bone sarcomas by [F-18]-fluorodeoxy-D-glucose positron emission tomography. Cancer 94:3277–3284

38. Hudson MM, Krasin MJ, Kaste SC (2004) PET imaging in pediatric Hodgkin's lymphoma. Pediatr Radiol 34:190–198

39. Montravers F, McNamara D, Landman-Parker J, Grahek D, Kerrou K, Younsi N, Wioland M, Leverger G, Talbot JN (2002) [(^{18})F]FDG in childhood lymphoma: clinical utility and impact on management. Eur J Nucl Med Mol Imaging 29:1155–1165

40. O'Hara SM, Donnelly LF, Coleman RE (1999) Pediatric body applications of FDG PET. AJR Am J Roentgenol 172:1019–1024

41. Shulkin BL (2004) PET imaging in pediatric oncology. Pediatr Radiol 34:199–204

42. Shulkin BL, Mitchell DS, Ungar DR, Prakash D, Dole MG, Castle VP, Hernandez RJ, Koeppe RA, Hutchinson RJ (1995) Neoplasms in a pediatric population:2-[F-18]-fluoro-2-deoxy-D-glucose PET studies. Radiology 194:495–500

43. Townsend DW, Cherry SR (2001) Combining anatomy and function: the path to true image fusion. Eur Radiol 11:1968–1974

44. Pfluger T, Vollmar C, Porn U, Schmid R, Dresel S, Leinsinger G, Schmid I, Winkler P, Fischer S, Hahn K (2002) Combined PET/MRI in cerebral and pediatric diagnostics. Der Nuklearmediziner 25:122–127

45. Hueltenschmidt B, Sautter-Bihl ML, Lang O, Maul FD, Fischer J, Mergenthaler HG, Bihl H (2001) Whole body positron emission tomography in the treatment of Hodgkin disease. Cancer 91:302–310

46. Torabi M, Aquino SL, Harisinghani MG (2004) Current concepts in lymph node imaging. J Nucl Med 45:1509–1518

47. Ilias I, Pacak K (2004) Current approaches and recommended algorithm for the diagnostic localization of pheochromocytoma. J Clin Endocrinol Metab 89:479–491

48. Korholz D, Kluge R, Wickmann L, Hirsch W, Luders H, Lotz I, Dannenberg C, Hasenclever D, Dorffel W, Sabri O (2003) Importance of F18-fluorodeoxy-D-2-glucose positron emission tomography (FDG-PET) for staging and therapy control of Hodgkin's lymphoma in childhood and adolescence – consequences for the GPOH-HD 2003 protocol. Onkologie 26:489–493

49. Popperl G, Lang S, Dagdelen O, Jager L, Tiling R, Hahn K, Tatsch K (2002) Correlation of FDG-PET and MRI/CT with histopathology in primary diagnosis, lymph node staging and diagnosis of recurrence of head and neck cancer. ROFO 174:714–120

50. Blockmans D, Knockaert D, Maes A, De Caestecker J, Stroobants S, Bobbaers H, Mortelmans L (2001) Clinical value of [(^{18})F]fluoro-deoxyglucose positron emission tomography for patients with fever of unknown origin. Clin Infect Dis 32:191–196

51. Kapucu LO, Meltzer CC, Townsend DW, Keenan RJ, Luketich JD (1998) Fluorine-18-fluorodeoxyglucose uptake in pneumonia. J Nucl Med 39:1267–1269

52. Kresnik E, Mikosch P, Gallowitsch HJ, Heinisch M, Lind P (2001) F-18 fluorodeoxyglucose positron emission tomography in the diagnosis of inflammatory bowel disease. Clin Nucl Med 26:867

53. Meller J, Becker W (2001) Nuclear medicine diagnosis of patients with fever of unknown origin (FUO). Nuklearmedizin 40:59–70

54. Weiner GM, Jenicke L, Buchert R, Bohuslavizki KH (2001) FDG PET for the localization diagnosis in inflammatory disease of unknown origin–two case reports. Nuklearmedizin 40:N35–N38

55. Barnett GH, Kormos DW, Steiner CP, Morris H (1993) Registration of EEG electrodes with three-dimensional neuroimaging using a frameless, armless stereotactic wand. Stereotact Funct Neurosurg 61:32–38

56. Winkler PA, Vollmar C, Krishnan KG, Pfluger T, Brückmann H, Noachtar S (2000) Usefulness of 3-D reconstructed images of the human cerebral cortex for localization of subdural electrodes in epilepsy surgery. Epilepsy Res 41:169–178

57. Carreras JL, Perez-Castejon MJ, Jimenez AM, Domper M, Montz R (2000) Neuroimaging in epilepsy. Advances in SPECT and PET in epilepsy. Rev Neurol 30:359–363

58. Matheja P, Kuwert T, Stodieck SR, Diehl B, Wolf K, Schuierer G, Ringelstein EB, Schober O (1998)

PET and SPECT in medically non-refractory complex partial seizures. Temporal asymmetries of glucose consumption, benzodiazepine receptor density, and blood flow. Nuklearmedizin 37:221–226

59. Noachtar S, Arnold S, Yousry TA, Bartenstein P, Werhahn KJ, Tatsch K (1998) Ictal technetium-99m ethyl cysteinate dimer single-photon emission tomographic findings and propagation of epileptic seizure activity in patients with extratemporal epilepsies. Eur J Nucl Med 25:166–172

60. Oliveira AJ, da Costa JC, Hilario LN, Anselmi OE, Palmini A (1999) Localization of the epileptogenic zone by ictal and interictal SPECT with ^{99m}Tc-ethyl cysteinate dimer in patients with medically refractory epilepsy. Epilepsia 40:693–702

61. Pfluger T, Vollmar C, Wismuller A, Dresel S, Berger F, Suntheim P, Leinsinger G, Hahn K (2000) Quantitative comparison of automatic and interactive methods for MRI-SPECT image registration of the brain based on 3-dimensional calculation of error. J Nucl Med 41:1823–1829

15 Cancer of Unknown Primary

L. S. Freudenberg, S. J. Rosenbaum-Krumme, A. Bockisch, W. Eberhardt, and A. Frilling

Recent Results in Cancer Research, Vol. 170
© Springer-Verlag Berlin Heidelberg 2008

15.1 Introduction

Cancer of unknown primary (CUP) is defined as malignancy without known origin at the time of the initial diagnosis, thus representing a heterogeneous group of tumors with varying clinical features. Between 0.5% and 7% of all cancer patients are diagnosed with cancer of an unknown primary tumor (van de Wous et al. 2002). Detected primary revealed lung cancer most often, followed by oropharynx carcinoma, nasopharynx, breast, colorectal, and esophagus carcinoma (Delgado-Bolton et al. 2003). Overall the primary tumor in CUP patients is detected in less than 40% of the patients by conventional diagnostic procedures, frequently after having performed many examinations in all patients. Moreover, even with autopsy the primary could only be detected in approximately 50%. Hypothesized reasons are a metastatic phenotype with a small size of the primary due to involution during the course of disease or an extremely slow growth rate, but none of the biological hypotheses is confirmed by results from the literature (Van de Wouw et al. 2003). As in many cases, patients present with obvious metastatic disease, in which the location of the primary lesion may never be found, the inability to do so prevents the optimization of therapeutic strategies, which is dependent on tumor differentiation, tumor location, and tumor stage as determined according to the TNM system (Greene 2002). Consequently, prognosis of CUP is generally unfavorable, with average survival of only a few months and an overall survival at 3 and 5 years of 11% and 6%, respectively (Abbruzzese et al. 1994; Daugaard et al. 1994).

The most frequent sites for metastatic disease from cancer of an unknown primary tumor are the lymph nodes of the supraclavicular and cervical regions. A meta-analysis conducted by Delgado Bolton et al. (2003) demonstrated that metastases of CUP are most often seen in cervical and supraclavicular lymph nodes, less frequently in the brain and bone with a histopathology of squamous cell carcinoma, adenocarcinoma, and undifferentiated carcinoma with descending frequency.

The diagnosis of CUP will trigger a comprehensive diagnostic work-up. Depending on histopathological analysis and in some cases tumor marker determination, the standard work-up of CUP is to some degree dependent on the spectrum of potential primaries. Primarily diagnostic procedures include general available and relatively inexpensive modalities such as ultrasonography, endoscopy, and CT. Unfortunately these morphologic imaging tools are burdened with low sensitivities and specificity: for example, CT-based diagnostic work-up of CUP patients has been shown to be rather limited in the identification of primary tumor sites in CUP patients, with sensitivities of less than 33% and a specificity of 65% (Rades et al. 2001b; Regelink et al. 2002; Di Martino 2000). In this context, MRI is gains clinical importance due to introduction of whole-body scanning, for example using a rolling table platform capable of moving the patient rapidly through the isocenter of the magnet bore (Lauenstein et al. 2004; Antoch et al. 2003). However, all these examinations are often inconclusive and generate discomfort for the patient. Furthermore, the individual diagnosis may add up to considerable costs and consume a great deal of time (Daugaard et al 1994). That is why a single diagnostic tool reaching the diagnosis quickly is desirable. As by definition the site of the primary tumor is unknown, the whole body needs to be investigated or at least a combination of areas under increased risk. In this situation, a high sensitivity is necessary, as the identification of the primary is essential for the course of the disease. On the other hand, limited specificity will end up with an unacceptably high number of false-positive findings and consequently unnecessary interventions.

In conclusion, CUP work-up requires a specific diagnostic procedure that sensitively screens the whole body – or at least the abdomen and thorax – or depending on the suspected site of the primary, also head and neck.

15.2   FDG-PET in CUP

Oncological positron emission tomography (PET) is based on the principles discovered by Warburg and co-workers (1930), i.e., tumors are hypermetabolic and may be distinguished from nonmalignant tissue by their elevated glucose metabolism. By means of radioactively labeled [^{18}F]-2-fluoro-2-deoxy-D-glucose (FDG), PET is able to image and quantify glucose metabolism in vivo (Engel et al. 1996; Lindholm et al. 1993). FDG is metabolized by the tumor cell but accumulates within the cell, as the hexokinase cannot process FDG. Thus FDG is an unspecific probe for detecting malignant tumor, the intensity of the FDG accumulation, and therefore the tumor/background ratio correlates positively with the power consumption of the tumor. High power consuming tumors that are likely to be more aggressive are detected with greater sensitivity. The average sensitivity of FDG-PET in oncological evalu-

ations is estimated at 84% (419 studies with 18,402 PET examinations) and the specificity at 88% (14,264 PET examinations) (Gambhir et al. 2001). The advantages of FDG-PET in comparison to conventional imaging methods are particularly evident in small growth and displacements, for example lymph nodes smaller than 1 cm, whole-body staging, and the differentiation of malignant and benign tissue (Knapp 1999; Reske et al. 2001).

Against this background, it is not surprising to find FDG-PET being the most efficient method capable of localizing unknown primary tumors in CUP to date. However, depending on the tumor entity, and the individual aggressiveness, a varying fraction of non-FDG-consuming tumors that are invisible in FDG-PET has to be expected. Therefore, in CUP the value of FDG-PET has to be judged depending on the expected primary. FDG-PET is especially sensitive in lymphoma, lung cancer, gastrointestinal tumors, malignant melanoma, and head and neck tumors.

Detection rates ranging from 19% to 100%, with a mean detection rate of 46.7%, have been described in the literature, as summarized in Table 15.1. Similarly, a meta-analysis by Gambhir and co-workers (2001) revealed an average FDG-PET sensitivity in CUP, with sensitivity and specificity 82% and 71% compared to CT with 33% and 64%, respectively. Another meta-analysis carried out by Delgado-Bolton et al. (2003) reported a detection rate of 43% (range, 8%–65%) and a sensitivity of 87% (range, 50%–100%) for FDG-PET based on 15 studies. These highly variable detection rates depend on the preselected patient populations. As until now, no consensus has been established on how routine clinical work-up should be done in patients with CUP, there is no standardization. This explains the reported differences in the accuracy for FDG-PET applied to the search for the primary tumor site. However, most studies claim that FDG-PET detects the primary tumor in 30%–60% of patients with negative results in the conventional diagnostic procedures (Fig. 15.1). If the primary is not located by FDG-PET, it is usually not detected in further follow-up because of the high sensitivity and specificity of FDG-PET in general (Lonneux et al. 2000).

Table 15.1 Sensitivity and specificity of FDG-PET in detection of CUP

Authors	Patients	FDG-PET			
	(n)	Sens. (%)	Spec. (%)	PPV (%)	NNV (%)
Schneider et al. 2006a	47	19	–	–	–
Pelosi et al. 2006	68	35	–	–	–
Schneider et al. 2006b	84	33	–	85	–
Scott et al. 2005	31	26	–	73	–
Freudenberg et al. 2005	21	57	–	–	–
Gutzeit et al. 2005	45	33	–	82	–
Nanni et al. 2005	21	57	–	–	–
Kolesnikov-Gauthier et al. 2004	24	25	–	55	–
Alberini et al. 2004	41	63	–	–	–
Mantaka et al. 2003	25	100	61	–	–
Johanson et al. 2002	42	24	–	–	–
Rades et al. 2001a	42	43	–	69	–
Rades et al. 2001b	52	40	–	67	–
Bohuslavizki et al. 2000	53	100	81	77	100
Lassen et al. 1999	20	–	–	69	–
Safa et al. 1999	14	75	80	60	89
Hanasono et al. 1999	20	70	60	64	67
Gerven et al. 1999	13	50	45	14	83
AAssar et al. 1999	15	100	63	70	100
Kole et al. 1998	29	70	–	–	–
Braams et al. 1997	13	80	–	–	–
Kole et al. 1995	19	67	–	–	–
Hubner et al. 1995	24	100	67	90	100
Summary	**808**	**46.7**	**80.5**	**69.6**	**92.6**

Sens, sensitivity; *Spec,* specificity; *PPV,* positive predictive value; *NNV,* negative predictive value

In patients with cervical CUP (Fig. 15.2), the primary detection rate is lower compared to other CUP patients. In a meta-analysis, Nieder t al. (2001) reported a tumor detection rate of 9%–25% with FDG-PET alone. Johanson et al. 2002) found a tumor detection rate of 24% in their study cohort of 42 patients with metastatic neck lesions of unknown primary site. These differences might to some degree be explained by difficulties when differentiating physiological FDG uptake from pathology in the head and neck area (Paulus et al. 1998).

Nevertheless, it must be emphasized that FDG-PET is superior to other imaging modalities in CUP patients. Given its diagnostic performance, the recommendation of several groups to employ FDG-PET as the imaging modality of choice in the diagnostic work-up of CUP patients is justified (Schieper et al. 1998). Consequently, the German Interdisciplinary Consensus conference on FDG-PET graded CUP primary diagnostics as a FDG-PET indication 1a, whereas Grade 1a indicates scientifically proven benefit and established clinical use (Reske et al. 2001).

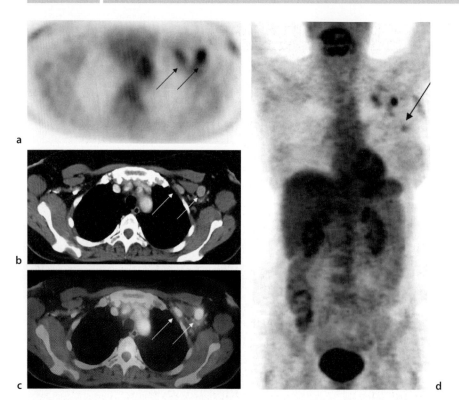

Fig. 15.1a–d. Female patient with history of palpable enlarged axillary lymph nodes whose histology revealed cancer of unknown primary. **a–c** Axial slices of the axillary area; **a** FDG-PET; **b** CT; **c** FDG-PET/CT. FDG-PET suspected breast cancer as primary, showing in addition pathologic FDG accumulation in the left axillary lymph nodes, accumulation in the left mamma (see *arrow* in the projection image **d** and corresponding axial slices of PET, CT, and PET/CT). Histology proved breast cancer, allowing adequate cancer therapy

15.3   Combined FDG-PET/CT

Although FDG-PET is a powerful tool in clinical oncology, one problem with the interpretation of PET data is the precise anatomical allocation of tracer enhancement due to often insufficient contrasting of anatomical structures in the PET image (Beyer et al. 2004). This, in turn, limits localization accuracy, which is important for targeted therapy. In diagnostic oncological imaging, however, precise anatomical allocation is especially important for planning surgical interventions or biopsy (Adams et al. 1998). As a consequence, visual correlation of CT and FDG-PET improves interpretation of both data sets in general (Büll et al. 2004; Reinartz et al. 2004). For image co-registration computer-assisted support appears helpful. However, in clinical routine acceptance of retrospective image fusion may be limited due to the complexity of retrospective co-registration algorithms and their limited accuracy for aligning areas of interest in independently acquired scans. Especially in the thorax and upper abdomen, nonlinear registration techniques are required to account for complex patient motion (Hutton et al. 2003). Most of these computer algorithms are only applicable to individual organs or limited whole-body areas. Due to the level of control necessary for the user, these algorithms are not suitable for obtaining maximum clinical throughput. The optimal solution for aligning functional and anatomical information across extended areas

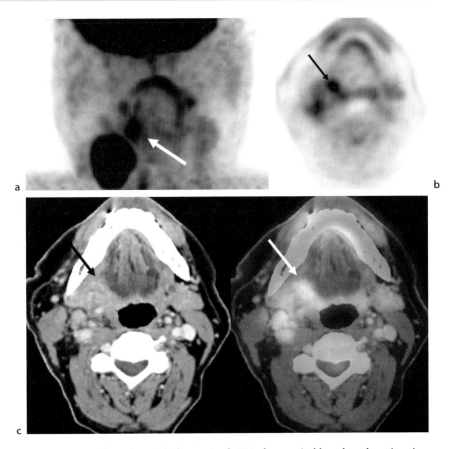

Fig. 15.2a–c. Male patient with diagnosis of CUP after cervical lymph node extirpation. FDG-PET/CT implemented to find the primary shows pathologic FDG accumulation oropharyngeal on the right side without definite corresponding lesion in the CT (see *arrow* in the projection image and corresponding axial slices of PET, CT, and PET/CT). In addition, further pathologic FDG accumulation is seen right cervical in terms of vital lymph node metastases. Hypopharyngeal cancer was diagnosed after PET/CT imaging and was proven by histology. Whole-body PET/CT revealed no additional distant metastases

(whole-body examination) in clinical routine is the simultaneous acquisition of functional (PET) and anatomical (CT) information using a single device, without the patient getting off the bed between scans. It has recently been shown that PET/CT is significantly more accurate in staging different malignant diseases compared with CT alone, PET alone, and side-by-side PET and CT (Antoch et al. 2004b).

Since PET/CT imaging systems providing accurately fused functional and morphological data in a single session became available in 2001, several studies have addressed the impact of FDG-PET/CT for detection of the primary tumor in patients with CUP. Two groups reported initial results of primary tumor detection in heterogeneous patient groups with cervical and extracervical metastases of unknown primary tumors (Gutzeit et al. 2005; Nanni et al. 2005). The tumor detection rate in the study reported by Gutzeit and co-workers (2005) was 33%, whereas the detection rate was 57% in the study reported by Nanni et al. (2005). It seems difficult to compare the results of these two studies and with our current results because of differences in study populations. For example, the study cohort of Nanni et al. (2005) included six patients with cervical metastases, whereas the cohort of Gutzeit et al. (2005) comprised 18 patients with cervical tumor spread (Fig. 15.3). Because of major differences between both tumor locations – cervical CUP and extracervical CUP – it seems difficult to compare the two tumor entities. Taking only the subgroup of cervical CUP patients from the study, the tumor detection rate was 32%. In another cohort from the same group, a tumor detection rate of 57% was reported in a patient population of 21 patients with cervical CUP using combined PET/CT (Freudenberg et al. 2005). This higher detection rate can be explained by different inclusion criteria, as patients were included who had not undergone blind biopsies of the nasopharynx, the tonsils and the base of the tongue.

Comparing results of FDG-PET/CT with FDG-PET alone or FDG-PET and CT read side-by-side, it was shown in all studies that FDG-PET/CT enhanced the diagnostic power with regard to the number of true-positive and false-positive findings due to exact ana-

tomical landmarks, suggesting an additional benefit compared to FDG-PET and CT read side by side. Furthermore, the simultaneous availability of CT data helped to reduce the number of false-positive FDG-PET findings. However, none of the studies showed a statistically significant improvement of diagnostic power compared to FDG-PET and CT read side by side. Nevertheless, in the authors view overall FDG-PET/CT seems to be advantageous for optimized primary tumor detection in CUP as well as for the guidance of any subsequent surgical intervention. To gain as much information as possible, interpretation of PET/CT should therefore be read by specialists in nuclear medicine and radiology.

Further studies will have to evaluate the exact impact of integrated FDG-PET/CT vs software fusion of the two modalities, keeping in mind that misregistration is not totally avoidable even with a combined PET/CT scanner especially in the thorax and upper abdomen (Beyer et al. 2004; Cohade et al. 2003). Finally the actual impact of more accurate tumor stag-

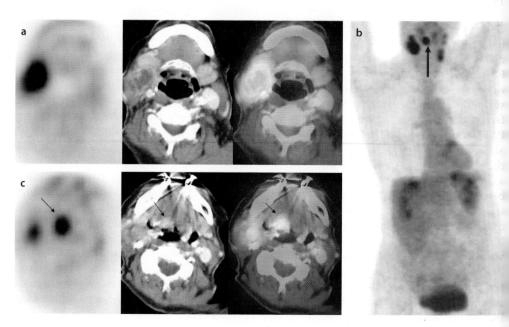

Fig. 15.3a–c Patient with right-side cervical swelling. Biopsy of the swelling (a) revealed CUP. In addition to pathologic FDG accumulation in the right cervical swelling, FDG-PET/CT shows pathologic accumulation in contralateral lymph nodes and in the oropharynx (see arrow in the projection image, **b**, and the corresponding axial slices of PET, CT, and PET/CT, **c**). Consequently, suspected oropharyngeal cancer was biopsy-proven

ing – beyond therapeutic decision making – on patient survival, will have to be determined in future studies.

15.3.1 Optimized PET/CT Protocol

Besides several advantages of PET/CT, one has to be aware of drawbacks such as artifacts of beam-hardening due to bones or metallic implants (Goerres et al. 2002a). Furthermore, local misregistration between the CT and the PET in integrated PET/CT and the use of CT contrast media may bias the PET tracer distribution following CT-based attenuation correction (Antoch et al. 2002). Consequently, protocol requirements for PET/CT with diagnostic CT also include special breathing protocols and alternative contrast application schemes to handle CT contrast agents appropriately. Using an optimized acquisition protocol significantly improves integrated PET/CT imaging and thus can further improve staging of CUP.

15.3.1.1 Breathing

Co-registration accuracy in combined PET/CT imaging is mainly impaired by respiration-induced mismatches between the CT and the PET. These artifacts are particularly severe when standard breath-hold techniques (e.g., scanning at maximum inspiration) are transferred directly from clinical CT to combined PET/CT without further adaptation (Beyer et al. 2004). Goerres et al. (2003) investigating the misregistration of pulmonary lesions with a combined PET/CT system found mismatches between PET and CT to be greatest when CT was performed during maximal inspiration of the patient, then ranging from 5 to 33 mm (Goerres et al. 2002b, 2003). Combined PET/CT scans during normal respiration show artifacts in the majority of cases as well. To reduce potential misregistration from differences in the breathing pattern between two complementary PET and CT data sets, our protocol uses a limited breath-hold technique: Patients are asked to hold their breath in normal expiration only for the time that the CT takes to cover the lower lung and liver, which is typically less than

15 s. Instructing the patient before the PET/CT examinations on the breath-hold command is essential to avoiding serious respiration artifacts (Beyer et al. 2003). When applying the limited breath-hold technique, the frequency of severe artifacts in the area of the diaphragm was reduced by half, and the spatial extent of respiration-induced artifacts can be reduced by at least 40% compared with the acquisition protocols without any breathing instructions (Beyer et al. 2003).

With the introduction of multi-row CT technology with up to 64 detector rows into PET/CT designs, the incidence of respiration artifacts in PET/CT examinations can further be reduced, even in patients who are unable to follow any breath-hold instructions. In PET/CT imaging in normally breathing patients, significant gains in diagnostic image quality can be expected from employing CT technology with six or more detector rows, because respiration-induced artifacts are reduced in both magnitude and prominence for PET/CT systems (Goerres et al. 2002b; Beyer et al. 2005a). In conclusion, special breathing protocols are effective and should be used for CT scans as part of combined imaging protocols using a dual-modality PET/CT tomograph.

15.3.1.2 Contrast Agents

Standard application of CT intravenous contrast agents in combined PET/CT may lead to high-density artifacts on CT and attenuation-corrected PET (Antoch et al. 2002). To avoid associated diagnostic pitfalls, a special contrast injection protocol is needed. Comparing different protocols, Beyer et al. found a reproducible high image quality in CT image and attenuation-corrected PET images without high-density image artifacts on either imaging modality using a dual-phase injection (80 and 60 ml at 3 and 1.5 ml/s, respectively) of contrast agent in the caudocranial direction with a 50-s delay (Beyer et al. 2005b). For intestinal delineation, a combination of 1,500 ml of water containing 0.2% locust bean gum and 2.5% mannitol has been shown to be superior to administration of barium and thus is routinely used in our institution (Antoch et al. 2004a).

15.4 Summary and Conclusion

FDG-PET has been proven to be very sensitive in detecting a large variety of carcinomas. The FDG accumulation in malignant tumors is quite stereotyped and often reflects the aggressiveness of the tumor. Therefore, FDG appears to be suitable to detect unknown primaries independent of the type of disease. Being unaware of the site of the primary and also being unaware of the intensity of glucose metabolism, the interpretation of FDG-PET images needs rules accepting a reduced specificity for the definition of malignancy. However, due to physiological FDG-uptake in the head and neck area, especially in lymphatic tissue and vocal cords, one has to accept a high rate of equivocal findings interpreting FDG-PET alone. In this situation, the use of dual-modality PET/CT is of particular value. It allows for correlating the suspicious or unclear PET finding directly with morphology and by that the rate of false-equivocal or false-positive findings is reduced. In addition, PET/CT can precisely define the site of the PET finding in terms of anatomy, helping to direct the surgeon. This characteristic is of different value depending on the location of the primary and tends to be of utmost importance in the head and neck area. Finally, CT by itself may contribute with the detection of PET-negative findings. Thus in conclusion, PET and PET/CT can help localize the primary in CUP in approximately 40% of all cases, even after a thorough work-up with a variety of other investigations.

References

AAssar OS, Fischbein NJ, Caputo GR, Kaplan MJ, Price DC, Singer MI, Dillon WP, Hawkins RA (1999) Metastatic head and neck cancer: role and usefulness of FDG PET in locating occult primary tumors. Radiology 210:177–181

Abbruzzese JL, Abbruzzese MC, Hess KR, Raber MN, Lenzi R, Frost P (1994) Unknown primary carcinoma: natural history and prognostic factors in 657 consecutive patients. J Clin Oncol 12:1272–1280

Adams S, Baum RP, Stuckensen T, Bitter K, Hor G (1998) Prospective comparison of ^{18}F-FDG PET with conventional imaging modalities (CT, MRI, US) in lymph node staging of head and neck cancer. Eur J Nucl Med 25:1255–1260

Alberini JL, Belhocine T, Hustinx R, Daenen F, Rigo P (2003) Whole-body positron emission tomography using fluorodeoxyglucose in patients with metastases of unknown primary tumours (CUP syndrome). Nucl Med Commun 24:1081–1086

Antoch G, Freudenberg LS, Egelhof T, Stattaus J, Jentzen W, Debatin JF, Bockisch A (2002) Focal tracer uptake: a potential artifact in contrast-enhanced dual-modality PET/CT scans. J Nucl Med 43:1339–1342

Antoch G, Kuehl H, Kanja J, Lauenstein TC, Schneemann H, Hauth E, Jentzen W, Beyer T, Goehde SC, Debatin JF (2004a) Dual-modality PET/CT scanning with negative oral contrast agent to avoid artifacts: introduction and evaluation. Radiology 230:879–885

Antoch G, Vogt FM, Freudenberg LS, Nazaradeh F, Goehde SC, Barkhausen J, Dahmen G, Bockisch A, Debatin JF, Ruehm SG (2003) Whole-body dual-modality PET/CT and whole-body MRI for tumor staging in oncology. JAMA 290:3199–3206

Antoch G, Saoudi N, Kuehl H, Dahmen G, Mueller SP, Beyer T, Bockisch A, Debatin JF, Freudenberg LS (2004b) Accuracy of whole-body dual-modality fluorine-18-2-fluoro-2-deoxy-D-glucose positron emission tomography and computed tomography (FDG-PET/CT) for tumor staging in solid tumors: comparison with CT and PET. J Clin Oncol 22:4357–4368

Beyer T, Antoch G, Blodgett T, Freudenberg LF, Akhurst T, Mueller S (2003) Dual-modality PET/CT imaging: the effect of respiratory motion on combined image quality in clinical oncology. Eur J Nucl Med Mol Imaging 30:588–596

Beyer T, Antoch G, Muller S, Egelhof T, Freudenberg LS, Debatin J, Bockisch A (2004) Acquisition protocol considerations for combined PET/CT imaging. J Nucl Med 45 [Suppl 1]:25S–35S

Beyer T, Antoch G, Bockisch A, Stattaus J (2005a) Optimized intravenous contrast administration for diagnostic whole-body ^{18}F-FDG PET/CT. J Nucl Med 46:429–435

Beyer T, Rosenbaum S, Veit P, Stattaus J, Muller SP, Difilippo FP, Schoder H, Mawlawi O, Roberts F, Bockisch A, Kuhl H (2005b) Respiration artifacts in whole-body ([18])F-FDG PET/CT studies with combined PET/CT tomographs employing spiral CT technology with 1 to 16 detector rows. Eur J Nucl Med Mol Imaging 32:1429–1439

Bohuslavizki KH, Klutmann S, Kroger S, Sonnemann U, Buchert R, Werner JA, Mester J, Clausen M (2000) FDG PET detection of unknown primary tumors. J Nucl Med 41:816–822

Braams JW, Pruim J, Kole AC, Nikkels PG, Vaalburg W, Vermey A, Roodenburg JL (1997) Detection of unknown primary head and neck tumors by positron emission tomography. Int J Oral Maxillofac Surg 26:112–115

Buell U, Wieres FJ, Schneider W, Reinartz P (2004) [18]FDG-PET in 733 consecutive patients with or without side-by-side CT evaluation: Analysis of 921 lesions. Nuklearmedizin 43:210–216

Cohade C, Osman M, Marshall LN, Wahl RN (2003) PET-CT: accuracy of PET and CT spatial registration of lung lesions. Eur J Nucl Med Mol Imaging 30: 721–726

Daugaard G (1994) Unknown primary tumours. Cancer Treatment Rev 20:119–147

Delgado-Bolton RC, Fernandez-Perez C, Gonzalez-Mate A, Carreras JL (2003) Meta-analysis of the performance of ^{18}F-FDG PET in primary tumor detection in unknown primary tumors. J Nucl Med 44:1301–1314

Di Martino E, Nowak B, Hassan HA, Hausmann R, Adam G, Buell U, Westhofen M (2000) Diagnosis and staging of head and neck cancer. Arch Otolaryngol Head Neck Surg 126:1457–1461

Engel H, Steinert H, Buck A, Berthold T, Huch Boni RA, von Schulthess GK (1996) Whole-body PET: physiologic and artifactual fluoro-deoxyglucose accumulations. J Nucl Med 37: 441–446

Freudenberg LS, Fischer M, Antoch G, Jentzen W, Gutzeit A, Rosenbaum SJ, Bockisch A, Egelhof T (2005) Dual modality of ^{18}F-fluorodeoxyglucose-positron emission tomography/computed tomography in patients with cervical carcinoma of unknown primary. Med Princ Pract 14:155–160

Gambhir SS, Czernin J, Schwimmer J, Silverman DH, Coleman RE, Phelps ME (2001) A tabulated summary of the FDG PET literature. J Nucl Med 42 [5 Suppl]:1–93

Goerres GW, Hany TF, Kamel E, von Schulthess GK, Buck A (2002a) Head and neck imaging with PET and PET/CT: artefacts from dental metallic implants. Eur J Nucl Med 29:367–370

Goerres GW, Kamel E, Heidelberg TN, Schwitter MR, Burger C, von Schulthess GK (2002b) PET/CT image co-registration in the thorax: influence of respiration. Eur J Nucl Med Mol Imaging 29:351–360

Goerres GW, Burger C, Schwitter MR, Heidelberg TN, Seifert B, von Schulthess GK (2003) PET/CT of the abdomen: optimizing the patient breathing pattern. Eur Radiol 13:734–739

Greene L (2002) AJCC cancer staging manual. Springer, New York

Greven KM, Keyes JW Jr, Williams DW III, McGuirt WF, Joyce WT III (1999) Occult primary tumors of the head and neck: lack of benefit from positron emission tomography imaging with 2-[F-18]fluoro-2-deoxy-D-glucose. Cancer 86:114–118

Hanasono MM, Kunda LD, Segall GM, Ku GH, Terris DJ (1999) Uses and limitations of FDG positron emission tomography in patients with head and neck cancer. Laryngoscope 109:880–885

Hutton BF, Braun M (2003) Software for image registration: algorithms, accuracy, efficacy . Sem Nucl Med 33:180–192

Johansen J, Eigtved A, Buchwald C, Theilgaard SA, Hansen HS (2002) Implication of ^{18}F-fluoro-2-deoxy-Dglucose positron emission tomography on management of carcinoma of unknown primary in the head and neck: a Danish cohort study. Laryngoscope 112:2009–2014

Knapp WH (1999) Leitlinie zur Tumordarstellung mit (F-18)-Fluordeoxyglukose (FDG). Nuklearmedizin 38: 267–269

Kole AC, Nieweg OE, Pruim J, Hoekstra HJ, Koops HS, Roodenburg JL, Vaalburg W, Vermey A (1998) Detection of unknown occult primary tumors using positron emission tomography. Cancer 82:1160–1166

Kolesnikov-Gauthier H, Levy E, Merlet P, Kirova J, Syrota A, Carpentier P, Meignan M, Piedbois P (2005) FDG PET in patients with cancer of an unknown primary. Nucl Med Commun 26:1059–1066

Lassen U, Daugaard G, Eigtved A, Damgaard K, Friberg L (1999) ^{18}F-FDG whole body positron emission tomography (PET) in patients with unknown primary tumours (UPT). Eur J Cancer 35:1076–1082

Lauenstein TC, Goehde SC, Herborn CU, Goyen M, Oberhoff C, Debatin JF, Ruehm SG, Barkhausen J (2004) Whole-body MR imaging: evaluation of patients for metastases. Radiology 233:139–148

Lindholm P, Minn H, Leskinen-Kallio S, Bergman J, Ruotsalainen U, Joensuu H (1993) Influence of the blood glucose concentration on FDG uptake in cancer – a PET study. J Nucl Med 34:1–6

Lonneux M, Reffad AM (2000) Metastases from unknown primary tumor: PET-FDG as initial diagnostic procedure? Clin Positron Imaging 3:137–141

Mantaka P, Baum RP, Hertel A, Adams S, Niessen A, Sengupta S, Hor G (2003) PET with 2-[F-18]-fluoro-2-deoxy-D-glucose (FDG) in patients with cancer of unknown primary (CUP): influence on patients' diagnostic and therapeutic management. Cancer Biother Radiopharm 18:47–58

Nanni C, Rubello D, Castellucci P, Farsad M, Franchi R, Toso S, Barile C, Rampin L, Nibale O, Fanti S (2005) Role of ^{18}F-FDG PET-CT imaging for the detection of an unknown primary tumour: preliminary results in 21 patients. Eur J Nucl Med Mol Imaging 32:589–592

Nieder C, Gregoire V, Ang KK (2001) Cervical lymph node metastases from occult squamous cell carcinoma: cut down a tree to get an apple? Int J Radiat Oncol Biol Phys 50:727–733

Paulus P, Sambon A, Vivegnis D, Hustinx R, Moreau P, Collignon J, Deneufbourg JM, Rigo P (1998) [18]FDG-PET for the assessment of primary head and neck tumors: clinical, computed tomography, and histopathological correlation in 38 patients. Laryngoscope 108:1578–1583

Pelosi E, Pennone M, Deandreis D, Douroukas A, Mancini M, Bisi G (2006) Role of whole body positron emission tomography/computed tomography scan with ^{18}F-fluorodeoxyglucose in patients with biopsy proven tumor metastases from unknown primary site. Q J Nucl Med Mol Imaging 50:15–22

Rades D, Kuhnel G, Wildfang I, Borner AR, Knapp W, Karstens JH (2001a) The value of positron emission tomography (PET) in the treatment of patients with cancer of unknown primary (CUP). Strahlenther Onkol 177:525–529

Rades D, Kuhnel G, Wildfang I, Borner AR, Schmoll HJ, Knapp W (2001b) Localised disease in cancer of unknown primary (CUP): the value of positron emission tomography (PET) for individual therapeutic management. Ann Oncol 12:1605–1609

Regelink G, Brouwer J, de Bree R, Pruim J, van der Laan BF, Vaalburg W, Hoekstra OS, Comans EF, Vissink A, Leemans CR, Roodenburg JL (2002) Detection of unknown primary tumors and distant metastases in patients with cervical metastases: value of FDG-PET versus conventional modalities. Eur J Nucl Med Mol Imaging 29:1024–1030

Reinartz P, Wieres FJ, Schneider W, Schur A, Buell U (2004) Side-by-side reading of PET and CT scans in oncology: which patients might profit from integrated PET/CT? Eur J Nucl Med Mol Imaging 31:1456–1461

Reske SN, Kotzerke J (2001) FDG-PET for clinical use. Results of the 3rd German Interdisciplinary Consensus Conference, «Onko-PET III», 21 July and 19 September 2000. Eur J Nucl Med 28:1707–1723

Safa AA, Tran LM, Rege S, Brown CV, Mandelkern MA, Wang MB, Sadeghi A, Juillard G (1999) The role of positron emission tomography in occult primary head and neck cancers. Cancer J Sci Am 5:214–218

Schiepers C, Hoh CK (1998) Positron emission tomography as a diagnostic tool in oncology. Eur Radiol 8:1481–1494

Schneider K, Aschoff P, Bihl H, Hagen R (2006a) The integrated PET/CT: technological advance in diagnostics of head and neck recurrences and CUP? Laryngorhinootologie 85:179–183

Schneider K, Hrasky A, Aschoff P, Bihl H, Hagen R (2006b) Significance of PET and integrated PET/CT in the diagnostics of occult primary tumors. Laryngorhinootologie. 85:819–823

Scott CL, Kudaba I, Stewart JM, Hicks RJ, Rischin D (2005) The utility of 2-deoxy-2-[F-18]fluoro-D-glucose positron emission tomography in the investigation of patients with disseminated carcinoma of unknown primary origin. Mol Imaging Biol 7:236–243

Van de Wouw AJ, Janssen-Heijnen ML, Coebergh JW, Hillen HF (2002) Epidemiology of unknown primary tumors: incidence and population-based survival of 1285 patients in Southeast Netherlands, 1984–1992. Eur J Cancer 38:409–413

Van de Wouw AJ, Jansen RL, Speel EJ, Hillen HF (2003) The unknown biology of the unknown primary tumour: a literature review. Ann Oncol 14:191–196

Warburg O, Wind F, Neglers E (1930) On the metabolism of tumors in the body. Constable, London, pp 254–270

16 FDG-PET in Paraneoplastic Syndromes

R. Linke and R. Voltz

Recent Results in Cancer Research, Vol. 170
© Springer-Verlag Berlin Heidelberg 2008

16.1 Definition, Etiology, Incidence

Paraneoplastic syndromes are defined as clinical syndromes involving nonmetastatic systemic effects that accompany malignant disease. In a broad sense, these syndromes are collections of symptoms that result from substances produced or induced by the tumor, and they occur remotely from the tumor itself. These syndromes may occur in 10%–15% of malignancies, and they may be the first or most prominent manifestation. However, this incidence could be underestimated and as many as 50% of cancer patients will have paraneoplastic symptoms at some time during their illness [37]. Paraneoplastic syndromes typically affect middle-aged to older people and are most common in patients with lung, ovarian, or breast cancer (Table 16.1). Although these syndromes are rare disorders, recognition is important because clinical manifestations of paraneoplastic syndromes may precede those of the underlying malignancy by months or even years [28, 34]. Early recognition followed by a search for the cause of the paraneoplastic symptoms facilitates preclinical detection and early treatment of the malignancy [1, 6, 9, 14].

Paraneoplastic syndromes are triggered by remote effects of tumor-derived factors, or by the immune system's response to cancer cells [6, 14]. Sometimes, when a tumor arises, the body may produce antibodies to fight it, by binding to and helping in the destruction of tumor cells. These antibodies are not only of diagnostic relevance (Table 16.2), but also point to an autoimmune pathogenesis of a number of paraneoplastic syndromes, as in some cases, these antibodies cross-react with normal tissues and destroy them, which may stimulate the onset of paraneoplastic symptoms [2, 21, 27, 31]. In contrast to patients with only clinically suspected paraneoplastic syndrome without known antibody status (Table 16.1), in patients with such an antibody, the likelihood of a tumor is close to 100% [1, 2, 23, 31].

However, not all paraneoplastic syndromes are associated with such antibodies but may result from production and release of physiologically active substances, or they may be idiopathic. Currently, the mechanisms of how cancers affect distant sites are not understood precisely. In fact, any tumor may produce hormones and protein hormone precursors, or a variety of enzymes and fetal proteins, or cytokines. More rarely, the tumor may interfere with normal metabolic pathways or steroid metabolism. The paraneoplastic symptoms may be endocrine, neuromuscular or musculoskeletal, cardiovascular, cutaneous, hematologic, gastrointestinal, renal, or miscellaneous in nature [36, 37].

Table 16.1. Probability of paraneoplastic etiology of some of the more frequent syndromes (adapted from [35, 37])

Paraneoplastic syndrome	Probability of paraneoplastic origin	Frequently underlying tumors
LEMS	60%	*SCLC*
Subacute cerebellar degeneration	50%	*SCLC*
Opsoclonus/myoclonus (infant)	50%	Neuroblastoma
SIADH	40%	*SCLC*, head and neck cancer
Dermatomyositis	30%	Ovarian, pancreatic cancer, *SCLC*
Hypercalcemia	20%	Breast-, renal-, ovarian cancer, *SCLC*
Opsoclonus/myoclonus (adult)	20%	Breast cancer
Limbic and/or brain stem encephalitis	20%	*SCLC*
Subacute sensory/sensorimotor neuropathy	15%	*SCLC*
Myasthenia gravis	15%	Thymoma
Encephalomyelitis (inflammation of brain/spinal cord)	10%	*SCLC*
Cushing's syndrome	10%	*SCLC*, pancreatic cancer
Vision problems	5%	*SCLC*
Stiff person syndrome	5%	Breast cancer

SIADH, syndrome of inappropriate antidiuretic hormone; *LEMS*, Lambert-Eaton myasthenic syndrome; *SCLC*, small cell lung cancer

Table 16.2 Selection of frequent antibodies in paraneoplastic syndromes (adapted from [34, 35])

Antibody	Typical tumors
Anti-Hu	*SCLC*, Neuroblastoma
Anti-Yo	Ovarian cancer
Anti Ma	Different tumors
Anti-Ma2	Testicular cancer, different tumors
Anti-Ri	Breast cancer
Anti-Tr	Hodgkin's disease
Anti-Ta	Testicular cancer

SCLC, small cell lung cancer

16.2   Symptoms

Nonspecific syndromes can precede the clinical manifestations of the tumor. Common nonspecific paraneoplastic symptoms are fever, anorexia, and cachexia [37]. Fever frequently is associated with lymphomas, acute leukemias, sarcomas, renal cell carcinomas, and digestive malignancies (including the liver). Although these nonspecific symptoms are the most common presentation of paraneoplastic syndromes, several clinical pictures may be observed, each one specifically simulating more common benign conditions. Because of their complexity and variety, the clinical pictures of paraneoplastic syndromes may vary greatly and may or may not be characteristic of a specific system. For example, paraneoplastic complications can mimic rheumatologic symptoms and paraneoplastic arthropathies arise as rheumatic polyarthritis or polymyalgia, particularly in patients with myelomas, lymphomas, acute leukemia, malignant histiocytosis, and tumors of the colon, pancreas, prostate, and CNS [36]. A well-known paraneoplastic phenomenon is the hypertrophic osteoarthropathy (Fig. 16.1), which may be observed in about 10% of patients with lung cancer or pleural mesothelioma [9].

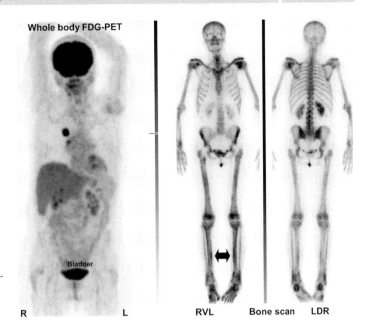

Fig. 16.1. Patient with lung cancer of the right lung (hot spot in the *whole body FDG-PET*) and hyperthropic osteoarthropathy. This well-known paraneoplastic phenomenon can be observed in up to 10% of patients with lung cancer but may also be associated with chronic lung disease or heart failure. The *bone scan* shows linear increased tracer uptake associated with the cortical margins reflecting periosteal bone deposition. This has been called the tramline or parallel stripe sign, best seen in distal femur and tibias (*arrow*)

Paraneoplastic endocrine syndromes are among the most common and best understood of the paraneoplastic syndromes [9, 14, 37]. Endocrine symptoms related to paraneoplastic syndromes usually resemble the more common endocrine disorders. There are many known and potential mediators of endocrine paraneoplastic syndromes, including ACTH or ACTH-like substances, ADH, parathyroid hormone-related protein, chorionic gonadotropin, renin, tumor necrosis factor, and cytokine growth factor. These syndromes include ectopic Cushing's syndrome, accompanied by hypokalemia, very high plasma adrenocorticotropic hormone (ACTH) levels, and increased serum and urine cortisol concentrations (Fig. 16.2), the syndrome of inappropriate antidiuretic hormone (SIADH), hypercalcemia, hypoglycemia, and oncogenic osteomalacia. Cushing's syndrome, SIADH, and hypercalcemia are the most common endocrine disorders linked to a malignancy (e.g., small cell lung cancer).

Paraneoplastic neurological syndromes (PNSs) account for approximately 10% of all nonmetastatic neurological complications in tumor patients [1, 18]. In roughly 60% of patients, highly specific antineuronal anti-bodies (Table 16.2) are found [1, 17, 18, 27]. Neurological symptoms generally develop in an acute or subacute fashion, over a period of days to weeks, and usually occur prior to the discovery of cancer [1, 18, 31], but can also occur at any time during the course of malignancy [37]. Symptoms may include fatigue, weakness, muscular pain, difficulty in walking and/or swallowing, memory loss, dementia with or without brain stem signs, rapid and irregular eye movements (opsoclonus) or ophthalmoplegia with vision problems, sensory neuropathy with sensory loss in the limbs or peripheral paresthesia with burning, numbness, or tingling sensations. Typical paraneoplastic syndromes involving the nervous system include are the Lambert-Eaton myasthenic syndrome (LEMS), encephalomyelitis (inflammation of the brain and spinal cord), myasthenia gravis, (subacute) cerebellar degeneration (symptoms: loss of coordination, slurred speech), limbic and/or brain stem encephalitis, stiff person syndrome, neuromyotonia, or myoclonus. The nervous system disability is usually severe and often more disabling than the local effects of the tumor itself [2, 3, 9, 11, 13, 17, 21, 31].

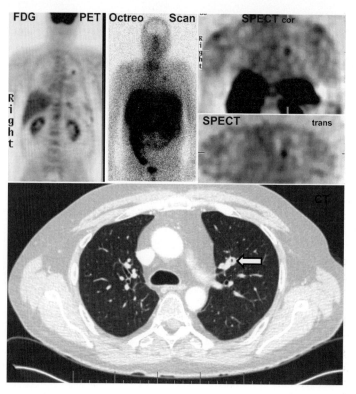

Fig. 16.2. Patient with suspected paraneoplastic Cushing's syndrome. Thoracic CT initially was interpreted as unsuspicious. *FDG-PET* and somatostatin receptor imaging (*octreo scan*) both demonstrated a focal increased tracer uptake in the left lung interpreted as malignant. The side-by-side reinterpretation of nuclear medicine modalities and CT revealed a circular wall thickening of a small bronchus, which was histologically confirmed as carcinoid infiltration by atypical lung resection

16.3   Treatment and Prognosis of Paraneoplastic Syndromes

The treatment for most paraneoplastic syndromes takes two approaches. The first is treatment of the underlying tumor with surgery in early-stage disease, radiation for inoperable disease, and chemotherapy for systemic or inoperable disease. The tumor therapy so far represents the most efficient therapeutic option [20]. However, probably due to the ongoing immune reaction, the tumors sometimes remain unusually small for a long time, which renders them difficult to diagnose [3, 16, 17, 33]. Therefore, the physician should search for cancer using the most sensitive technology available.

The second approach is to suppress the mediator causing the syndrome. Even with treatment, irreversible damage to the target organ can occur [37]. Therefore, the prognosis for patients with paraneoplastic syndromes depends on the specific type of the paraneoplastic syndrome and the progression of the underlying cancer. Endocrine symptoms or neurological disorders without cell damage or neuronal loss, such as LEMS, myasthenia gravis, or opsoclonus/myoclonus, can recover once the causal insult is removed. Disorders such as cerebellar degeneration, encephalomyelitis, limbic and/or brain stem encephalitis are usually associated with neuronal damage. Because they evolve subacutely and treatment is often delayed, neurons die, making recovery much more difficult. In order to speed up tumor diagnosis in patients with paraneoplastic syndromes, the use of whole-body positron emission tomography (PET) with [18]fluorine fluoro-2-deoxy-glucose (FDG) has been suggested.

16.4 The Role of FDG-PET in the Search for a Tumor

To rule out tumor in the majority of patients and detect a neoplastic lesion in the remaining patients, extensive diagnostic examination including panendoscopy, whole-body computed tomography (CT), MRI, or other, i.e. more invasive procedures (bronchial lavage, mediastinoscopy, or thoracotomy), are necessary [6]. The type of the paraneoplastic syndrome (Table 16.1) or a specific antibody (Table 16.2) may give a lead to the possible tumor site.

A number of paraneoplastic syndromes may be caused by small cell lung cancer (SCLC). In suspected lung cancer, CT is the procedure of choice for initial staging, because of its high sensitivity for peripherally localized lesions [8, 26]. However, the false-positive rate of CT lung scanning may be very high [26, 31, 32]. In a series of 1,035 current or former smokers, a prevalence of 29% of pulmonary nodules was reported in a 2-year screening period using single-slice spiral CT [26]. Another screening trial using the more sensitive multislice CT identified uncalcified pulmonary nodules in 1,049 of 1,520 patients at risk for lung cancer (69%) in a period of 3 years [31]. However, in each of these studies, 93% and 98% of these nodules, respectively, were benign, and therefore, false-positive for cancer [26,31]. In centrally, mediastinally localized lung tumors, the sensitivity of CT is substantially lower than in the periphery [8]. The only CT finding suggestive of mediastinal lymph node involvement in SCLC is nodal size and deformation. In general, the smaller the nodal diameter used to distinguish normal and abnormal nodes, the higher the sensitivity and the lower the specificity of CT. When using 1 cm as the upper limit of normal, sensitivity and specificity of CT is roughly 60% [8, 24]. However, in anti-Hu associated paraneoplastic syndromes, metastases of SCLC are often limited to the mediastinal lymph nodes [1, 3, 22]. For instance, in a study on patients with antibody-positive paraneoplastic neurological syndromes, 80% of patients with SCLC presented with a centrally/mediastinally localized cancer. In these patients FDG-PET was positive in 100%, while sensitivity of CT scanning was 50% [22].

Consequently, in patients with paraneoplastic symptoms, FDG-PET as an additional staging method is beginning to be advocated, in order to increase sensitivity and specificity of CT [26]. In a first series of 15 patients with anti-Hu antibodies, a SCLC was detected in 12 of 15 patients using CT scan or chest x-ray. In the remaining three patients, an FDG-PET revealed the diagnosis [1]. In all five of their patients with paraneoplastic syndromes, Crotty et al. [9] detected the malignant tumor site in the lung with FDG-PET. In all cases, SCLC was confirmed by biopsy. Another study looked into 43 patients with a clinically suspected paraneoplastic syndrome [25]. The a priori probability in this patient group having a paraneoplastic syndrome lies in between 5% and 60% (see Table 16.1). A pathological glucose hypermetabolism was detected by FDG-PET in 16 of 43 (37%) patients; in seven patients the tumor was confirmed histologically. In a well-defined group of patients harboring a paraneoplastic antibody in their serum, a pathological FDG-PET – the histologically confirmed malignant tumor– was found at higher rate of 77% (10/13) [22].

Even if SCLC is frequently involved in paraneoplastic complications, many other tumor types can trigger paraneoplastic symptoms. Most of these tumors, especially gynecological cancers, such as breast cancer, ovarian cancer, and cervical cancer, are now recognized as good indications for imaging with FDG-PET [3, 4, 24]. In breast cancer, mammography and MRI are the methods of choice for searching for the primary, but FDG-PET may help to localize the tumor in unexpected locations. For excluding an abdominal tumor, abdominal and pelvic CT is an established procedure, although CT has only moderate sensitivity and specificity for diagnosing small abdominal tumors with bowel or lymph node involvement [3, 15, 22, 24]. Figure 16.3 presents an example of a patient with an anti-Ma-antibody-positive paraneoplastic subacute sensorimotor neuropathy. CT of the neck, thorax, and abdomen initially were not suspicious of a tumor, but FDG-PET demonstrated an area with pathologically increased glucose metabolism in the upper abdomen next to the liver and the stomach. In retrospect, knowing the pathological FDG-PET finding,

Whole body FDG-PET

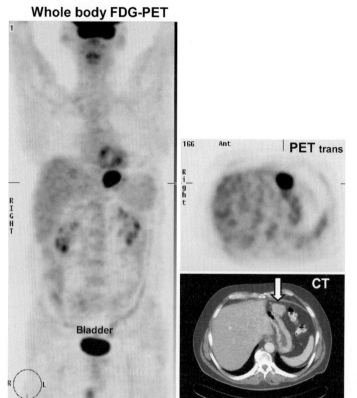

Fig. 16.3. *Whole-body FDG-PET* and corresponding transaxial slices of contrast-enhanced *CT* and *FDG-PET* of an anti-Ma-antibody-positive patient and suspected paraneoplastic subacute sensorimotor neuropathy. In this patient, a recurrent melanoma was suspected since in 1993 a melanoma of the right neck was surgically removed. *CT* of neck, thorax, and abdomen were not suspicious of a tumor. *FDG-PET* demonstrated an area with pathologically increased glucose metabolism in the upper abdomen next to the liver and the stomach (surgery confirmed a metastasis of a melanoma). The corresponding mass, which was retrospectively visualized on *CT* with knowledge of the pathological *FDG-PET* finding, initially had been interpreted as part of the left liver lobe

the corresponding mass could be visualized on CT and removed by surgery and a melanoma metastasis was confirmed by histology. This example emphasizes the usefulness of FDG-PET when searching for a malignant tumor.

In a comparison between CT and FDG-PET for diagnosis of tumor or tumor recurrence in patients with a variety of paraneoplastic syndromes, a significantly higher sensitivity (77% vs 23%) and accuracy (85% vs 46%) with FDG-PET compared to CT was demonstrated [22]. However, the most reliable results were obtained if both tests were combined (sensitivity, 100%; accuracy, 92%). Furthermore, a combination of FDG-PET and CT may contribute to accurately distinguishing a true tumor or recurrence from benign lesions or physiologic or inflammatory uptake [22, 35]. For example, inflammatory lesions in the bowel or in joints or FDG uptake in brown fat ought to be considered within the differential diagnosis of hot

spots in FDG-PET, but may cause false-positive results when searching for a malignant tumor [1, 3, 26, 30]. A combined interpretation of PET and CT imaging allows for precise localization of increased FDG uptake and distinction between benign increased tracer uptake and malignant findings [30].

False-negative results are infrequent with FDG-PET and may correspond to tumors with a diameter clearly less than 1 cm or slow growth [1, 24, 26]. A specific pathological entity of neoplasms, which often grow slowly and have low metabolic activity but may cause paraneoplastic syndromes are neuroendocrine tumors, i.e., carcinoid tumors or neuroblastomas. These tumors often are not FDG avid on PET, and therefore additional nuclear medicine techniques, such as somatostatin receptor imaging or MIBG scintigraphy or morphological imaging with CT or MRI may be more promising for diagnosis and staging.

16.5 The Role of PET in Cerebral Imaging

Central nerval or cerebellar dysfunction is much more likely to be caused by brain metastasis than subacute paraneoplastic degeneration or inflammation [37]. PET with FDG is not the modality of choice for the detection or exclusion of brain metastases. The sensitivity of FDG-PET in the detection of metastatic brain lesions is low, because the surrounding normal brain tissue has a high glucose uptake [5]. CT and/or MRI remain the standard imaging test to stage the brain [35] and usually establish the diagnosis by demonstrating the presence of a metastatic lesion.

Typically, in paraneoplastic encephalitis, brain MRI shows an unspecific hyperintensity in the temporal and medial regions on T2-weighted images, but involvement of other areas, for example, insula and basal ganglia, has also been reported. Brain PET using FDG may show hypermetabolism in these areas during the active phase of inflammatory disease [5]. Cerebellar or cortical atrophy with consecutive hypometabolism in FDG-PET are findings that may occur in later stages of disease. In a very early paraneoplastic inflammation, MRI or CT may show no abnormality, while FDG hypermetabolism is present [5]. Consequently, a normal MRI or CT of the brain does not exclude a paraneoplastic origin of symptoms.

In Figure 16.4 a patient with anti-Hu associated paraneoplastic encephalomyelitis is presented. This patient presented initially with symptoms and signs compatible with optic neuritis misdiagnosed as multiple sclerosis. Early-appearing epileptic seizures and the atypical

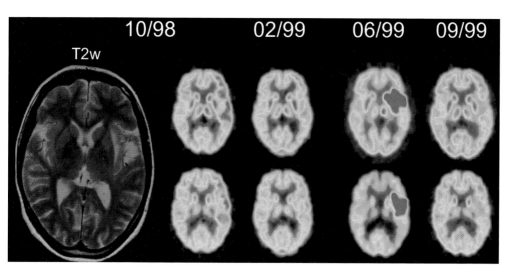

Fig. 16.4. Cerebral MRI and FDG-PET in a patient with adult neuroblastoma and anti-Hu-positive encephalitis: The MRI (*T2-weighted sequence*) shows cortical and subcortical laminar hyperintensity involving the left insula and left parietal cortex without gadolinium enhancement. Correspondingly, FDG-PET revealed hypermetabolism of the left insula and the left parietal cortex, reflecting epileptic and/or encephalitic activity (*second row, 10/98*). After resection of the tumor (histologically confirmed adult neuroblastoma) and after chemotherapy, the hypermetabolism of left cortex decreased (*third row, 02/99*) and the EEG revealed no more epileptic seizures. Four months later, the neurological symptoms started to deteriorate again quickly. Reoccurrence of focal seizures was noted; in parallel, cerebral FDG-PET again demonstrated a substantial increase in hypermetabolism in the left insula and striatum (*fourth row, 06/99*). Due to otherwise unexplained worsening of neurological symptoms, a neuroblastoma relapse was suspected and was confirmed in an abdominal CT scan. After the second surgery, the neurological symptoms improved rapidly within a few days, and the glucose metabolism of the left insula and striatum decreased (*fifth row, 02/99*). The rapid clinical improvement after tumor surgery observed in this patient demonstrates that tumor therapy is very effective in positively influencing the ongoing autoimmune reaction

presentation on PET and MRI, however, led to further diagnostic procedures and the subsequent diagnosis of a malignant tumor. As tumor therapy remains the mainstay of treatment for paraneoplastic encephalomyelitis, early diagnosis of the initial tumor is of utmost clinical importance. Successful tumor treatment leads to remission of symptoms and metabolic activity [5]. Furthermore, otherwise unexplained worsening of neurological symptoms and an increase in metabolic activity in circumscribed cortical regions may herald a tumor recurrence. Sequential changes in FDG metabolism have been shown in different types of encephalitis, with FDG hypermetabolism seen in the acute phase but hypometabolism seen in later stages, while abnormal signal intensity was seen on both early- and late-stage MR imaging studies. Therefore, PET imaging appears to be more sensitive in detecting the exact phase of the inflammatory process and offers greater specificity for staging encephalitis [29]. This fact may warrant the elective inclusion of the brain in routine whole-body FDG PET in patients with suspected paraneoplastic syndrome.

16.6   Summary

Paraneoplastic syndromes are rare disorders, but recognition is important because clinical manifestations of paraneoplastic syndromes may precede those of the underlying malignancy by months or even years. As tumor therapy still is the mainstay of treatment for paraneoplastic syndromes, early diagnosis of the initial tumor or its recurrence is of utmost clinical importance. For finding the associated tumor, the combined use of FDG-PET and CT seems to have the highest sensitivity and may contribute to accurately distinguishing a true tumor or recurrence from benign lesions or physiologic or inflammatory uptake. Further, this approach helps localize the tumor for further management of the patient such as surgery or more invasive diagnostic procedures. Cerebral FDG-PET proved to confirm paraneoplastic encephalitis and may help monitor tumor therapy.

References

1. Antoine JC, Cinotti L, Tilikete C et al (2000) [^{18}F]fluorodeoxyglucose positron emission tomography in the diagnosis of cancer in patients with paraneoplastic neurological syndrome and anti-Hu antibodies. Ann Neurol 48:105–108
2. Bataller L, Dalmau J (2003) Paraneoplastic neurologic syndromes: approaches to diagnosis and treatment. Semin Neurol 23:215–224
3. Bataller L, Dalmau JO (2004) Paraneoplastic disorders of the central nervous system: update on diagnostic criteria and treatment. Semin Neurol 24:461–471
4. Belhocine T, De Barsy C, Hustinx R et al (2002) Usefulness of ^{18}F-FDG-PET in the post-therapy surveillance of endometrial carcinoma. Eur J Nucl Med Mol Imaging 29:1132–1139
5. Belhocine T, Weiner SM, Brink I et al (2005) A plea for the elective inclusion of the brain in routine whole-body FDG PET. Eur J Nucl Med Mol Imaging 32:251–256
6. Berner U, Menzel C, Rinne D et al (2003) Paraneoplastic syndromes: detection of malignant tumors using [(^{18})F]FDG-PET. Q J Nucl Med 47:85–89
7. Bombardieri E, Seregni E, Villano C et al (2004) Position of nuclear medicine techniques in the diagnostic work-up of neuroendocrine tumors. Q J Nucl Mol Imaging 48:150–163
8. Bonomo L, Ciccotosto C, Guidotti A et al (1996) Lung cancer staging: the role of computed tomography and magnetic resonance imaging. Eur J Radiol 23:35–45
9. Crotty E, Patz EF (2001) FDG-PET imaging in patients with paraneoplastic syndromes and suspected small cell lung cancer. J Thorac Imaging 16:89–93
10. Dalmau J, Graus F, Rosenblum MK et al (1992) Anti-Hu-associated paraneoplastic encephalomyelitis/sensory neuronopathy. A clinical study of 71 patients. Medicine 71:59–72
11. Dalmau J, Graus F, Cheung N-KV et al (1995) Major histocompatability proteins, anti-Hu antibodies, and paraneoplastic encephalomyelitis in neuroblastoma and small cell lung cancer. Cancer 75:99–109
12. Darnell RB (2004) Paraneoplastic neurologic disorders: windows into neuronal function and tumor immunity. Arch Neurol 61:30–32
13. Dreessen J, Jeanjean AP, Sindic CJ (2004) Paraneoplastic limbic encephalitis: diagnostic relevance of CSF analysis and total body PET scanning. Acta Neurol Belg 104:57–63
14. Enck RE (2004) Paraneoplastic syndromes. Am J Hosp Palliat Care 21:85–86
15. Frings M, Antoch G, Knorn P et al (2005) Strategies in detection of the primary tumor in anti-Yo-associated paraneoplastic cerebellar degeneration. J Neurol 252:197–201
16. Graus F, Dalmau J, Rene R et al (1997) Anti-Hu antibodies in patients with small-cell lung cancer: association with complete response to therapy and improved survival. J Clin Oncol 15:2866–2872

17. Graus F, Dalmau J, Valldeoriola F et al (1997) Immunological characterization of a neuronal antibody (anti-Tr) associated with paraneoplastic cerebellar degeneration and Hodgkin's disease. J Neuroimmunol 74:55–61
18. Graus F, Keime-Guibert F, Rene R et al (2001) Anti-Hu-associated paraneoplastic encephalomyelitis: analysis of 200 patients. Brain 124:1138–1148
19. Gultekin SH, Rosenfeld MR, Voltz R et al (2000) Paraneoplastic limbic encephalitis: neurological symptoms, immunological findings and tumour association in 50 patients. Brain 123:1481–1494
20. Keime-Guibert F, Graus F, Broet P et al (1999) Clinical outcome of patients with anti-Hu-associated encephalomyelitis after treatment of the tumor. Neurology 53:1719–1723
21. Lang B, Dale RC, Vincent A (2003) New autoantibody mediated disorders of the central nervous system. Curr Opin Neurol 16:351–357
22. Linke R, Schroeder M, Helmberger T et al (2004) Antibody-positive paraneoplastic neurological syndromes: value of CT and PET for tumor diagnosis. Neurology 63:282–286
23. Lucchinetti CF, Kimmel DW, Lennon VA (1998) Paraneoplastic and oncologic profiles of patients seropositive for type 1 antineuronal nuclear autoantibodies. Neurology 50:652–657
24. March DE, Wechsler RJ, Kurtz AB et al (1991) CT-pathologic correlation of axillary lymph nodes in breast carcinoma. J Comput Assist Tomogr 15:440–444
25. Rees JH, Hain SF, Johnson MR et al (2001) The role of [18F]fluoro-2-deoxyglucose-FDG-PET scanning in the diagnosis of paraneoplastic neurological disorders. Brain 124:2223–2231
26. Pastorino U, Bellomi M, Landoni C et al (2003) Early lung-cancer detection with spiral CT and positron emission tomography in heavy smokers: 2-year results. Lancet 362:593–597
27. Pittock SJ, Kryzer TJ, Lennon VA (2004) Paraneoplastic antibodies coexist and predict cancer, not neurological syndrome. Ann Neurol 56:715–719
28. Posner JB (1995) Paraneoplastic syndromes. In: Posner JB (ed) Neurologic complications of cancer. Contemporary Neurological Series. FA Davis, Philadelphia, pp 353–385
29. Provenzale JM, Barboriak DP, Coleman RE (1998) Limbic encephalitis: comparison of FDG PET and MR imaging findings. AJR Am J Roentgenol 170:1659–1660
30. Rousseau C, Bourbouloux E, Campion L et al (2006) Brown fat in breast cancer patients: analysis of serial (18)F-FDG PET/CT scans. Eur J Nucl Med Mol Imaging 33:785–791
31. Swensen SJ, Jett JR, Hartman TE et al (2003) Lung cancer screening with CT: Mayo clinic experience. Radiology 226:756–761
32. Swensen SJ (2003) Screening for cancer with computed tomography. BMJ 326:894–895
33. Voltz R, Dalmau J, Posner JB et al (1998) T-cell receptor analysis in anti-Hu associated paraneoplastic encephalomyelitis. Neurology 51:1146–1150
34. Voltz R (2002) Paraneoplastic neurological syndromes: an update on diagnosis, pathogenesis and therapy. Lancet Neurol 1:294–305
35. Voltz R, Linke R (2004) Bildgebung bei paraneoplastischen neurologischen Erkrankungen. In: Zettl U, Mix E (ed) Bildgebung in der klinischen Neuroimmunologie. Thieme Verlag, pp 194–200
36. Wiese W, Alansari H, Tranchida P et al (2004) Paraneoplastic polyarthritis in an ovarian teratoma. J Rheumatol 31:1854–1857
37. Zumsteg MM, Casperson DS (1998) Paraneoplastic syndromes in metastatic disease. Semin Oncol Nurs 14:220–229

17 PET and PET/CT with F-18 Fluoride in Bone Metastases

H. Palmedo, C. Grohé, Y. Ko, and S. Tasci

Recent Results in Cancer Research, Vol. 170
© Springer-Verlag Berlin Heidelberg 2008

17.1 Background

17.1.1 Lung Cancer

Lung cancer is the most common malignant tumor of the male patient [1]. In Germany, 29,000 men died of lung cancer in the year 1995. The mortality rate has decreased slightly in the last few decades to 45 cases per 100,000 inhabitants. For women, lung cancer represents the third most common malignant tumor, increasing steadily over the last few decades. Therefore, the standardized mortality rate has reached a level of 9.6 cases per 100,000 inhabitants per year for the year 1995 [1].

Because of its different biological properties, lung cancer is classified as belonging to the group of non-small cell lung cancer (NSCLC), with a frequency of approximately 76%, or to the group of small cell lung cancer (SCLC), diagnosed in about 21% of cases [2, 3]. An exact staging of any lung cancer following the TNM classification is essential to stage relevant-therapy planning [4]. Besides the histopathological diagnosis of the primary tumor, imaging is indispensable for the staging of the mediastinum, the liver, the skeleton and the adrenal glands. For small cell lung cancer, patients with limited disease (stage I–IIIb) must be distinguished from patients with extensive disease (presence of distant metastases) [5].

The probability of having distant metastases is correlated with the T- and the N-stage of the tumor. Distant metastases will be found in 20%–40% of patients with the early stage I–II (T1–2 cancer with N0 or with N1 = ipsilateral-hilus lymph node). However, this patient group only accounts for roughly 25% of all lung cancers [6–10]. For all lung cancers, the most frequent locations of distant metastases are the liver, bones, bone marrow, lymph nodes, brain, and adrenal glands [11, 12]. In patients with SCLC, distant metastases and therefore extensive disease is present in 45%–60% of cases at the time of primary diagnosis [13]. In patients with a higher stage of disease, bone marrow disease is found three to four times as often for SCLC as for NSCLC [14]. Consequently, lung cancer tends to metastasize to the bones at a very early stage, demonstrating the need for diagnostic workup at this time.

Although different staging examinations such as bone scintigraphy are performed, it must be assumed that patients showing no evidence of metastases at the time of imaging also frequently present an advanced stage of disease. For lung cancer, an imaging modality detecting osseous metastases as early as possible with high diagnostic accuracy is required for the following reasons:

- Clearly bone metastases have a high prognostic relevance for all types of lung cancer [16–18]. The broad range of the 5-year survival in stage I (50%–80%) and stage II (35%–60%) may result from very early development of osseous metastases. Moreover, early detection of bone metastases could be helpful for the planning and evaluation of therapy by enabling the clinician to build special subgroups of patients.

- Mainly for NSCLC (rarely in SCLC patients), curative surgery is only indicated if bone metastases have been excluded [15]. If bone metastases were detected at an early stage a high-risk operation could be avoided for these patients. Additionally, early detection would mean better patient selection, which would result in an improvement of the survival rate after curative therapy.
- Neoadjuvant chemotherapy of lung cancer for stage III (mainly IIIa) patients could be a curative approach if followed by surgical tumor elimination. Also in this patient group, exclusion of metastatic bone disease is extremely important [19].
- It is necessary to determine the exact extent of bone disease to localize regions with a high fracture risk that are appropriate for external beam radiotherapy.
- In patients with SCLC, the evidence of osseous metastases will modify the chemotherapeutic regimen. In patients in whom bone disease has been excluded, aggressive chemotherapy has shown some advantage in patient survival [20, 21].

17.1.2 Prostate Cancer

Prostate cancer is the second leading cause for cancer-related mortality in men [22]. In the year 1994, mortality reached a level of 30 cases per 100,000 male inhabitants, and the incidence has steadily increased over the last few years [23]. The mean age at diagnosis is approximately 70 years.

Depending on the stage, prostate cancer generally metastasizes in the locoregional lymph nodes of the pelvis. Subsequently, tumor extension follows the lymphatic vessels to the retroperitoneal and para-aortal region or disseminates into bones, lung, and liver [24, 25]. Typically, prostate cancer generates osteoblastic bone metastases that are mainly located in the vertebral column (lumbar region), pelvis, and ribs [24].

The exact TNM staging of prostate cancer, which is a precondition for adequate therapy planning, is a particular problem. Approximately 50%–60% of the preoperatively T1- and T2-staged tumors that have been operated on in curative intention are identified as advanced T3 cancers later on and therefore have been understaged [26, 27].

To determine the T stage of the tumor, a digital rectal examination (DRE), transrectal sonography (TRS), and PSA measurement are performed. The understaging rate for DRE and TRS was found to lie at a level of 60% and 38%, respectively [28, 29]. The measurement of PSA has been integrated as a valuable parameter in the diagnostic work-up and the follow-up of prostate cancer patients [30]. There is a positive correlation between clinical and pathological stage and the extent of the tumor disease [31]. However, a significant overlap with regard to PSA measurements exists between malignant and benign tumors of the prostate because benign prostate tumors produce also PSA [32]. Therefore, when evaluating the PSA value, one has to take into account different factors such as the volume of the prostate gland. PSA is reliable to differentiate T2 from T3 tumors [33]. Consequently, prostatovesiculectomy continues to be the gold standard to determine the T stage in prostate cancer.

A similar situation can be found for the lymph node staging. In spite of PSA measurements and modern imaging modalities such as sonography, computer tomography, MRI, and PET, pelvic lymphadenectomy is the only exact staging method for the lymph nodes [34]. Controversy continues on which patients require pelvic lymphadenectomy [35, 36].

If local tumor growth is present (maximal T2) curative therapy by radical prostatectomy or external beam radiation is possible [37–40]. Roughly 50%–60% of patients have T1–2 stage cancer. If advanced local tumor (pT3) or lymph node or bone metastases are present the disease is considered a systemic cancer requiring a palliative therapy regimen [41]. The incidences of distant metastases at T1–2 and stage T3 are 20% and 40%, respectively [42]. Since a strong correlation between the PSA value and the frequency of bone metastases has been proven, bone scintigraphy is recommended only for prostate cancer patients with PSA values over 10 ng/ml [43].

Early detection of metastatic bone diseases in prostate cancer is extremely important at the time of primary diagnosis because a decision must be made on whether palliative or curative (radical prostatectomy or external beam radiation) treatment is the most appropriate for the patient. In this context, it is important to recall that in spite of systematic biopsies of the prostate gland, 30%–50% of pT3 tumors are operated on because they had been staged as T2 tumors before surgery [44, 45]. The number of operated T3 patients could be reduced if early detection of bone metastases was possible preoperatively. Moreover, it is helpful if the exact extent of bone disease can be defined to plan potential external beam radiotherapy.

17.1.3 Breast Cancer

Carcinoma of the breast represents the most common malignant tumor in women [46, 47]. Every ninth woman in the modern countries of the Western world will develop breast cancer during her lifetime. The incidence in western and northern Europe is approximately 70–100 cases per 100,000 women and mortality lies at 29 per 100,000. Disease will appear mainly in women between 45 and 65 years of age. For women 35–45 years of age, breast cancer is the leading cause of death [48].

The dynamics of tumor growth differ from breast tumor to breast tumor and the time for a tumor to double in volume lies between 23 and 209 days [49]. It has been observed that 75% of tumors first metastasize via the lymphatic vessels and subsequently develop distant metastases via the blood vessels [50]. However, in roughly 25% of patients it must be assumed that tumor cells spread out primarily via the blood vessels because patients demonstrate distant metastases without having lymphatic

disease. The preferred locations for breast cancer metastases are the lungs, liver and bones [51]. The size of the primary tumor correlates strongly with the probability of having lymph node and distant metastases [52, 53]. Given the aforementioned biological behavior of early hematological spread of some of the breast cancers, small tumors 1–2 cm in size also generate distant metastases in 25% of cases during the course of disease [53]. In contrast, in 10% of breast tumors 8 cm or larger, distant metastases are missing and, in 25% of patients with axillary lymph node metastases at the time of primary diagnosis, no distant metastases will appear [52]. This makes it clear that the predictive value of the tumor size alone is of limited value.

Most patients discover breast cancer on their own during self-examination of the breasts, detecting tumors with a mean diameter of 2 cm [54, 55]. Mammography screening is able to detect occult breast carcinoma and has led to an increase in the detection rate and the surgical treatment of such early cancers [56–58]. Still, in a patient with a solid breast cancer, a clinically detectable distant metastasis must be assumed in about 30% of patients at the time of primary diagnosis [59]. One of the first locations often concerned is the skeleton [60]. Bone marrow involvement (proof of cancer cells) in T1/T2 tumors and in T3/T4 tumors can be found in 22% and 40% of cases, respectively [61]. At the time of primary diagnosis, bone scintigraphy demonstrates metastatic disease in approximately 2%–3% of patients, whereas this rate increases up to 30% in patients with recurrent disease [62, 63]. Frequently, osseous metastases are observed in patients with well-differentiated estrogen-positive tumors [64].

The early detection of bone metastases in breast cancer at the time of primary staging is important because the result will influence the further therapeutic management of the patient. Consequently, the surgeon will confine the graft to a purely palliative treatment such as tumorectomy or mastectomy if osseous disease is present. Moreover, in patients who only have distant metastases confined to the bone, often hormonal treatment is preferred instead of chemotherapy [65]. In combination with chemotherapy, the administration of bisphosphonates inhibits activity of osteoclasts and results in a delay of progression and extension of bone metastases [66–68]. In patients with newly diagnosed local recurrence, it is important to exclude osseous metastases because a curative approach is possible in this patient group [69, 70]. For the palliative treatment strategy, it is valuable to determine the exact extent of bone disease to be able to monitor therapy success and to apply external beam radiotherapy. This question is also important in patients with a singular sternal metastases in whom surgical resection is considered [71]. It is not clear if early detection of bone metastases can prolong survival in patients in whom no further organs are affected. Currently, the oncologic community recommends screening for bone metastases only in high-risk or symptomatic patients.

17.2   Conventional Screening for Bone Metastases

The method of choice for screening bone metastases in lung, prostate, and breast cancer is bone scintigraphy. This imaging modality has the advantage that the whole body is examined within a relatively short time period [72]. Bone scintigraphy including SPECT imaging has a high sensitivity for detecting metastatic bone disease. Moreover, the administration of technetium-labeled phosphonates does not have any side effects except for a low radiation burden. One disadvantage of bone scintigraphy is its limited specificity that regularly necessitates further modalities such as x-ray imaging. It has been shown that MRI detects more osteolytic metastatic lesions in the vertebra column than planar scintigraphy. However, in these studies, no systematic SPECT imaging was performed. This seems to be important because there is evidence that SPECT increases sensitivity for detecting bone metastases in the vertebra column and the pelvis. With regard to the ribs, the sternum, and the skull, bone scintigraphy revealed the highest sensitivity of all imaging modalities.

17.3   PET and PET-CT with F-18 Sodium Fluoride for Metastatic Bone Disease

F-18 sodium fluoride (NaF-18) is a new PET tracer that is currently being investigated for imaging metastatic bone disease. Similar to the use of technetium-99m-labeled phosphonates, NaF-18 can visualize bone metabolism. However, in comparison to whole-body scintigraphy, PET with NaF-18 delivers high-resolution cross-sectional imaging of the whole body (Fig. 17.1).

F-18 sodium fluoride has been used earlier for conventional bone scintigraphy [74–80]. When new technetium-99m-labeled radiopharmaceuticals were introduced into clinical routine, NaF-18 scintigraphy was dropped because it had worse physical characteristics for the gamma camera. Since positron emission tomography was introduced as a routine clinical procedure, NaF-18 has gained new interest. One underlying reason for this is the high spatial resolution of PET [73], which is approximately 5 mm, whereas the spatial resolution of single photon emission computer tomography (SPECT) lies between 1 cm and 1.5 cm [75]. A further advantage of NaF-18 is that its bone uptake in regions of pathologically elevated bone metabolism is clearly higher than that of technetium-99m-labeled phosphonates [76]. Moreover, it has been shown that the absolute tracer uptake in normal bone of NaF-18 is twice as high as that of the phosphonates [77]. These properties of NaF-18 result in an enhanced image contrast of metastasis to normal bone and, consequently, lead to a better visualization and detection rate for PET. Additionally, tracer elimination from the vascular compartment is more rapid for NaF-18 than for the polyphosphonates [76]. Therefore, the time interval between injection of the agent and start of acquisition can be shortened when using NaF-18.

Preliminary results with NaF-18 PET are very encouraging [72, 81–84]. Schirrmeister et al. conducted a study in breast cancer patients comparing the diagnostic accuracy for detecting osseous metastases between F-18 PET and planar whole body scintigraphy [72]. In this study, MRI was used as a gold standard refer-

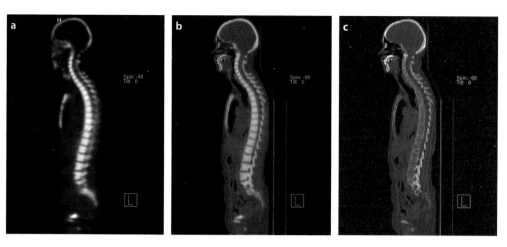

Fig. 17.1a–c. A 60-year-old patient with carcinoma of the breast who was examined by integrated PET/CT for primary staging. Sagittal slices of (**a**) pure PET image, (**b**) fusion image, and (**c**) pure CT image (bone window) are visualized showing a normal finding. Note the good resolution of F-18 sodium fluoride PET depicting all vertebrae of the spinal column

ence method. The authors found that the extent of metastatic bone disease was underestimated in 11 of 17 patients by bone scintigraphy but correctly identified in all patients by F-18 PET (identical with MRI results). Furthermore, F-18 PET revealed bone metastases in three patients with negative scintigraphy. The authors concluded that F-18 PET had an impact on clinical patient management in 18% of the cases. However, one shortcoming of study was that bone SPECT was not compared to F-18 bone PET. We do not know whether the three false-negative bone scans would have been true-positive with bone SPECT. This can be supposed as there is evidence that SPECT detects more metastases than planar bone scintigraphy. In spite of these considerations, bone PET still has the advantage of delivering whole-body cross-sectional images within a short time interval and with a better anatomical resolution.

Comparing bone scintigraphy with FDG-PET in breast cancer, Lonneux et al. showed that in 33 patients with normal bone scintigraphy, bone marrow infiltration could be demonstrated with a high sensitivity by FDG-PET [85]. Some studies proved that bone scintigraphy and FDG-PET have similar sensitivity in detecting breast cancer bone metastases but that specificity is significantly higher with

FDG-PET [86, 87]. There are data giving evidence that FDG-PET is more sensitive than bone scintigraphy in diagnosing small osteolytic bone and bone marrow metastases. In osteoblastic metastases, however, scintigraphy with phosphonates was more accurate than FDG-PET. It is known that breast cancer generates predominantly osteolytic metastases, but also mixed osteolytic-osteoblastic disease can occur. Therefore, neither bone scintigraphy nor FDG-PET can be exclusively favored for the detection of bone metastases. FDG-PET has the advantage of also delivering staging information about other organs such as liver, lung, and lymph nodes. Special attention must be paid to previous treatment because recent chemotherapy or continuing hormonal therapy often reduces FDG-uptake. In this situation, the staging of the disease by FDG-PET does not make sense, as it is rather imaging the presence of active tumor tissue for therapy monitoring. The authors recommended performing FDG-PET/CT as a perioperative primary staging method for all organ systems. If only the skeletal system is to be examined for metastatic disease, we consider F-18 fluoride PET the best examination (Fig. 17.2); however, no comparative study between F-18 fluoride PET and FDG-PET has been published so far. It must be assumed

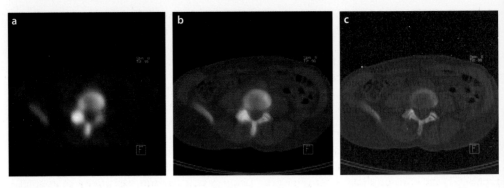

Fig. 17.2a–c. Same patient as in Fig. 17.1. Focal accumulation of F-18 sodium fluoride was detected in the lumbar vertebra 4. By fusion of PET and CT images, the tracer uptake can be located in the right small intervertebral joint L4/5, indicating degenerative disease and excluding a bone metastasis. Transversal slices of (**a**) pure PET image, (**b**) fusion image, and (**c**) pure CT image (*bone window*) are shown

that bone PET might also miss small bone marrow metastases that are visible on FDG-PET.

For lung cancer patients, there are also few prospective studies comparing bone scintigraphy and F-18 fluoride-PET. Schirrmeister and colleagues included 53 patients with SCLC or with NSCLC, prospectively performing planar bone scintigraphy, SPECT, and bone-PET with F-18 fluoride. Twelve patients had bone metastases. Planar bone scintigraphy, SPECT, and F-18 fluoride PET produced six, one, and no false-negative findings, respectively. The ROC curve analysis (mirroring diagnostic accuracy) showed that F-18 PET had the highest value; however, it was not significantly better than bone SPECT. In all but one patient, bone scintigraphy with SPECT diagnosed metastatic disease with the same sensitivity as bone PET. The authors concluded that bone PET is the most accurate method but is costly and not always readily available. They propose that a practicable and cost-effective strategy with a significant effect on patient management is the combination of planar bone scintigraphy with SPECT, complemented by MRI for unclear lesions. We also investigated 40 lung cancer patients with planar bone scintigraphy and SPECT and F-18 fluoride PET and correlated the findings with MRI of the spine serving as the gold standard. We found a higher sensitivity of bone PET and bone SPECT in comparison with planar bone scintigraphy. In four patients with predominantly osteoblastic metastases,

F-18 fluoride revealed bone disease in spite of a false-negative MRI. These findings were confirmed by clinical follow-up. However, in three patients with osteolytic metastases, MRI was more accurate than F-18 fluoride PET and bone SPECT.

Comparing bone scintigraphy and FDG-PET, there are contradictory results [88–89]. In a study of 100 patients, Marom et al. found that sensitivity for FDG-PET (92%) was higher than that for bone scintigraphy (50%) [88]. In contrast to these findings, other groups report that bone scintigraphy had a higher sensitivity than FDG-PET (84% vs 67%) but a lower specificity (84% vs 96%). The reason for these discrepancies might be the different metabolism of osteosclerotic and osteolytic metastases, as already mentioned above. Garcia et al. detected more osteosclerotic metastases on bone scintigraphy than in FDG-PET, whereas lytic metastases were better visualized by FDG-PET than by bone scans [89].

It seems that FDG-PET is the best technique for preoperative whole-body staging of lung cancer (including the detection of bone disease). When FDG-PET is negative and/or bone metastases are suspected, it is useful to perform an additional bone SPECT or bone PET.

In prostate cancer, we generally find osteoblastic bone lesion. Urologists recommend using bone scintigraphy in preoperative management only in patients with PSA levels over 10–20 ng/ml. In patients with rising PSA value after radical prostatectomy or radiation therapy, bone scintigraphy is requested in approximately 70% of cases for follow-up. It seems that F-18 fluoride has the potential to detect bone disease due to prostate cancer earlier than bone scintigraphy. Even-Sapir et al. investigated 44 patients with high-risk prostate cancer prospectively with planar bone scintigraphy, SPECT, bone PET, and bone PET/CT [90]. In 24 patients who also had whole-body bone SPECT, sensitivity was 100% for PET and PET/CT, 92% for SPECT, and 70% for planar bone scintigraphy. Specificity was 100% for PET/CT, 82% for PET and SPECT, and 64% for planar scintigraphy. The authors conclude that PET/CT with F-18 fluoride is a highly accurate modality for detection of bone metastases in high-risk prostate cancer patients. It is more specific than F-18 fluoride PET alone and more sensitive and specific than planar and bone SPECT. Looking at these data, we can learn that bone SPECT should be performed whenever possible in patients showing an abnormality as well as in prostate cancer patients with no accumulation on planar images. Furthermore, F-18 fluoride PET should replace bone scintigraphy whenever available. Ideally, patients should receive PET/CT with F-18 fluoride because it combines high sensitivity with high specificity. It seems possible to detect bone metastases in prostate cancer patients at an earlier stage of disease and probably at a lower PSA level. Data to confirm this is still lacking. Bone metastases as well as lymph node metastases can be detected by F-18 cholin PET in prostate cancer patients. F-18 cholin is a very promising radiopharmaceutical for prostate cancer. Comparative studies between F-18 cholin and F-18 fluoride for the detection of bone metastases are not available. Therefore, the author would recommend using F-18 fluoride if the question is exclusively the presence of osseous metastases.

It also seems important to stress a number of methodical points. If possible, SPECT should always be performed in addition to planar imaging. SPECT can increase specificity. By roughly localizing a focal accumulation, differentiation between degenerative and metastatic lesions can often be made. Also, the sensitivity of SPECT is higher than that of planar imaging. This means for our everyday clinical practice that SPECT is to be performed also (and especially) in patients showing a normal bone SPECT. Several studies have demonstrated that additional metastases can be detected in this situation by SPECT. The same is true for F-18 PET, which clearly delivers better anatomical resolution than SPECT. Whereas the diagnostic gain is huge if planar scintigraphy is compared with bone-PET, it is less important if SPECT and F-18 are compared. In prostate and lung cancer patients, sensitivity of bone-PET was slightly higher than that of bone-SPECT.

New camera devices consist of a combined nuclear camera and CT camera part, providing the advantage of defining exactly the location of a focal accumulation on SPECT or PET images (Fig. 17.3). Preliminary studies show that PET/CT as well as SPECT/CT is able to increase specificity of bone SPECT and bone PET significantly (Fig. 17.4). These results are very encouraging.

Another new approach for the detection of bone metastases is whole-body MRI. However, sensitivity for metastatic disease in the skull, the sternum, and the ribs was lower than that of planar bone scintigraphy [91]. In the spine, some studies have shown that planar bone scintigraphy detects fewer metastatic lesions than MRI [92, 93]. However, there is no comparison of MRI with bone SPECT or bone PET. Furthermore, these studies investigated very heterogeneous patient groups and therefore did not differentiate between tumor type and or the osteolytic and osteoblastic type. Some studies used MRI for the gold standard in the spine when comparing F-18 bone PET with planar bone scintigraphy and bone SPECT. Schirrmeister reported that F-18 PET detected all breast cancer bone metastases that were found by special spine-focused MRI. The authors concluded that sensitivity of F-18 bone PET is at least as high as that of MRI in the spine. Since MRI performed less well than nuclear imaging in the skull, sternum, and ribs, and since there is no study proving an advantage of MRI over bone SPECT or over bone PET in the spine, the author would not recommend whole-body MRI as a screening method for bone metastases.

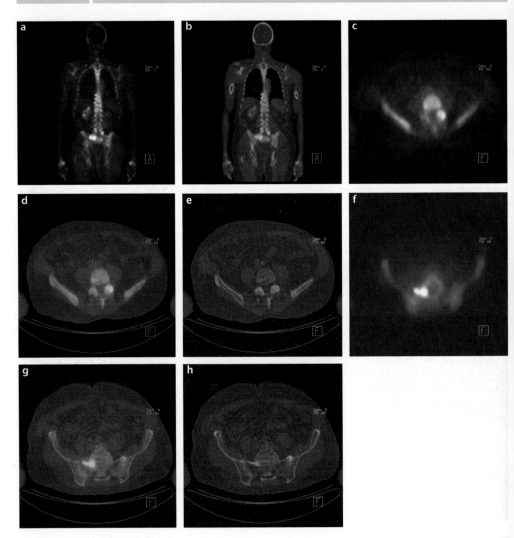

Fig 17.3a–h. Patient with lung cancer who complained about lumbar pain and was investigated with integrated PET/CT for primary staging. The coronal slice shows two foci of tracer uptake, one in the lower lumbar spine on the left side and one in the sacroiliac region on the right side (**a** PET image, **b** fusion image). These findings could correspond to metastatic osseous disease as well as to degenerative changes of the intervertebral and sacroiliac joints. Transverse slices of the lumbar focus [**c** pure PET image, **d** fusion image, and **e** pure CT image (*bone window*)] show that tracer uptake is located in the left small intervertebral joint L4/5, indicating degenerative disease. Transverse slices of the sacroiliac region [**f** pure PET image, **g** fusion image, and **h** pure CT image (*bone window*)] demonstrate that tracer uptake is only located in the right massa lateralis of the sacrum with no sign of degenerative changes in CT images. This finding indicates metastatic bone disease, which was later confirmed by MRI and histology

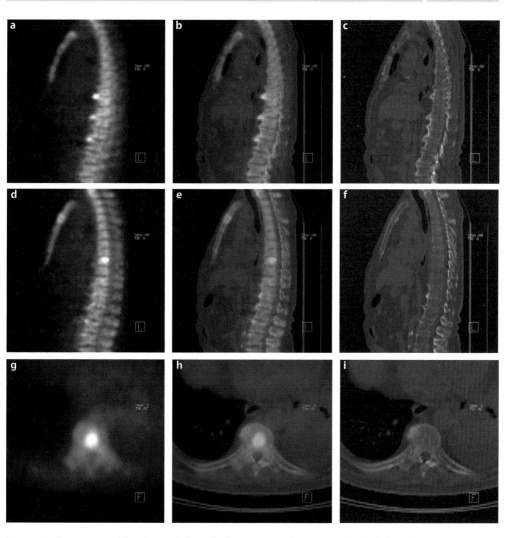

Fig. 17.4a–i. A 64-year-old patient with bronchial carcinoma who presented with diffuse back pain was investigated with integrated PET/CT for restaging purposes. The sagittal slices [**a** pure PET image, **b** fusion image, and **c** pure CT image (*bone window*)] demonstrate multiple F-18 sodium-fluoride foci in the ventral part of the thoracic vertebrae, indicating spondylarthrosis of the vertebral column. However, one focal uptake in the thoracic vertebra 9 was suspicious for malignancy [sagittal slices of **d** pure PET image, **e** fusion image, and **f** pure CT image (*bone window*)]. Transverse slices [**g** pure PET image, **h** fusion image, and **i** pure CT image (*bone window*)] show that the focal accumulation is exactly located on an osteolytic region with circumferential hyperostosis. This is a clear finding corresponding to pronounced degenerative changes (Schmorl nodule) and not to metastatic bone disease

References

1. Becker N, Wahrendorf J (1998) Krebsatlas der Bundesrepublik Deutschland 1981–1990. Springer, Berlin New York Heidelberg
2. Schalhorn A (1985) Bronchialkarzinom: Möglichkeiten und Grenzen der Chemotherapie. Fortschr Med 103:309–311
3. Schalhorn A (1985) Bronchialkarzinom: Möglichkeiten und Grenzen der Chemotherapie. Fortschr Med 103:453–456
4. Sobin LH, Wittekind C (1997) TNM classification of malignant tumors, 5th edn. Wiley-Liss, New York
5. Stahel RA, Ginsberg R, Havemann K et al (1989) Staging and prognostic factors in small cell lung cancer: a consensus report. Lung Cancer 5:119–126
6. Stuschke M, Heilmann HP (1996) Lunge und Mediastinum. In: Scherer E, Sack H (eds) Strahlentherapie. Springer, Berlin New York Heidelberg
7. Holmes EC (1989) Surgical adjuvant therapy of NSCLC. J Surg Oncol 42 [Suppl 1]:26–33
8. Dosoretz D, Galmarini D, Rubenstein JH et al (1993) Local control in medically inoperable lung cancer: analysis of its importance in outcome and factors determining the probability of tumor eradication. Int J Radiat Oncol Biol Phys 27:507–516
9. Noordijk EM, van der Poest, Hermans J, Wever AMJ, Leer JWH (1988) Radiotherapy as an alternative to surgery in elderly patients with resectable lung cancer. Radiother Oncol 13:83–89
10. Sandler HM, Curran WJ, Turrisi AT (1990) The influence of tumor size and pre-treatment staging on outcome following radiation therapy alone for stage I NSCLC. Int J Radiat Oncol Biol Phys 10:9–13
11. Bülzebruck H, Danzer B, Hilkemeier G et al (1998) Metastasierung und Prognose des kleinzelligen Bronchialkarzinoms. Onkologe 4:1039–1047
12. Line D, Deeley TJ (1971) The necropsy findings in carcinoma of the bronchus. Br J Dis Chest 65:238
13. Wolf M (1998) Kleinzelliges Bronchialkarzinom: Klinische Präsentation, Diagnostik und prognostische Faktoren. Onkologe 4:1005–1018
14. Hansen HH, Muggia FM (1972) Staging of inoperable patients with bronchogenic carcinoma with special reference to bone marrow and peritoneoscopy. Cancer 30:1395–1401
15. Schalhorn A, Sunder-Plassmann L (2000) Maligne Tumoren der Thorakal- und Mediastinalorgane. In: Wilmanns W, Huhn D, Wilms K (eds) Internistische Onkologie. Thieme, Stuttgart, pp 617–642
16. Bonomi PD, Finkelstein DM, Ruckdeschel JC et al (1989) Combination chemotherapy vs. single agents followed by combinations chemotherapy in stage IV NSCLC: a study of the eastern cooperative oncology group. J Clin Oncol 7:1602–1613
17. Drings P, Becker H, Bülzebruck H, Manke HG, Tessen HW (1990) Chemotherapie des fortgeschrittenen nichtkleinzelligen Bronchialkarzinoms mit Ifosfamid und Etoposid. Tumordiagn Ther 11:79–84
18. Spiegelman D, Maurer H, Ware JH (1989) Prognostic factors in SCLC: an analysis of 1521 patients. J Clin Oncol 7:344–354
19. Rosell R, Lopez-Cabrerizo MP, Astudillo J (1997) Preoperative chemotherapy for stage IIIA NSCLC. Curr Opin Oncol 9:149–155
20. Albain KS, Crowley JJ, Leblanc M, Livingston RB (1990) Determinants of improved outcome in SCLC: an analysis of the 2580 patients – Southwest Oncology Group data base. J Clin Oncol 8:1563–1574
21. Manegold C, Bülzebruck H, Drings P, Vogt-Moykopf I (1989) Prognostische Faktoren beim kleinzelligen Bronchialkarzinom. Onkologe 12:240–245
22. Golz R, Störkel S (1999) Anatomie und Pathologie des Prostatakarzinom. In: Hinkelbein W, Miller K, Wiegel T (eds) Prostatakarzinom. Springer, Berlin New York Heidelberg
23. Statistisches Bundesamt (1994) Gesundheitswesen. Fachserie 12, Reihe 4 Todesursachen in Deutschland, Wiesbaden
24. Saitoh H, Hida M, Shimbo T et al (1984) Metastatic patterns of prostatic cancer. Cancer 54:3078–3084
25. De la Monte SM, Moore GW, Hutchins GM (1986) Metastatic behaviour of prostate cancer. Cancer 58:985–993
26. Ravery V, Schmid HP, Toublanc M, Boccon-Gibod L (1996) Is the percentage of cancer in biopsy cores predictive of extracapsular disease in T1-T2 prostate cancer? Cancer 78:1079–1084
27. Badalament RA, Miller MC, Peller PA et al (1996) An algorithm for predicting nonorgan confined prostate cancer using the results obtained from sexant core biopsies with prostate specific antigen level. J Urol 156:1375–1380
28. Breul J, Binder K, Hartung R (1991) Fehler bei der präoperativen Bestimmung des lokalen Tumorstadiums bei der radikalen Prostatektomie. In: Hartung R, Kropp A (eds) Urologische Beckenchirurgie. Springer, Berlin New York Heidelberg, pp 271–298
29. Rorvik J, Halvorsen OJ, Servoll E, Haukaas S (1994) Transrectal ultrasonography to assess local extent of prostatic cancer before radical prostatectomy. Br J Urol 73:65–69
30. Partin A, Yoo J, Carter HB (1990) PSA in the staging of localized prostate cancer: influence of tumor differentiation tumor volume and benign hyperplasia. J Urol 143:747–756
31 Kleer E, Oesterlin JE (1993) PSA and staging of localized prostate cancer. Urol Clin North Am 20:695–705
32. Catalona WJ, Smith DS, Ratliff TL Basler JW et al (1991) Measurement of PSA in serum as a screening test for prostate cancer. N Engl J Med 324:1156–1161
33. Wirth MP, Frohmüller HGW (1992) PSA and prostate acid phosphatase in the detection of early prostate cancer and the prediction of regional lymph node metastases. Eur Urol 22:27–32
34. Shreve PD, Grossman HB, Gross MD, Wahl RL (1996) Metastatic prostate cancer: initial findings of PET with F-18 fluoro-D-glucose. Radiology 199:751–756

35. Partin AW, Kattan MW, Subong EN et. al (1997) Combination of PSA, clinical stage, and Gleason Score to predict pathological stage of localized prostate cancer. JAMA 277:1445–1451

36. Klän R, Meier T, Knispel HH, Wegner HE, Miller K (1995) Laparoscopic pelvic lymphadenectomy in prostatic cancer. Urol Int 55:78–83

37. Catalona WJ, Smith DJ (1994) 5-year tumor recurrence rates after anatomical radical retropubic prostatectomy for prostate cancer. J Urol 152:1837–1842

38. Ohori M, Goag JR, Wheeler TM et al (1994) Can radical prostatectomy alter the progression of poorly differentiated prostate cancer? J Urol 152:1843–1849

39. Hanks GE, LeeWR, Haulon MS et al (1996) Conformal technique dose escalation for prostate cancer. Int J RadiatOncol Biol Phys 35:861–868

40. Zietman AL, Shipley WU (1993) Randomized trials in loco-regionally confined prostate cancer: past present and future. Semin Radiat Oncol 3:210–220

41. Epstein JI, Pizov G, Walsh PC (1993) Correlation of pathologic findings with progression after radical retropubic prostatectomy. Cancer 71:3586–3589

42. Perez CA, Hanks GE, Leibel SA et al (1993) Localized carcinoma of the prostate (stages T1, T2 and T3). Cancer 72:3156–3173

43. Chybowski FM, Keller JL, Bergstrahl EJ, Oesterling JE (1991) Predicting radionuclide bone scan finding in patients with newly diagnosed untreated prostate cancer. J Urol 145:313–318

44 Andriole GL, Kavoussi LR, Torrence JR (1988) Transrectal ultrasonography in the diagnosis and staging of the carcinoma of the prostate. J Urol 140:758–760

45. Noldus J, Stamey TA (1996) Limitations of serum PSA in predicting peripheral and transition zone cancer volumes as measured by correlation coefficients. J Urol 155:232–237

46. Kelsey JL, Gammon MD (1991) The epidemiology of breast cancer. Cancer 41:146–65

47. Sondik EJ (1994) Breast cancer trends. Incidence, mortality and survival. Cancer 74:995–999

48. Possinger K, Große Y (2000) Mammakarzinome und gynäkologische Tumoren. In: Wilmanns W, Huhn D, Wilms K (eds) Internistische Onkologie Thieme, Stuttgart, pp 452–508

49. Spratt JS, Donegan WL. Cancer of the breast. Saunders Philadelphia 1979.

50. Tabar l, Grad A, Holmberg LH et al (1985) Reduction in mortality from breast cancer after mass screening with mammography. Lancet 1:829

51. Boag JW, Jaybittle JL, Fowler JR (1971) The number of patinets required in a clinical trial. Brit J Radiol 44:122

52. Smart CR, Myers MH, Gloeckler LA (1978) Implications from SEER data on breast cancer management. Cancer 41:787–789

53. Koscielny SM, Tubiana M, Le MG et al (1984) Breast cancer. Relationship between the size of the primary tumor and the probability of metastatic dissemination. Br J Cancer 49:709

54. Donegan WL Epidemiology. In: Donegan WL, Spratt JS (eds) Cancer of the breast. Saunders, Philadelphia, pp 39–46

55. Foster RS Jr, Lang SP, Costanza MC et al (1978) Breast self-examination practices and breast cancer stage. New Engl J Med 299:265–270

56. Andersson I (1988) Mammographic screening and mortality from breast cancer: Malmö mammographic screening trial. BMJ 297 943–948

57. Frisell J, Eklund G, Hellström L et al (1991) Randomized study of mammography screening – preliminary report on mortality in the Stockholm trial. Breast Cancer Res Treat 18:49–56

58. Miller AB, Baines CJ, To T et al (1992) Canada national breast screening study. Can Med Assoc J 147:1459–1488

59. Meuret G (1995) Grundlagen des Mammakarzinoms. In: Meuret G (ed) Mammakarzinom. Thieme, Stuttgart, pp 1–21

60. Clark GM, Sledge GW, Osborne CK, McGuire WL (1987) Survival from first recurrence: relative importance of prognostic factors in 1015 breast cancer patients. J Clin Oncol 5:55–61

61. Come SE, Schnipper LE (1991) Myelophtisisanemia and other aspects of bone marrow involvement. In: Harris JR, Hellman S, Henderson IC, Kinne DW (eds) Breast diseases. Lippincott, Philadelphia, pp 761–766

62. Perez DJ, Powles TJ, Milan J et al (1983) Detection of breast carcinoma metastases in bone: relative merits of x-rays and skeletal scintigraphy. Lancet 2:613–616

63. Rossing N, Munck O, Nielsen SP et al (1982) What do early bone scans tell about breast cancer patients? Eur J Cancer Clin Oncol 18:629–636

64. Kamby C, Bruun Rasmussen B, Kristensen B (1991) Prognostic indicators of metastatic bone disease in human breast cancer. Cancer 68:2045–2050

65. Muss HB (1992) Endocrine therapy for advanced breast cancer: a review. Breast Cancer Res Treat 21:15–26

66. Diel IJ, Solomayer EF, Costa SD et al (1998) Reduction in new metastases in breast cancer with adjuvant clodronate treatment. N Engl J Med 339:357–363

67. Conte N, Giannessi PG, Latreille J et al (1994) Delayed progression of bone metastases with pamidronate therapy in breast cancer patients: a randomized, multicenter phase III trial. Br J Cancer 70: 554–558

68. Van Holten-Verzantvoort ATM, Hermans J et al (1996) Does supportive pamodronate treatment prevent or delay the first manifestation of bone metastases in breast cancer patients. Eur J Cancer 32:450–454

69. Aberizk WJ, Silver B, Henderson IC et al (1986) The use of radiotherapy for treatment of isolated locoregional recurrence of breast carcinoma after mastectomy. Cancer 58:1214–1218

70. Janjan NA, McNeese MD, Buzdar AU et al (1986) Management of locoregional recurrent breast cancer. Cancer 58:1552–1556

71. Noguchi S, Miyauchi K, Nishizawa Y et al (1987) Results of surgical treatment for sternal metastases in breast cancer. Cancer 60:2524–2531

72. Schirrmeister H, Guhlmann A, Kotzerke J et al (1999) Early detection and accurate description of extent of metastatic bone disease in breast cancer with fluoride ion and positron emission tomography. J Clin Oncol 17:2381–2389

73. Gambhir SS, Czernin J, Schwimmer J et al (2001) A tabulated summary of the FDG-PET literature. J Nucl Med 42:1S–93S

74. Blau M, Nagler W, Bender MA (1962) A new isotope for bone scanning. J Nucl Med 3:332–334

75. Cook G, Fogelman I (2001) The role of positron emission tomography in skeletal disease. Semin Nucl Med 1:50–61

76. Hawkins RA, Choi Y, Huang SC et al (1992) Evaluation of the skeletal kinetics of fluorine-18-fluoride ion with PET. J Nucl Med 33:633–642

77. Hoh CK, Hawkins RA, Dahlbom M et al (1993) Whole body skeletal imaging with F-18 fluoride ion and PET. J Comp Assist Tomogr 17:34–41

78. Mc Neil BJ et al (1973) Fluroine-18 bone scintigraphy in children with osteosarcoma or Ewing's sarcoma. Radiology 109:627–631

79. Buck AC et al (1975) Serial fluorine-18 bone scans in the follow-up of carcinoma of the prostate. Br J Urol 47:287–294

80. Rosenfield N, Treves S (1974) Osseous and extraosseous uptake of fluorine-18 and techentium-99m polyphosphate in children with neuroblastoma. Radiology 111:127–133

81. Schirrmeister H, Rentschler M, Kotzerke J et al (1998) Skeletal imaging with F-18 NaF PET and comparison with planar scintigraphy. Fortschr Röntgenstr 168:451–456

82. Schirrmeister H, Guhlmann CA, Diederichs CG, Träger H, Reske SN (1999) Planar bone imaging vs. F-18 PET in patients with cancer of the prostate, thyroid and lung. J Nucl Med 40:1623–1629

83. Schirrmeister H, Glatting G, Hetzel J, Nussle K, Arslandemir C, Buck AK, Dziuk K, Gabelmann A, Reske SN, Hetzel M (2001) Prospective evaluation of the clinical value of planar bone scans, SPECT, and (^{18})F-labeled NaF PET in newly diagnosed lung cancer. J Nucl Med 42:1800–1804

84. Palmedo H, Schaible R, Textor J, Ko Y, Grohé C, von Mallek D, Ezziddin S, Reinhardt MJ, Biersack HJ (2002) PET with ^{18}F Fluoride compared to bone scintigraphy in the diagnosis of bone metastases: results of a prospective study. J Nucl Med [Suppl]:1150–1151

85. Lonneux M, Borbath II, Berliere M, Kirkove C, Pauwels S (2000) The place of whole-body PET FDG for the diagnosis of distant recurrence of breast cancer. Clin Positron Imaging 3:45–49

86. Ohta M, Tokuda Y, Suzuki Y, Kubota M, Makuuchi H, Tajima T, Nasu S, Suzuki Y, Yasuda S, Shohtsu A (2001) Whole body PET for the evaluation of bony metastases in patients with breast cancer: comparison with 99Tcm-MDP bone scintigraphy. Nucl Med Commun 22:875–879

87. Yang SN, Liang JA, Lin FJ, Kao CH, Lin CC, Lee CC (2002) Comparing whole body (^{18})F-2-deoxyglucose positron emission tomography and technetium-99m methylene diphosphonate bone scan to detect bone metastases in patients with breast cancer. J Cancer Res Clin Oncol 128:325–328

88. Marom EM, McAdams HP, Erasmus JJ, Goodman PC, Culhane DK, Coleman RE, Herndon JE, Patz EF Jr (1999) Staging non-small cell lung cancer with whole-body PET. Radiology 212:803–809

89. Garcia JR, Simo M, Perez G, Soler M, Lopez S, Setoain X, Lomena F (2003) ^{99m}Tc-MDP bone scintigraphy and ^{18}F-FDG positron emission tomography in lung and prostate cancer patients: different affinity between lytic and sclerotic bone metastases. Eur J Nucl Med Mol Imaging 30:1714.

90. Even-Sapir E, Metser U, Mishani E, Lievshitz G, Lerman H, Leibovitch I (2006) The detection of bone metastases in patients with high-risk prostate cancer: ^{99m}Tc-MDP planar bone scintigraphy, single- and multi-field-of-view SPECT, ^{18}F-fluoride PET, and ^{18}F-fluoride PET/CT. J Nucl Med 47:287–297

91. Buscombe JR, Holloway B, Roche N, Bombardieri E (2004) Position of nuclear medicine modalities in the diagnostic work-up of breast cancer. Q J Nucl Med Mol Imaging 48:109–118

92. Ghanem N, Altehoefer C, Kelly T, Lohrmann C, Winterer J, Schafer O, Bley TA, Moser E, Langer M (2006) Whole-body MRI in comparison to skeletal scintigraphy in detection of skeletal metastases in patients with solid tumors. In Vivo 20:173–182

93. Frat A, Agildere M, Gencoglu A, Cakir B, Akin O, Akcali Z, Aktas A (2006) Value of whole-body turbo short tau inversion recovery magnetic resonance imaging with panoramic table for detecting bone metastases: comparison with 99MTc-methylene diphosphonate scintigraphy. J Comput Assist Tomogr 30:151–156

18 Receptor PET/CT Imaging of Neuroendocrine Tumors

R. P. Baum, V. Prasad, M. Hommann, and D. Hörsch

Recent Results in Cancer Research, Vol. 170
© Springer-Verlag Berlin Heidelberg 2008

This chapter is dedicated to Gustav Hör, Professor Emeritus and former Director of the Department of Nuclear Medicine, University of Frankfurt/Main, on the occasion of his 75th birthday.

18.1 Introduction

Neuroendocrine tumors (NETs) are a heterogeneous group of neoplasms which are characterized by their endocrine metabolism and histology pattern. The diversity of NETs can be judged with the different names [carcinoid tumor, APUDoma gastroenteropancreatic (GEP) tumor, islet cell tumor, neuroendocrine tumor, and neuroendocrine carcinoma] that have been put forward for describing these endocrine tumors (Solcia et al. 2000). Oberndorfer (1907) first described the term "carcinoid tumor" for the "endocrine tumor originating in small intestine and characterized by slow growth and late metastases". Previously, NETs have also been called APUDomas (for amine precursor uptake and decarboxylation) and were suspected of originating from the neural crest. However, the peptide-secreting cells of the tumors are not derived from the neuroectodermal unit (Jensen 2005). Subsequently, the origin of these tumors was traced to pluripotent stem cells or differentiated neuroendocrine cells (Li and Beheshti 2005). The slow growth of these tumors makes it very diffi-

cult to localize the site of the tumor in the early stage (Baum and Hofmann 2004; Kaltsas et al. 2004). Localization is essential to select the optimal currently available management protocols (including curative surgery, cytoreductive surgery, and antiproliferative tumor treatment) and for predicting the patient's prognosis (Jensen 2005). The various compounds produced by these tumors, along with their characteristic symptoms – although useful in the diagnosis of the disease – do not help much in solving a clinician's dilemma to decide upon the best treatment regime. Conventional imaging modalities such as ultrasonography (USG), CT scan, magnetic resonance imaging (MRI), although useful for detecting the number of lesions and other anatomical details, do not give information on the functional status of the tumor, which is essential for defining the prognosis (Li and Beheshti 2005).

These issues and the discovery of overexpression of receptors for peptide hormones in cancerous tissue in the mid 1980s led to the gradual upsurge in the role of nuclear medicine procedures in the diagnostic algorithm for NET. The biokinetics of peptides, unlike radiolabeled monoclonal antibodies, are favorable because of fast clearance, rapid tissue penetration and low antigenicity (Krenning et al. 2004). Many different radiolabeled peptide analogs, for example, somatostatin, cholecystokinin (CCK), bombesin, substance P, gastrin, vasoactive intestinal peptides (VIP), and neuropeptide (NP)-Y have been used for the evaluation of receptor expression on tumor cells (Behr and Behe 2002; Behr et al. 1998, 2001; Blum et al. 2000; Krenning et al. 1989, 1992, 1993; Kwekkeboom et al. 2000; Reubi et al. 1997, 2000a, 2001a, 2002; van Hagen et al. 1996; Virgolini et al. 1995, 1996, 1998; Weiner and Thakur 2002). Amongst the somatostatin analogs, 111In-DTPA-octreotide (DTPA-OC) was approved by the Food and Drug Administration (FDA) for scintigraphy of patients with neuroendocrine tumors. Various other radiopharmaceuticals have been used successfully for the diagnosis of NET, especially metastasized NETs. This article will focus mainly on the role of receptor PET and PET/CT along with different peptides currently used in the diagnosis of NET. The clinical symptoms and the role of other diagnostic modalities (conventional imaging as well as basic nuclear medicine procedures) will be highlighted briefly.

18.2   Pathology and Clinical Course of NETs

The incidence of neuroendocrine tumors is reported to be low; however, because of the indolent nature of the tumor, it is expected that many of the patients do not get diagnosed during their lifetime. Although NET can occur at many places in the body, the most common sites are the bronchus/lungs and the gastroenteropancreatic tract; other less common sites are skin, adrenal glands, thyroid, and genital tract (Jensen 2005). The definition of NET encompasses a wide variety of tumors, for example, gastroenteropancreatic NETs (GEPs), neuroblastoma, multiple endocrine neoplasia (MEN), pheochromocytoma, medullary thyroid carcinoma, small cell lung cancer, and others. Traditionally, NETs are classified according to the site of origin (foregut, midgut, and hindgut) as the tumors originating from the same site share functional manifestations, histochemistry, and secretory granules (Jensen 2005). Based upon histopathology, WHO has defined a separate classification to the NETs (Schmitt-Gräff et al. 2000; Solcia et al. 2000). Approximately 70% of carcinoid tumors origi-

nating from GI tissue are found in the following three sites: bronchus, jejunoileum, or colon/rectum. The carcinoid tumors and other tumors originating from the pancreas commonly show a malignant behavior. Other than insulinomas, in which fewer than 10% are malignant, nearly 50%–100% of pancreatic NET show a malignant behavior. Among the NETs of the GI tract, the incidence of metastases is highest in jejunoileum (58%), followed by lung/bronchus (6%) and rectum (4%) (Jensen 2005).

NETs consist of monotonous sheets of small round cell nuclei and are characterized by their propensity to being stained with silver and to markers of neuroendocrine tissues (e.g., chromogranin, neuron-specific enolase, and synaptophysin) using immunohistochemical methods. On electron microscopy, these tumors possess numerous membrane-bound neurosecretory granules containing various hormones and biogenic amines. The secretion of these into the blood gives rise to various typical clinical syndromes (Jensen 2005).

NETs have also been classified according to the presence or absence of clinical syndromes into functional/nonfunctional NETs (Jensen 2005). Nonfunctional NETs comprise nearly 33%–50% of all NETs. The symptoms present in this subset of patients with a NET are largely related to the mass effect of the tumor. Many times they are detected occasionally, often at a late stage when the tumor is already metastasized. In the group of functional NETs, the most common symptoms are diarrhea, flushing, pain, asthma/wheezing, pellagra, carcinoid heart disease such as endocardial fibrosis (Jensen 2005). There are numerous factors that influence the survival and prognosis of the patients among which the presence of liver metastases is the single most important factor. A correlation has been found between the size of the primary tumor and the chances of metastases in small intestinal carcinoids. Metastases to liver occurred in 15%–25% of tumors if the tumor diameter was smaller than 1 cm, in 58%–80% if it was 1–2 cm, and in more than 75% if the tumor size was larger than 2 cm (Jensen 2005). All these factors make it essential to have a correct diagnostic algorithm before selecting a particular treatment regime.

18.3 Diagnosis

The diagnosis of NET begins with a detailed history and thorough clinical examination. The characteristic history of flushing and intractable diarrhea warrants biochemical evaluation, which starts with measuring serum serotonin or the metabolite in the urine (5-hydroxy indole acid). Other NET markers, such as chromogranin A and neuron-specific enolase (NSE), are measured in serum. Generally these markers are elevated in carcinoid tumors. In case gastrinoma is suspected (history of abdominal pain, diarrhea, and gastroesophageal reflux disease), the fasting gastrin level should be measured. If the diagnosis of insulinoma is suspected, elevated insulin levels are found in fasting condition. C-peptide and serum glucose levels are also measured. In case pheochromocytoma is suspected, metanephrines, catecholamines, and their metabolites should be measured in the blood and urine (Jensen 2005).

After the evaluation of biochemical markers, the next step in the diagnostic algorithm is to determine the site of the primary tumor. Chest x-ray should be performed specifically if a thoracic origin of the tumor is suspected (Bombardieri et al. 2004). The role of USG in diagnosis of NET is variable and depends largely on the site of disease. USG has very high diagnostic accuracy for detection of liver metastases. If a gastric or pancreatic primary tumor is suspected, endoscopic USG should be used. Sometimes, for assessment of tumor vascularity, color Doppler and power Doppler USG are used in conjunction with CT.

CT and MRI are used for morphologic delineation of the tumor. CT is essential for preoperative staging. It is also used in patient follow-up. The accurate measurement of tumor size and extent can be evaluated using three-dimensional reconstruction. MRI is the method of choice in the study of cervical masses. MRI is also useful in intracranial lesions, intraspinal lesions and for detection of bone marrow involvement (Bombardieri et al. 2004). However, in spite of giving a perfect anatomical information of the tumors, these morphologic imaging methodologies are of limited use for determining the functional tumor status. This is the field where nuclear medicine procedures, with its armamentarium of radiopharmaceuticals, yields essential information in addition to morphological parameters. One significant advantage of nuclear medicine imaging techniques is the possibility of performing a whole-body scan in a single study.

18.4 Radionuclide Imaging of NETs

Radionuclide imaging has been used for the diagnosis of NET for many years. However, only in the last decade, PET and PET/CT, using specific radiopharmaceuticals, have gained a special role in the diagnostic work-up of NET patients.

18.4.1 Radiopharmaceuticals Used in Conventional Nuclear Medicine

18.4.1.1 ^{131}I-MIBG and ^{123}I-MIBG

Metaiodobenzylguanidine (MIBG), a functional and structural analog of norepinephrine, tagged with the gamma-emitting radionuclide ^{123}I or ^{131}I, is used to localize neuroblastomas, pheochromocytomas, and paragangliomas (Berglund et al. 2001; Castellani et al. 2000; Shapiro et al. 1985, 1989). [123]I is preferred over ^{131}I because of the better physical characteristics, higher photon efficiency, and the possibility of performing a high-quality SPECT study. The tumor uptake of MIBG is inhibited by several drugs such as tricyclic antidepressants, sympathomimetics, and certain antihypertensive/cardiovascular drugs which must be paused prior to imaging with ^{123}I-MIBG or ^{131}I MIBG (Khafagi et al. 1989; Solanki et al. 1992).

Peptide-Based Radiopharmaceuticals for Diagnosis of NETs

Radiolabeled peptides have been used for targeting specific receptors on neuroendocrine tumors or over 15 years now (Krenning et al. 1989, 1990, 1992). The overexpression of peptide receptors in various tumor cells opened a new chapter in the field of molecular imaging. Peptides have better pharmacokinetic properties and no (or very low) antigenicity as compared to monoclonal antibodies, making them an ideal ligand for receptor-based scintigraphy. Somatostatin, a cyclic peptide hormone, or somatostatin analogs labeled with different radionuclides, is an example of these peptides that have been used with high efficiency in the diagnosis of NETs.

18.4.1.2 Somatostatin Receptor-Based Peptides

There are two naturally occurring bioactive forms of somatostatins: somatostatin-14 and somatostatin-28. The receptors of somatostatin are normally expressed in different parts of the body (e.g., in the pituitary, thyroid gland, pancreas, and GI tract). The primary action of this peptide hormone is the inhibition of hormone secretion and modulation of neurotransmission and cell proliferation through specific G-protein-coupled receptors (Wild et al. 2003). Five different types of somatostatin receptor proteins have been cloned (sstr1–5). Some of these receptors are overexpressed in NETs, which enables their visualization and localization with radiometal chelator conjugates of somatostatin analogs (Wild et al. 2003). Most of the tumors that have been studied with radiolabeled somatostatin analogues mainly express sstr2; however, recent results have shown that sstr1 and sstr3–5 are also expressed on many tumors to varying degrees (Reubi et al. 2001b). In neuroendocrine tumors of mid-gut origin, sstr2 is expressed maximally (95%) followed by sstr1 (80%) and sstr5 (75%) (Jensen 2005). The first radiolabeled somatostatin analog to be approved for the scintigraphy of NET was ^{111}In-DTPA- D-Phe1-octreotide (OctreoScan, ^{111}In-pentetreotide) (Krenning et al. 1989, 1990, 1992). Results have shown that this radiopharmaceutical is ideally suited for localizing primary and metastatic NET (Krenning et al. 1993; Lebtahi et al. 2002). The ^{99m}Tc-labeled somatostatin analogs such as ^{99m}Tc-depreotide, ^{99m}Tc-vapreotide, ^{99m}Tc-P829, and ^{99m}Tc-EDDA-HYNIC-TOC are also used

(Decristoforo et al. 2000; Lebtahi et al. 2002; Virgolini 2000). ^{99m}Tc-EDDA-HYNIC-TOC (Fig. 18.1) has been shown to be superior to ^{111}In-pentetreotide for the detection of sstr-positive tumors (Decristoforo et al. 2000). In an effort to find somatostatin analogs with higher affinity for certain sstr subreceptors, the next generation of somatostatin analogs, DOTA-TOC (1,4,7,10-tetraazacyclododecane-1,4,7,10-tetraacetic acid Tyr[3] octreotide) was developed and labeled with different radionuclides for imaging as well as for therapy (de Jong et al. 1997; Otte et al. 1998, 1999; Paganelli et al. 2001; Pershagen 1998; Stolz et al. 1998; Waldherr et al. 2002). Replacement of the alcohol group at the C-terminus of the peptide by a carboxylic acid group results in the formation of DOTA-D-Phe1-Tyr[3]-Thr[8]-octreotide (DOTA-TATE), which has the highest affinity for the sstr2 receptor (Kwekkeboom et al. 2001; Reubi et al. 2000c, Antunes et al. 2007). However, the binding affinity to other sstr receptors has been less than expected; binding to sstr5 is low, to sstr3 is negligible, and there is no or very little affinity to sstr1 and sstr4 (Wild et al. 2003, Antunes et al. 2007). ^{111}In-DOTA-lanreotide (LAN; D-2-Nal-Cys-tyr-D-Trp-Lys-Val-Thr-NH$_2$) was found to be superior to ^{111}In-DTPA-octreotide for the detection of primary pancreatic adenocarcinomas (Raderer et al. 1998). However, the claim of Raderer et al. that 111In-DOTA-lanreotide targets sstr2–5 with higher affinity and sstr1 with lower affinity was not confirmed by Reubi et al. (2000c).

Next in the development were the third-generation somatostatin analogs such as DOTA-NOC (DOTA-1-Nal[3]-octreotide), which was the result of an amino acid exchange at position 3 of octreotide. This compound has been shown to have improved affinity for sstr2 and higher affinity to sstr3 and sstr5 (Wild et al. 2003), resulting in coverage of a wider spectrum of sstr (pansomatostatin analog) and thereby improve the diagnosis of NET and various other somatostatin receptor-expressing tumors, for example malignant pheochromocytoma (Fig. 18.2), paraganglioma, and glomus tumors. After receptor binding, ^{68}Ga-DOTA-NOC/DOTA-TOC is internalized

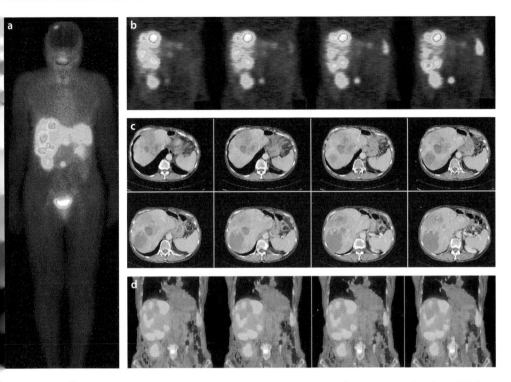

Fig. 18.1a–d. ^{99m}Tc EDDA Hynic TOC whole-body scan: (**a** anterior view 1 h postinjection) and SPECT slices (**b** coronal view 2 h p.i.) demonstrating multiple liver metastases of a bronchus carcinoid operated 17 years before. In addition, bone metastases in the lumbar spine and in the skull are seen. **c** and **d** show the transaxial CT and coronal PET slices of the same patient using Ga-68 DOTA-NOC with intense accumulation of the somatostatin analog in the liver metastases

into the tumor cells with minimal washout of the peptides from the tumor cells thereafter (Henze et al. 2001, 2004, 2005). Other somatostatin analogs labeled with various radionuclides have been used for scintigraphy of sstr-positive tumors with variable success (Rufini et al. 2006). New somatostatin analogs that are in the preclinical stage of development are DOTA-NOC-ATE (DOTA-1Nal^3,Thr^8)-octeotide and DOTA-BOC and DOTA-BOC-ATE (DOTA, BzThi^3, Thr^8)-octreotide. Radiolabeled with 111In, they have been shown to have high affinity for sstr2, sstr3, and sstr5 and intermediate affinity to sstr4 (Ginj et al. 2005).

Also, SSTR antagonists such as (NH(2)-CO-c(DCys-Phe-Tyr-DAgl(8)(Me,2-naphthoyl)-Lys-Thr-Phe-Cys)-OH (sst(3)-ODN-8) and (sst(2)-ANT) have been labeled with ^{111}In.

Their superiority over SSTR agonists (in the mouse model) for in vivo targeting of SSTR2- and SSTR3-rich tumors, as shown by the group of Reubi (Ginj et al. 2006; Reubi et al. 2000b) has resulted in a paradigm shift and they are now being considered for tumor diagnosis.

18.4.1.3 Radiolabeled Vasoactive Intestinal Peptide and Other Peptides for Diagnosis of NETs

VIP, a 28 amino acid peptide, initially isolated from porcine intestine, radiolabeled with either ^{99m}Tc or I-123, has also been used for imaging NETs. Two subtypes of VIP receptors (VIPAC1 and VIPAC2) have been described. VIP receptors, predominantly VIPAC1, is expressed in the majority of common tumors: breast, prostate, lung, pancreas, colon, stomach, liver, and blad-

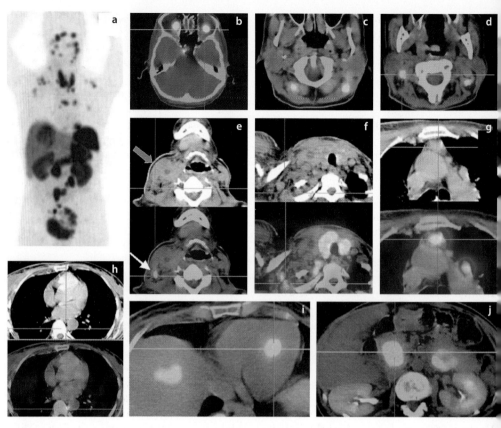

Fig. 18.2a–j. Heavily metastasizing, recurrent bilateral malignant pheochromocytoma: maximum intensity projection (MIP) image (**a**) and selected transversal Ga-68 DOTA-NOC PET/CT slices showing bilateral retro-bulbar metastases (**b**) and subcutaneous (**c**) and cervical lymph node lesions (**d**). Specific uptake can be seen in a small lymph node metastasis in the right neck (**e**, *white arrow*), whereas a large parajugular abscess shows only blood pool activity (red arrow; see also CT scan). Further metastases are detected in the thyroid and in supraclavicular (**f**) as well as in mediastinal/para-aortic (**g**) lymph nodes and in a very small (Ø <5 mm) prevertebral lesion (**h**). PET/CT also revealed a previously unknown myocardial metastasis (**i**) and strong uptake in multiple abdominal lesion (para-aortic lymph node metastases (**j**) and in a local recurrence)

der carcinomas. Leiomyomas predominantly express VPAC2 receptors, whereas paraganglimas, glial tumors, neuroblastomas, pituitary adenomas, pheochromocytomas, and endometrial carcinomas most commonly express VPAC1 receptors. Although only a few results have been published to date, their main indication is probably in the GEP neuroendocrine tumors (Moody et al. 2003; Reubi and Waser 2003; Thakur et al. 2000; Virgolini et al. 1994, 1995).

Other peptides that have been used for receptor scintigraphy of NET are cholecystokinin (CCK-B), gastrin, and bombesin (gastrin-releasing peptide) (Rufini et al. 2006). The experience with some of these radiolabeled peptides have been encouraging, but limited (Behe et al. 2003; Behr et al. 1998, 1999; Breeman et al. 1999; Kwekkeboom et al. 2000; Reubi et al. 1998).

18.4.1.4 Other Radiopharmaceuticals Used in Nuclear Medicine for Imaging NETs

^{99m}Tc-sestamibi and ^{99m}Tc-tetrofosmin have also been used for imaging melanomas and small cell lung cancer but without much clinical success (Bombardieri et al. 2001; Takekawa et al. 1999). ^{99m}Tc-DMSA was previously used frequently in medullary carcinoma thyroid (Ohta et al. 1984).

18.4.2 PET Radiopharmaceuticals

In spite of so many different radiopharmaceuticals used for the diagnosis, staging, and follow-up of NET patients with gamma camera-based scintigraphy, there has always been a compelling need to generate newer PET radiopharmaceuticals because of the superiority of PET imaging over gamma camera imaging. ^{18}F-FDG ^{18}F-fluoro-2-deoxy-d-glucose, 11C-5-HTP, ^{11}C-5-hydroxy-l-tryptophan, ^{18}F/^{11}C-DOPA, ^{18}F-fluoro-phenylalanine, ^{68}Ga-DOTA-TOC/^{68}Ga DOTA-NOC, ^{64}Cu-TETA-octreotide (TETA= 1,4,8,11-tetraazacyclotetradecane-N′, N″, N‴, N⁗-tetraectic acid), and Gluc-Lys ^{18}F-FP-TOCA (Nα-(1-deoxy-d-fructosyl)-Nε-(2-(^{18}F)fluoropropionyl)-Lys⁰-Tyr³-octreotate, are some of the radiopharmaceuticals that have been used for imaging NET. The clinical results will be discussed separately. However, ^{68}Ga needs special emphasis as it is heralded as a major breakthrough in the field of imaging for NET. ^{68}Ga is readily available from a generator (^{68}Ge/^{68}Ga generator), making it less expensive and easier to handle as compared to other positron-emitting radionuclides (Maecke et al. 2005) such as ^{18}F and ^{11}C, which require an onsite cyclotron. ^{68}Ge, the parent in the generator, is accelerator-produced (on Ga^{2}O^3 targets by a (p,2n) reaction) with a physical half-life of 270.8 days. ^{68}Ga has a half-life of 68 min and decays mainly by positron emission (89%). The concept of using a ^{68}Ge/^{68}Ga generator and a cold kit formulation was already proposed in 1993 (Deutsch 1993). Since then, several groups have been actively involved in the development of a better generator version and ^{68}Ga-labeled peptides. Until now, several ^{68}Ga peptides have been tested clinically for imaging somatostatin, melanocortin, and bombesin receptor-expressing tumors (Hofmann et al. 2001; Baum et al. 2007).

18.5 Radionuclide Imaging Methods

18.5.1 Single Photon Emission Computed Tomography vs Planar Imaging

The major disadvantage of planar imaging is the lack of precise localization of the tumor site as it is two-dimensional. Single photon emission computed tomography (SPECT) has the advantage of 3D reconstruction and thus assists in better localization. Several studies have shown that SPECT is more sensitive to planar imaging for detection of deep-seated tumors.

18.5.2 SPECT vs PET

One disadvantage of SPECT imaging is that quantification is very difficult and not routinely performed in practice. Objective methods for follow-up of cancer patients under strict guidelines (such as EORTC, RECIST, WHO) are essential for better patient management. In our experience, this is best carried out using PET/CT. The higher resolution of PET images is also a significant advantage compared to SPECT. The only limiting factor with PET is the higher cost of the equipment, making SPECT the most commonly used imaging method in oncology in various countries (especially in less developed or developing countries). The maintenance of cyclotron units and the implementation of good manufacturing practices has made the running cost of a fully functional PET–cyclotron unit very high and beyond the reach of many developing countries. This is where the in-house positron emitting radionuclide generators, because of their low cost and easy availability, will play an important role in the future.

18.5.3 SPECT Versus SPECT/CT and PET vs PET/CT

Nuclear medicine imaging in general lacks sufficient anatomical details. The addition of CT to SPECT or PET data helps in the precise localization of tumors. In addition, the present generation of gamma cameras/PET scanners have an embedded CT in the gantry, which makes it possible to perform contrast-enhanced CT with high resolution. In one sitting, it is possible to obtain both anatomical information and functional information. Indeed, PET/CT is already being heralded as the next-generation imaging methodology.

18.6 Clinical Indications for PET or PET/CT in NETs

Based upon our own PET/CT experience and the review of the literature, the following indications are important:
- Diagnosis and staging of NET.
- Defining the prognosis of patients (under investigation).
- Follow-up of patients after surgery.
- Follow-up of patients after somatostatin analog therapy.
- Choosing the appropriate therapeutic regime for PRRT (under investigation).
- Predicting the response after PRRT.
- PET/CT can be used for choosing the best therapy monitoring protocol for NET (molecular vs anatomical imaging).

18.7 Clinical Studies

18.7.1 ^{18}F-FDG PET

^{18}F-FDG PET is increasingly being used for various oncological indications. ^{18}F-FDG is useful for evaluating tumor hexokinase activity, which is increased in tumor cells because of the accelerated rate of glycolysis. ^{18}F-FDG PET is primarily used in tumors for the purpose of diagnosis, staging, restaging, and evaluation of the response to treatment. The main use of FDG-PET in diagnosis of NETs depends on the grade of differentiation and/or aggressiveness of NETs (Adams et al. 1998; Eriksson et al. 2000; Pasquali et al. 1998; Scanga et al. 2004; Sundin et al. 2004; Zhao et al. 2002).

A study comparing 111In-pentetreotide somatostatin receptor scintigraphy (SS-R),[18]F-FDG PET, and ^{99m}Tc(V)DMSA scintigraphy (dual radionuclide technique, DNS = SS-R+ ^{99m}Tc(V)DMSA) in patients with GEP and medullary thyroid carcinoma (Adams et al. 1998) has shown that FDG-PET is more sensitive than SS-R in picking up less differentiated GEP tumors (Figs. 18.3–18.5) but is less sensitive than SS-R in the detection of differentiated GEP tumors. In patients with recurrent MTC and rapidly increasing CEA levels, FDG-PET was found to be superior to DNS. Based on these observations, the authors of the study concluded that ^{18}F-FDG PET should be performed only if SS-R or DNS studies were negative. In another study conducted on 16 patients with NET (Pasquali et al. 1998), FDG uptake in NETs was related to the aggressiveness and rapid growth of the tumor and denoted worse prognosis. It was also concluded in the study that FDG-PET contributes to better staging of the advanced diseases as compared to CT scan and SS-R. In a multicenter study, FDG-PET was found to be a useful method for the staging and follow-up of patients, as it has the highest lesion detection probability for MTC tissues as compared to other imaging modalities such as ^{99m}Tc(V) DMSA, SS-R,CT, etc. (Diehl et al. 2001). In NET of the pancreatic-duodenal region, FDG PET was found to have the potential to change the treatment protocol in 17% of patients. FDG-PET was proved to be the second-line technique in pancreatic-duodenal region NETs. The authors of the study found that FDG-PET was best suited for patients suspected of having malignant tumor or having a pancreatic mass greater than 2 cm or MEN I cases with at least one visible lesion. FDG-PET was found not to be useful in duodenal tumors, benign insulinomas, and small single pancreatic neuroendocrine lesions (Pasquali et al. 2004).

However, in spite of these successful results, one major limitation of FDG as a tumor marker is that it is not completely specific for tumors. FDG is known to accumulate in inflammatory lesions also, thereby increasing the false-positivity rate.

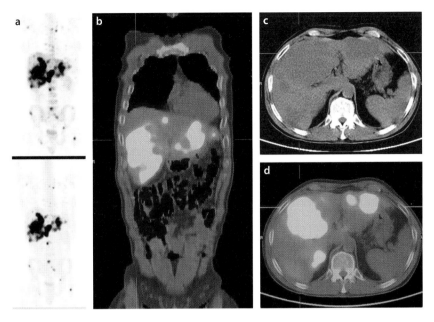

Fig. 18.3a–d. F-18 FDG PET/CT in a 43-year-old patient with neuroendocrine pancreatic cancer (proliferation rate <10%, synaptophysin and chromogranin A staining positive) diagnosed 4 months earlier. MIP image (**a**), coronal PET/CT fusion image (**b**), CT (**c**), and transversal PET/CT fusion image (**d**) demonstrate multiple FDG-avid metastases before therapy

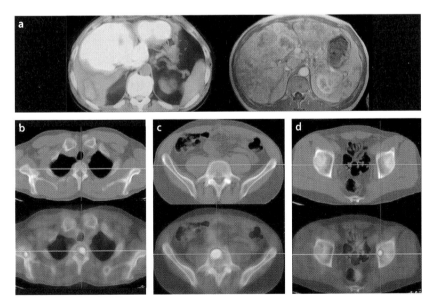

Fig. 18.4a–d. Same patient as described in Figure 18.3. Extensive, bilobar liver metastases (**a**) as shown by F-18 FDG-PET/CT (upper left row, highest glucose metabolism in segment VII with an standard uptake value (SUV) of 29.1) and MRI (upper right image). Hypermetabolic bone metastases are detected by FDG-PET in the thoracic spine and in the right scapula (**b**), in the lumbar spine in L5 (**c**), and in the left acetabulum (**d**), whereas the CT scan is still normal (i.e., the lesions are located mainly in the bone marrow)

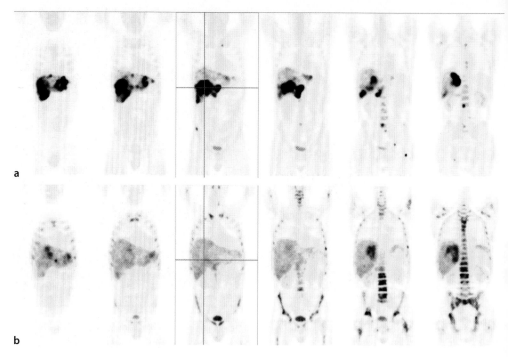

Fig. 18.5a,b. Same patient as described in Figure 18.3. F-18 FDG PET/CT (coronal slices) before (**a**) and after (**b**) combined peptide receptor radiotherapy (PRRT, 2 cycles of Y-90 DOTA-TATE, total administered activity 7.5 GBq) and chemotherapy (TCE scheme, Taxol, carboplatin, etoposide) with impressive metabolic response after combined treatment. Note activation of normal bone marrow in the spine after G-CSF therapy (upper right panel **b**)

18.7.2 ^{18}F-DOPA PET

NETs are known to accumulate and decarboxylate 5'-hydroxytryptamine and l-3,4-dihydroxyphenylalanine (l-DOPA) (Pearse 1969). An increase in the activity of l-DOPA decarboxylase is one of the hallmarks of NETs (Baylin et al. 1980; Berger et al. 1984; Gazdar et al. 1988). The first study that demonstrated the utility of 11C-DOPA in the detection of pancreatic tumor was conducted by Ahlstrom et al. (1995). ^{18}F-FDOPA PET has also been found to be useful in advanced NET. One study found that ^{18}F-FDOPA performs better than SS-R scintigraphy in visualizing NETs. The authors also proposed that ^{18}F-FDOPA performs better than CT in detection of bone lesions (Becherer et al. 2004). However, in small cell lung cancer, ^{18}F-FDOPA was found

to be of no use, whereas ^{18}F FDG PET had a significant role (Jacob et al. 2003). In patients with pheochromocytoma, both ^{18}F-FDOPA PET and MRI were found to be superior to ^{131}I MIBG study with sensitivity and specificity of 100% (Hoegerle et al. 2002). However, this study cannot be taken as a reference study because the imaging method (^{131}I MIBG scintigraphy) with which the PET study and MRI study was compared is not the current gold standard (SS-R) for the detection of NETs.

The potential limitation of [18]FDOPA-PET is the normally high uptake in the duodenum and pancreas (Fig. 18.6), which might cause problems in localization of tumors in these regions. Apart from this, the nonspecific accumulation of [18]FDOPA in the intestine is a potential source of false-positive interpretations.

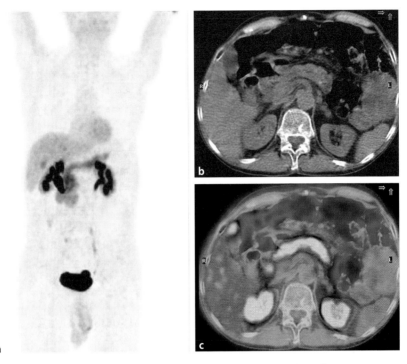

Fig. 18.6a–c. F-18 DOPA PET/CT showing physiological high uptake in the pancreas: MIP image (**a**), CT scan (**b**), and PET/CT fusion image (**c**). (Image courtesy of Stefano Fanti, University of Bologna)

18.7.3 ¹¹C-5-HTP

In a study comparing 5-HTP-PET with CT and somatostatin receptor scintigraphy in patients with carcinoid and endocrine pancreatic tumors, 5-HTP-PET was found to be superior to CT and somatostatin receptor scintigraphy for tumor visualization. Many small, previously overlooked lesions were diagnosed by ¹¹C-5-HTP-PET (Eriksson et al. 2000; Orlefors et al. 1998).

18.7.4 ⁶⁸Ga-DOTANOC/DOTATOC Receptor PET/CT

Somatostatin receptor scintigraphy has been validated as the most specific tool for the detection of NETs and is used extensively for the follow-up of patients after receiving somatostatin analog therapy. However, some of the

studies that have compared nonsomatostatin PET radiopharmaceuticals and SS-R have found that, in some cases, the PET study was more sensitive in picking up tumor lesions. This may be attributed to the decreased sensitivity of gamma camera imaging methods as compared to PET. This fact plus the need to evaluate the effect of rapidly progressive role of peptide receptor therapy based on somatostatin analog made scientists work toward finding a positron emitting radionuclide that could be tagged with somatostatin analogs. The ability to tag somatostatin analogs with ⁶⁸Ga has revolutionized the role of PET in diagnosis, staging, and therapy monitoring of patients with receptor-positive NETs. One of the advantages of the ⁶⁸Ga-DOTANOC/DOTATOC PET or PET/CT study over ¹¹¹In-octreotide scintigraphy is better visualization of deep-seated lesions, which are difficult to be seen on planar and SPECT images (Kwekkeboom et al. 1994). The normal physiologic distribution along with the SUVmax value has been calculated by these authors (Baum and Prasad 2006). This information is essential for proper interpretation of images as well as for defining a cut-off value for malignant lesions. In a preliminary clinical study, Hofmann et al. (2001) showed that ^{68}Ga-DOTATOC is superior to ^{111}In-octreotide SPECT (CT was taken as the reference for comparison) in detecting upper abdominal metastases. Kowalski et al. (2003) also showed that in comparison to the [^{111}In]-DTPAOC-scan, ^{68}Ga-DOTATOC PET appears to be superior, especially in detecting small tumors or tumors bearing only a low density of somatostatin receptors (SSTRs). Apart from this, ^{68}Ga-DOTATOC PET has also been envisaged to have a potential role in the small cell lung cancer, as it is known to express soma-

tostatin receptor and thus is a potential candidate for PRRT with ^{90}Y-DOTATOC/DOTATATE (Maecke et al. 2005). In unpublished data in more than 800 ^{68}Ga-DOTANOC PET/CT studies conducted by the authors of this article to date, it was found that:

- ^{68}Ga-DOTANOC PET was able to pick up many lesions which could not be picked up by CT (Fig. 18.7).
- ^{68}Ga-DOTANOC PET is of significant value in therapy monitoring (Figs. 18.8, 18.9) of patients with NET (total number of patients treated, n=358) having received PRRT.
- PET/CT provides additional information about the tumor as compared to PET study alone.
- ^{68}Ga-DOTA-NOC PET/CT is a useful adjunct in deciding the amount of radioactivity to be administered for PRRT.

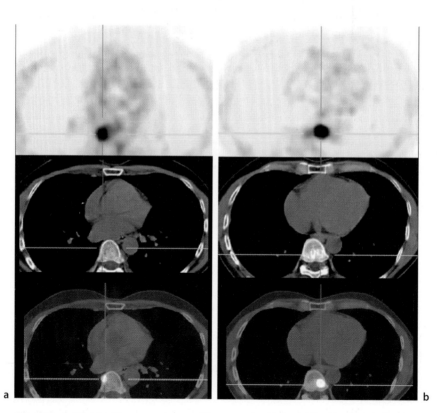

a   b

Fig. 18.7a,b. Vertebral bone metastases of ileum carcinoid. Osteoblastic, receptor-positive lesion on CT in one thoracic vertebra (**a**), whereas another lesion, with strong, focal SMS-receptor expression on Ga-68 DOTA-NOC-PET, is invisible on CT scan (**b**)

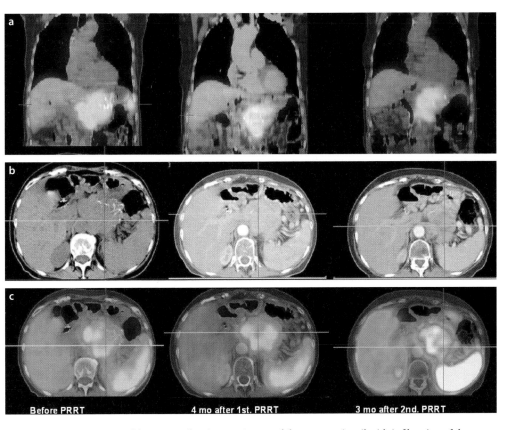

Fig. 18.8a–c. Large, inoperable neuroendocrine carcinoma of the pancreatic tail with infiltration of the stomach. Ga-68 DOTA-NOC receptor PET/CT (**a** coronal PET slices, **b** transversal CT slices, and **c** fused images before intra-arterial PRRT using Y-90 DOTA-TATE, 4 months after the first treatment, and 3 months after the second intra-arterial therapy) showing high but heterogeneous SMS-receptor expression. Before treatment, the 66-year-old patient needed multiple blood transfusions despite intense conventional treatment, including chemotherapy and Sandostatin. After the second PRRT, the bleeding stopped completely

In an intraindividual study comparing the diagnostic efficacy of ^{68}Ga DOTA-NOC and ^{68}Ga DOTA–TATE, our group (Antunes et al. 2007) demonstrated for the first time that ^{68}Ga DOTA-NOC is superior to ^{68}Ga DOTA–TATE. Koukouraki et al. (2006) found that based on the pharmacokinetic data of ^{68}Ga-DOTA-TOC, it is possible to separate the blood background activity from the receptor binding, which is potentially a very significant observation as it may help in optimizing the planning of ^{90}Y-DOTA-TOC therapy.

In summary, among several advantages of ^{68}Ga-somatostatin analogs over other nonsomatostatin analog-based PET radiopharmaceuticals for the detection and staging of NETs, the most important ones are kit formulation, easy availability, higher specificity, and the ability to monitor therapy and follow-up of NET patients.

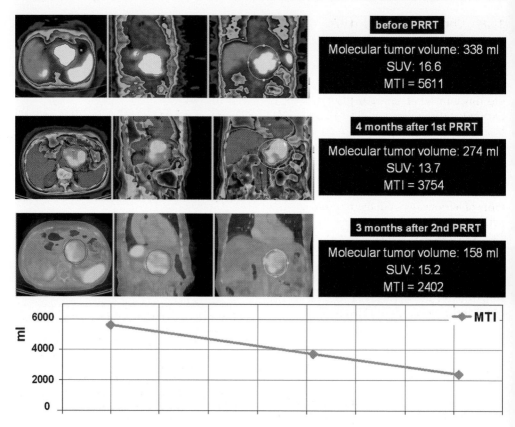

Fig. 18.9. Molecular imaging for measuring response after therapy by calculating the molecular tumor index using ROI technique and Ga-68 DOTA-NOC receptor PET/CT. Metabolic/molecular tumor index (MTI) = molecular tumor volume (MTV) multiplied by SUV. The significant decrease in MTI over time correlated with the improvement of the patient's clinical symptoms

18.7.5 Gluc-Lys ((^{18}F)FP)-TOCA PET

The success of ^{68}G-DOTA-TOC/DOTA-NOC has encouraged the use of ^{18}F as the radioligand for somatostatin analogs. Gluc-Lys ((^{18}F)FP)-TOCA is a recently developed ^{18}F-labeled somatostatin analog. A preliminary comparative study found that Gluc-Lys ((^{18}F)FP)-TOCA PET is superior to a 111In-DTPA-octreotide scan in the diagnosis of NETs. In the same study (based on a literature survey), it was stressed that Gluc-Lys ((^{18}F)FP)-TOCA PET is comparable with ^{68}Ga-DOTA-TOC/DOTA-NOC PET findings in NETs (Meisetschlager et al. 2006).

18.7.6 ^{64}Cu-TETA-Octreotide PET

^{64}Cu (half-life, 12.7 h; β+ 0.653 MeV [17.4%]; β–, 0.579 MeV [39%], 43.6% electron capture) is being investigated and has shown good potential as a positron emitting radionuclide for PET imaging and radiotherapy (Anderson et al. 2001; Lewis et al. 1999; Wang et al. 2003). The possibility of performing dosimetry for PRRT based on ^{64}Cu is another big advantage. In a preliminary study ^{64}Cu-TETA-octreotide PET has been found to have high sensitivity as well as favorable dosimetry and pharmacokinetics (Anderson et al. 2001).

18.8 Conclusion and Future Directions

Somatostatin receptor scintigraphy has revolutionized the diagnosis of NET. The rapidly growing number of new radiopharmaceuticals and the greater understanding of the molecular basis of NETs has helped tremendously in the management of patients with neuroendocrine tumors. Future studies with receptor PET/CT need to be directed toward optimizing the therapeutic dose for PRRT of NETs. The possibility of performing both therapy and imaging with the same radiopharmaceutical (e.g., using ^{64}Cu-TETA-octreotide) could be an advantage over the currently used PET radiopharmaceuticals. Novel somatostatin analogs need to be rigorously tested for high affinity toward sstr subtypes and may enable even better treatment of NETs then what is possible today.

References

Adams S, Baum R, Rink T, Schumm-Drager PM, Usadel KH, Hor G (1998) Limited value of fluorine-18 fluorodeoxyglucose positron emission tomography for the imaging of neuroendocrine tumours. Eur J Nucl Med 25:79–83

Ahlstrom H, Eriksson B, Bergstrom M, Bjurling P, Langstrom B, Oberg K (1995) Pancreatic neuroendocrine tumors: diagnosis with PET. Radiology 195:333–337

Anderson CJ, Dehdashti F, Cutler PD, Schwarz SW, Laforest R, Bass LA, Lewis JS, McCarthy DW (2001) ^{64}Cu-TETA-octreotide as a PET imaging agent for patients with neuroendocrine tumors. J Nucl Med 42:213–221

Antunes P, Ginj M, Zhang H, Waser B, Baum RP, Reubi JC, Maecke H (2007) Are radiogallium-labelled DOTA-conjugated somatostatin superior to those labelled with other radiometals? Eur J Nucl Med Mol Imaging 34:982–993

Baum RP, Hofmann M (2004) Nuklearmedizinische Diagnostik neuroendokriner tumoren. Onkologe 10:598–610

Baum RP, Prasad V (2007) Molecular imaging of neuroendocrine tumors using Ga-68 DOTA-NOC receptor PET/CT semiquantitative analyses after 1,257 studies (EPOS). European Congress of Radiology 2007, Vienna, Austria

Baylin SB, Abeloff MD, Goodwin G, Carney DN, Gazdar AF (1980) Activities of L-dopa decarboxylase and diamine oxidase (histaminase) in human lung cancers and decarboxylase as a marker for small (oat) cell cancer in cell culture. Cancer Res 40:1990–1994

Becherer A, Szabo M, Karanikas G, Wunderbaldinger P, Angelberger P, Raderer M, Kurtaran A, Dudczak R, Kletter K (2004) Imaging of advanced neuroendocrine tumors with (^{18}F-FDOPA PET. J Nucl Med 45:1161–1167

Behe M, Becker W, Gotthardt M, Angerstein C, Behr TM (2003) Improved kinetic stability of DTPA-dGlu as compared with conventional monofunctional DTPA in chelating indium and yttrium: preclinical and initial clinical evaluation of radiometal labelled minigastrin derivatives. Eur J Nucl Med Mol Imaging 30:1140–1146

Behr TM, Behe MP (2002) Cholecystokinin-B/gastrin receptor-targeting peptides for staging and therapy of medullary thyroid cancer and other cholecystokinin-B receptor-expressing malignancies. Semin Nucl Med 32:97–109

Behr TM, Jenner N, Radetzky S, Behe M, Gratz S, Yuckent S, Raue F, Becker W (1998) Targeting of cholecystokinin-B/gastrin receptors in vivo: preclinical and initial clinical evaluation of the diagnostic and therapeutic potential of radiolabelled gastrin. Eur J Nucl Med 25:424–430

Behr TM, Behe M, Angerstein C, Gratz S, Mach R, Hagemann L, Jenner N, Stiehler M, Frank-Raue K, Raue F, Becker W (1999) Cholecystokinin-B/gastrin receptor binding peptides: preclinical development and evaluation of their diagnostic and therapeutic potential. Clin Cancer Res 5:3124s–3138s

Behr TM, Gotthardt M, Barth A, Behe M (2001) Imaging tumors with peptide-based radioligands. Q J Nucl Med 45:189–200

Berger CL, de Bustros A, Roos BA, Leong SS, Mendelsohn G, Gesell MS, Baylin SB (1984) Human medullary thyroid carcinoma in culture provides a model relating growth dynamics, endocrine cell differentiation, and tumor progression. J Clin Endocrinol Metab 59:338–343

Berglund AS, Hulthen UL, Manhem P, Thorsson O, Wollmer P, Tornquist C (2001) Metaiodobenzylguanidine (MIBG) scintigraphy and computed tomography (CT) in clinical practice. Primary and secondary evaluation for localization of phaeochromocytomas. J Intern Med 249:247–251

Blum J, Handmaker H, Lister-James J, Rinne N (2000) A multicenter trial with a somatostatin analog (99m)Tc depreotide in the evaluation of solitary pulmonary nodules. Chest 117:1232–1238

Bombardieri E, Maccauro M, De Deckere E, Savelli G, Chiti A (2001) Nuclear medicine imaging of neuroendocrine tumours. Ann Oncol 12 [Suppl 2]:S51–S61

Bombardieri E, Seregni E, Villano C, Chiti A, Bajetta E (2004) Position of nuclear medicine techniques in the diagnostic work-up of neuroendocrine tumors. Q J Nucl Med Mol Imaging 48:150–163

Breeman WA, De Jong M, Bernard BF, Kwekkeboom DJ, Srinivasan A, van der Pluijm ME, Hofland LJ, Visser

TJ, Krenning EP (1999) Pre-clinical evaluation of [(^{111})In-DTPA-Pro(1), Tyr(4)]bombesin, a new radioligand for bombesin-receptor scintigraphy. Int J Cancer 83:657–663

Castellani MR, Chiti A, Seregni E, Bombardieri E (2000) Role of ^{131}I-metaiodobenzylguanidine (MIBG) in the treatment of neuroendocrine tumours. Experience of the National Cancer Institute of Milan. Q J Nucl Med 44:77–87

De Jong M, Bakker WH, Krenning EP, Breeman WA, van der Pluijm ME, Bernard BF, Visser TJ, Jermann E, Behe M, Powell P, Macke HR (1997) Yttrium-90 and indium-111 labelling, receptor binding and biodistribution of [DOTA0,d-Phe^1,Tyr^3]octreotide, a promising somatostatin analogue for radionuclide therapy. Eur J Nucl Med 24:368–371

Decristoforo C, Melendez-Alafort L, Sosabowski JK, Mather SJ (2000) ^{99m}Tc-HYNIC-[Tyr^3]-octreotide for imaging somatostatin-receptor-positive tumors: preclinical evaluation and comparison with ^{111}In-octreotide. J Nucl Med 41:1114–1119

Deutsch E (1993) Clinical PET: its time has come? J Nucl Med 34:1132–1133

Diehl M, Risse JH, Brandt-Mainz K, Dietlein M, Bohuslavizki KH, Matheja P, Lange H, Bredow J, Korber C, Grunwald F (2001) Fluorine-18 fluorodeoxyglucose positron emission tomography in medullary thyroid cancer: results of a multicentre study. Eur J Nucl Med 28:1671–1676

Eriksson B, Bergstrom M, Orlefors H, Sundin A, Oberg K, Langstrom B (2000) Use of PET in neuroendocrine tumors. In vivo applications and in vitro studies. Q J Nucl Med 44:68–76

Gazdar AF, Helman LJ, Israel MA, Russell EK, Linnoila RI, Mulshine JL, Schuller HM, Park JG (1988) Expression of neuroendocrine cell markers L-dopa decarboxylase, chromogranin A, and dense core granules in human tumors of endocrine and nonendocrine origin. Cancer Res 48:4078–4082

Ginj M, Chen J, Walter MA, Eltschinger V, Reubi JC, Maecke HR (2005) Preclinical evaluation of new and highly potent analogues of octreotide for predictive imaging and targeted radiotherapy. Clin Cancer Res 11:1136–1145

Ginj M, Zhang H, Waser B, Cescato R, Wild D, Wang X, Erchegyi J, Rivier J, Macke HR, Reubi JC (2006) Radiolabeled somatostatin receptor antagonists are preferable to agonists for in vivo peptide receptor targeting of tumors. Proc Natl Acad Sci U S A 103:16436–16441

Henze M, Schuhmacher J, Hipp P, Kowalski J, Becker DW, Doll J, Macke HR, Hofmann M, Debus J, Haberkorn U (2001) PET imaging of somatostatin receptors using [^{68}GA]DOTA-D-Phe1-Tyr^3-octreotide: first results in patients with meningiomas. J Nucl Med 42:1053–1056

Henze M, Schuhmacher J, Dimitrakopoulou-Strauss A, Strauss LG, Macke HR, Eisenhut M, Haberkorn U (2004) Exceptional increase in somatostatin receptor expression in pancreatic neuroendocrine tumour, visualised with (^{68}Ga-DOTATOC PET. Eur J Nucl Med Mol Imaging 31:466

Henze M, Dimitrakopoulou-Strauss A, Milker-Zabel S, Schuhmacher J, Strauss LG, Doll J, Macke HR, Eisenhut M, Debus J, Haberkorn U (2005) Characterization of ^{68}Ga-DOTA-D-Phe^1-Tyr^3-octreotide kinetics in patients with meningiomas. J Nucl Med 46:763–769

Hoegerle S, Nitzsche E, Altehoefer C, Ghanem N, Manz T, Brink I, Reincke M, Moser E, Neumann HP (2002) Pheochromocytomas: detection with ^{18}F DOPA whole body PET: initial results. Radiology 222:507–512

Hofmann M, Maecke H, Borner R, Weckesser E, Schoffski P, Oei L, Schumacher J, Henze M, Heppeler A, Meyer J, Knapp H (2001) Biokinetics and imaging with the somatostatin receptor PET radioligand (^{68})Ga-DOTATOC: preliminary data. Eur J Nucl Med 28:1751–1757

Jacob T, Grahek D, Younsi N, Kerrou K, Aide N, Montravers F, Balogova S, Colombet C, De Beco V, Talbot JN (2003) Positron emission tomography with [(^{18})F]FDOPA and [(^{18})F]FDG in the imaging of small cell lung carcinoma: preliminary results. Eur J Nucl Med Mol Imaging 30:1266–1269

Jensen RT (2005) Endocrine tumors of the gastrointestinal tract and pancreas. In: Kasper DL, Fauci AS, Longo DL et al. (eds) Harrison's principles of internal medicine. McGraw-Hill, New York, pp 2221–2231

Kaltsas GA, Besser GM, Grossman AB (2004) The diagnosis and medical management of advanced neuroendocrine tumors. Endocr Rev 25:458–511

Khafagi FA, Shapiro B, Fig LM, Mallette S, Sisson JC (1989) Labetalol reduces iodine-131 MIBG uptake by pheochromocytoma and normal tissues. J Nucl Med 30:481–489

Koukouraki S, Strauss L, Georgoulias V, Schuhmacher J, Haberkorn U, Karkavitsas N, Dimitrakopoulou-Strauss A (2006) Evaluation of the pharmacokinetics of ^{68}Ga-DOTATOC in patients with metastatic neuroendocrine tumours scheduled for ^{90}Y-DOTATOC therapy. Eur J Nucl Med Mol Imaging 33:460–466

Kowalski J, Henze M, Schuhmacher J, Macke HR, Hofmann M, Haberkorn U (2003) Evaluation of positron emission tomography imaging using [^{68}Ga]-DOTA-D Phe(^{1})-Tyr(^{3})-Octreotide in comparison to [^{111}In]-DTPAOC SPECT. First results in patients with neuroendocrine tumors. Mol Imaging Biol 5:42–48

Krenning EP, Bakker WH, Breeman WA, Koper JW, Kooij PP, Ausema L, Lameris JS, Reubi JC, Lamberts SW (1989) Localisation of endocrine-related tumours with radioiodinated analogue of somatostatin. Lancet 1:242–244

Krenning EP, Bakker WH, Lamberts SW (1990) Receptor scintigraphy with somatostatin analog in oncology. Ned Tijdschr Geneeskd 134:1077–1080

Krenning EP, Bakker WH, Kooij PP, Breeman WA, Oei HY, de Jong M, Reubi JC, Visser TJ, Bruns C, Kwekkeboom DJ et al (1992) Somatostatin receptor scintigraphy with indium-111-DTPA-D-Phe-1-octreotide in man:

metabolism, dosimetry and comparison with iodine-123-Tyr-3-octreotide. J Nucl Med 33:652–658

Krenning EP, Kwekkeboom DJ, Bakker WH, Breeman WA, Kooij PP, Oei HY, van Hagen M, Postema PT, de Jong M, Reubi JC et al (1993) Somatostatin receptor scintigraphy with [^{111}In-DTPA-D-Phe^1]- and [^{123}I-Tyr^3]-octreotide: the Rotterdam experience with more than 1000 patients. Eur J Nucl Med 20:716–731

Krenning EP, Kwekkeboom DJ, Valkema R, Pauwels S, Kvols LK, De Jong M (2004) Peptide receptor radionuclide therapy. Ann N Y Acad Sci 1014:234–245

Kwekkeboom DJ, Kho GS, Lamberts SW, Reubi JC, Laissue JA, Krenning EP (1994) The value of octreotide scintigraphy in patients with lung cancer. Eur J Nucl Med 21:1106–1113

Kwekkeboom DJ, Bakker WH, Kooij PP, Erion J, Srinivasan A, de Jong M, Reubi JC, Krenning EP (2000) Cholecystokinin receptor imaging using an octapeptide DTPA-CCK analogue in patients with medullary thyroid carcinoma. Eur J Nucl Med 27:1312–1317

Kwekkeboom DJ, Bakker WH, Kooij PP, Konijnenberg MW, Srinivasan A, Erion JL, Schmidt MA, Bugaj JL, de Jong M, Krenning EP (2001) [^{177}Lu-DOTAOTyr^3]octreotate: comparison with [^{111}In-DTPAo]octreotide in patients. Eur J Nucl Med 28:1319–1325

Lebtahi R, Le Cloirec J, Houzard C, Daou D, Sobhani I, Sassolas G, Mignon M, Bourguet P, Le Guludec D (2002) Detection of neuroendocrine tumors: ^{99m}Tc-P829 scintigraphy compared with 111In-pentetreotide scintigraphy. J Nucl Med 43:889–895

Lewis JS, Lewis MR, Cutler PD, Srinivasan A, Schmidt MA, Schwarz SW, Morris MM, Miller JP, Anderson CJ (1999) Radiotherapy and dosimetry of ^{64}Cu-TETA-Tyr^3-octreotate in a somatostatin receptor-positive, tumor-bearing rat model. Clin Cancer Res 5:3608–3616

Li S, Beheshti M (2005) The radionuclide molecular imaging and therapy of neuroendocrine tumors. Curr Cancer Drug Targets 5:139–148

Maecke HR, Hofmann M, Haberkorn U (2005) (^{68})Ga-labeled peptides in tumor imaging. J Nucl Med 46 [Suppl 1]:172S–178S

Meisetschlager G, Poethko T, Stahl A, Wolf I, Scheidhauer K, Schottelius M, Herz M, Wester HJ, Schwaiger M (2006) Gluc-Lys([^{18}F]FP)-TOCA PET in patients with SSTR-positive tumors: biodistribution and diagnostic evaluation compared with [^{111}In]DTPA-octreotide. J Nucl Med 47:566–573

Moody TW, Hill JM, Jensen RT (2003) VIP as a trophic factor in the CNS and cancer cells. Peptides 24:163–177

Oberndorfer S (1907) Karzinoide tumoren des dünndarms. Frankf Z Pathol 1:426–429

Ohta H, Yamamoto K, Endo K, Mori T, Hamanaka D, Shimazu A, Ikekubo K, Makimoto K, Iida Y, Konishi J et al (1984) A new imaging agent for medullary carcinoma of the thyroid. J Nucl Med 25:323–325

Orlefors H, Sundin A, Ahlstrom H, Bjurling P, Bergstrom M, Lilja A, Langstrom B, Oberg K, Eriksson B (1998) Positron emission tomography with 5-hydroxytryprophan in neuroendocrine tumors. J Clin Oncol 16:2534–2541

Otte A, Mueller-Brand J, Dellas S, Nitzsche EU, Herrmann R, Maecke HR (1998) Yttrium-90-labelled somatostatin-analogue for cancer treatment. Lancet 351:417–478

Otte A, Herrmann R, Heppeler A, Behe M, Jermann E, Powell P, Maecke HR, Muller J (1999) Yttrium-90 DOTATOC: first clinical results. Eur J Nucl Med 26:1439–1447

Paganelli G, Zoboli S, Cremonesi M, Bodei L, Ferrari M, Grana C, Bartolomei M, Orsi F, De Cicco C, Macke HR, Chinol M, de Braud F (2001) Receptor-mediated radiotherapy with ^{90}Y-DOTA-D-Phe^1-Tyr^3-octreotide. Eur J Nucl Med 28:426–434

Pasquali C, Rubello D, Sperti C, Gasparoni P, Liessi G, Chierichetti F, Ferlin G, Pedrazzoli S (1998) Neuroendocrine tumor imaging: can ^{18}F-fluorodeoxyglucose positron emission tomography detect tumors with poor prognosis and aggressive behavior? World J Surg 22:588–592

Pasquali C, Sperti C, Scappin S, Lunardi C, Chierichetti F, Liessi G, Pedrazzoli S (2004) Role and indications of fluorodeoxyglucose positron emission tomography (FDG-PET) in neuroendocrine pancreatico-duodenal tumors. J Pancreas 6 [5 Suppl]:528–529

Pearse AG (1969) The cytochemistry and ultrastructure of polypeptide hormone-producing cells of the APUD series and the embryologic, physiological and pathologic implications of the concept. J Histochem Cytochem 17:303–313

Pershagen G (1998) Environmental epidemiology in public health. Lancet 352:417

Raderer M, Pangerl T, Leimer M, Valencak J, Kurtaran A, Hamilton G, Scheithauer W, Virgolini I (1998) Expression of human somatostatin receptor subtype 3 in pancreatic cancer in vitro and in vivo. J Natl Cancer Inst 90:1666–1668

Reubi JC, Waser B (2003) Concomitant expression of several peptide receptors in neuroendocrine tumours: molecular basis for in vivo multireceptor tumour targeting. Eur J Nucl Med Mol Imaging 30:781–793

Reubi JC, Schaer JC, Waser B (1997) Cholecystokinin (CCK)-A and CCK-B/gastrin receptors in human tumors. Cancer Res 57:1377–1386

Reubi JC, Waser B, Schaer JC, Laederach U, Erion J, Srinivasan A, Schmidt MA, Bugaj JE (1998) Unsulfated DTPA- and DOTA-CCK analogs as specific high-affinity ligands for CCK-B receptor-expressing human and rat tissues in vitro and in vivo. Eur J Nucl Med 25:481–490

Reubi JC, Gugger M, Waser B, Schaer JC (2001a) Y(1)-mediated effect of neuropeptide Y in cancer: breast carcinomas as targets. Cancer Res 61:4636–4641

Reubi JC, Waser B, Schaer JC, Laissue JA (2001b) Somatostatin receptor sst1-sst5 expression in normal and neoplastic human tissues using receptor autoradiography with subtype-selective ligands. Eur J Nucl Med 28:836–846

Reubi JC, Laderach U, Waser B, Gebbers JO, Robberecht P, Laissue JA (2000a) Vasoactive intestinal peptide/pituitary adenylate cyclase-activating peptide receptor subtypes in human tumors and their tissues of origin. Cancer Res 60:3105–3112

Reubi JC, Schaer JC, Wenger S, Hoeger C, Erchegyi J, Waser B, Rivier J (2000b) SST3-selective potent peptidic somatostatin receptor antagonists. Proc Natl Acad Sci U S A 97:13973–3978

Reubi JC, Schar JC, Waser B, Wenger S, Heppeler A, Schmitt JS, Macke HR (2000c) Affinity profiles for human somatostatin receptor subtypes SST1-SST5 of somatostatin radiotracers selected for scintigraphic and radiotherapeutic use. Eur J Nucl Med 27:273–282

Reubi C, Gugger M, Waser B (2002) Co-expressed peptide receptors in breast cancer as a molecular basis for in vivo multireceptor tumour targeting. Eur J Nucl Med Mol Imaging 29:855–862

Rufini V, Calcagni ML, Baum RP (2006) Imaging of neuroendocrine tumors. Semin Nucl Med 36:228–247

Scanga DR, Martin WH, Delbeke D (2004) Value of FDG PET imaging in the management of patients with thyroid, neuroendocrine, and neural crest tumors. Clin Nucl Med 29:86–90

Schmitt-Gräff A, Hezel B, Wiedenmann B (2000) Pathologisch-diagnostische Aspekte neuroendokriner tumoren des Gastrointestinal trakts. Onkologe 6:613–623

Shapiro B, Copp JE, Sisson JC, Eyre PL, Wallis J, Beierwaltes WH (1985) Iodine-131 metaiodobenzylguanidine for the locating of suspected pheochromocytoma: experience in 400 cases. J Nucl Med 26:576–585

Shapiro B, Fig LM, Gross MD, Khafagi F (1989) Radiochemical diagnosis of adrenal disease. Crit Rev Clin Lab Sci 27:265–298

Solanki KK, Bomanji J, Moyes J, Mather SJ, Trainer PJ, Britton KE (1992) A pharmacological guide to medicines which interfere with the biodistribution of radiolabelled meta-iodobenzylguanidine (MIBG) Nucl Med Commun 13:513–521

Solcia E, Kloppel G, Sobin LH (2000) Histological typing of tumors. International Histological Classification of Tumors in collaboration with 9 pathologists from 4 countries (WH OP PW H. Organisation, ed.) Springer Berlin New York Heidelberg

Stolz B, Weckbecker G, Smith-Jones PM, Albert R, Raulf F, Bruns C (1998) The somatostatin receptor-targeted radiotherapeutic [^{90}Y-DOTA-DPhe^1, Tyr^3]octreotide (^{90}Y-SMT 487) eradicates experimental rat pancreatic CA 20948 tumours. Eur J Nucl Med 25:668–674

Sundin A, Eriksson B, Bergstrom M, Langstrom B, Oberg K, Orlefors H (2004) PET in the diagnosis of neuroendocrine tumors. Ann N Y Acad Sci 1014:246–257

Takekawa H, Shinano H, Tsukamoto E, Koseki Y, Ikeno T, Miller F, Kawakami Y (1999) Technetium-99m-tetrofosmin imaging of lung cancer: relationship with histopathology. Ann Nucl Med 13:71–75

Thakur ML, Marcus CS, Saeed S, Pallela V, Minami C, Diggles L, Le Pham H, Ahdoot R, Kalinowski EA (2000) ^{99m}Tc-labeled vasoactive intestinal peptide analog for rapid localization of tumors in humans. J Nucl Med 41:107–110

Van Hagen PM, Breeman WA, Reubi JC, Postema PT, van den Anker-Lugtenburg PJ, Kwekkeboom DJ, Laissue J, Waser B, Lamberts SW, Visser TJ, Krenning EP (1996) Visualization of the thymus by substance P receptor scintigraphy in man. Eur J Nucl Med 23:1508–1513

Virgolini I (2000) Peptide imaging. Springer, Berlin New York Heidelberg

Virgolini I, Raderer M, Kurtaran A, Angelberger P, Banyai S, Yang Q, Li S, Banyai M, Pidlich J, Niederle B, Scheithauer W, Valent P (1994) Vasoactive intestinal peptide-receptor imaging for the localization of intestinal adenocarcinomas and endocrine tumors. N Engl J Med 331:1116–1121

Virgolini I, Kurtaran A, Raderer M, Leimer M, Angelberger P, Havlik E, Li S, Scheithauer W, Niederle B, Valent P et al (1995) Vasoactive intestinal peptide receptor scintigraphy. J Nucl Med 36:1732–1739

Virgolini I, Raderer M, Kurtaran A, Angelberger P, Yang Q, Radosavljevic M, Leimer M, Kaserer K, Li SR, Kornek G, Hubsch P, Niederle B, Pidlich J, Scheithauer W, Valent P (1996) ^{123}I-vasoactive intestinal peptide (VIP) receptor scanning: update of imaging results in patients with adenocarcinomas and endocrine tumors of the gastrointestinal tract. Nucl Med Biol 23:685–692

Virgolini I, Szilvasi I, Kurtaran A, Angelberger P, Raderer M, Havlik E, Vorbeck F, Bischof C, Leimer M, Dorner G, Kletter K, Niederle B, Scheithauer W, Smith-Jones P (1998) Indium-111-DOTA-lanreotide: biodistribution, safety and radiation absorbed dose in tumor patients. J Nucl Med 39:1928–1936

Waldherr C, Pless M, Maecke HR, Schumacher T, Crazzolara A, Nitzsche EU, Haldemann A, Mueller-Brand J (2002) Tumor response and clinical benefit in neuroendocrine tumors after 7.4 GBq (^{90}Y)-DOTATOC. J Nucl Med 43:610–616

Wang M, Caruano AL, Lewis MR, Meyer LA, VanderWaal RP, Anderson CJ (2003) Subcellular localization of radiolabeled somatostatin analogues: implications for targeted radiotherapy of cancer. Cancer Res 63:6864–6869

Weiner RE, Thakur ML (2002) Radiolabeled peptides in the diagnosis and therapy of oncological diseases. Appl Radiat Isot 57:749–763

Wild D, Schmitt JS, Ginj M, Macke HR, Bernard BF, Krenning E, De Jong M, Wenger S, Reubi JC (2003) DOTA-NOC, a high-affinity ligand of somatostatin receptor subtypes 2:3 and 5 for labelling with various radiometals. Eur J Nucl Med Mol Imaging 30:1338–1347

Zhao DS, Valdivia AY, Li Y, Blaufox MD (2002) ^{18}F-fluorodeoxyglucose positron emission tomography in small-cell lung cancer. Semin Nucl Med 32:272–275

19   PET and PET/CT in Radiotherapy

S. Könemann and M. Weckesser

Recent Results in Cancer Research, Vol. 170
© Springer-Verlag Berlin Heidelberg 2008

Many aspects have to be considered in planning, applying, and following up radiotherapy procedures. This field poses a major challenge for diagnostic techniques. The first goal in the definition of multimodal oncological therapy concepts is to identify the patients who benefit from a definitive or adjuvant radiotherapy. After the decision for radiotherapy, the sequential process of radiotherapy planning and application has to be initiated. The basic principle is the exploitation of the therapeutic ratio, i.e., obtaining a high tumor dose and maximal protection of the surrounding normal tissue at risk. Computed tomography (CT) is an integral part of radiotherapy planning. Aside from its diagnostic value of tumor and neighboring normal tissue identification, the radiographic density matrix of CT is the basis for calculating the three-dimensional dose distribution. Positron emission tomography (PET) is not yet established as a standard in radio-oncological concept and procedure. The implementation of hybrid instruments, in which CT and PET are constructively united, can define the potential advantages of PET in view of therapeutic decisions and optimize radiotherapy treatment concepts.

Evident questions that are raised as a result of combined anatomic-metabolic imaging, are the influences this technique has on staging of malignant disease, the additional information provided, and the definition of the gross tumor volume (GTV) and the planning target volume (PTV). Furthermore, it is worth asking whether additional metabolic imaging can improve the evaluation of individual radiation sensitivity or resistance. Re-evaluation based on metabolic imaging during and after treatment for monitoring or restaging is of potential clinical relevance as well. Moreover, which specific advantages can be obtained using constructional integrated PET and CT must be investigated, especially in view of employee time management efficiency and fusion precision.

In the following, the possible influence of PET on radiotherapy is discussed, under special consideration of combined PET/CT, focusing on the evaluation of glucose metabolism, as assessed with F-18-labeled deoxyglucose (FDG). The potential of other molecular probes is also discussed.

19.1   Indication for Radiotherapy

The therapeutic approach is defined predominantly by tumor stage. This is especially true for radiation therapy with curative intention, yet can also be considered for palliative therapy concepts in order to avoid or reduce complications caused by tumor growth. In the case of therapy concepts with curative intention, adjuvant and definitive treatment situations must be distinguished.

Accurate staging is prerequisite for curative radiation therapy. Undetected distant metastases or locoregional lymph node manifestations can be the reason for therapy failure. Understaging can lead to erroneous indication decisions for radiation therapy or inadequate radiotherapy planning.

For many tumor entities, it has been shown that FDG-PET may detect unknown distant metastases and lymph node manifestations. Therefore, an important contribution to tumor staging is to be expected [26]. A good example is non-small cell lung cancer (NSCLC), which has been intensively studied with PET. A meta-analysis could show the advantage of FDG-PET in detecting mediastinal lymph nodes compared to conventional diagnostic methods. Several studies show the impact of lymph node staging with FDG-PET on therapeutic strategies. Furthermore, FDG-PET may detect previously unsuspected distant metastases, thus challenging a curative therapy concept [6, 10, 13, 31].

In the case of lung cancer, several studies are available that show that the combined implementation of FDG-PET and CT in a hybrid system for staging is superior to the single techniques [2, 19]. Optimized staging, based for example on additional FDG-PET findings, may influence radio-oncologic consultation and intention of therapy. The influence of FDG-PET results on the indication for radiotherapy was examined in a prospective study with 153 patients [20]. The therapy intention was changed from curative to palliative for 30% of the patients. The reasons for this decision were mostly unexpected distant metastases (18%) or locoregional tumor spread (12%). In individual cases, an unexpected favorable tumor extent was observed and a surgical intervention was initiated. The authors conclude that the influence of FDG-PET findings on the therapeutic approach is even larger in radiotherapy than for surgical procedures. It should be remembered that in case of curative radiotherapy concepts a higher probability of potential side effects is accepted than in a palliative approach. If no increase in life expectancy can be achieved, the improvement of quality of life is the major objective.

19.2 Definition of the Tumor and Planning Target Volumes

A prerequisite for sufficient radiotherapy is an adequately high-dose distribution in planning target volume (PTV) and a low exposure of surrounding normal tissue at risk. This is especially the case for less radiosensitive tumors with a clear dose-effect relation. Innovative diagnostic procedures are particularly useful in these treatment situations and will gain further significance with the introduction of new radiation therapy planning methods. Precise tumor identification is a prerequisite for advanced conformal radiation techniques such as intensity modulated radiation therapy (IMRT).

PET with FDG for tumor imaging has been studied for a number of tumor entities. Two examples are non-small cell lung cancer and head and neck tumors. In particular functionally inoperable or locally advanced nonmetastasized tumors are suggested for curative defined radiotherapy. Details for indications for radiotherapy are available in the guidelines of the "Informationszentrum für Standards in der Onkologie" (ISTO) of the German Cancer Society [33]. The limited surgical options result not only from the tumor size and co-morbidity (functional inoperability), but also from the vicinity of vital normal organ structures. In these situations, the morbidity associated to the surgical intervention must be discussed in view of the lower side effects and potential cure of a definitive radio- (chemo-) therapy. Since tumor growth is usually associated with an increased glucose metabolism, metabolic information must be included in radiotherapy planning.

A recently published review reports on the implementation of FDG-PET for definition of PTV of lung cancer [3, 21]. In addition to the effect on therapeutic intention, as described above, a considerable modification of the target volume can result from FDG-PET findings. Protecting the radiation-exposed tissue of non-involved structures leads to PET-based radiation planning. Examples are ventilation disturbances and atelectases in patients with lung cancer. If there is no additional pneumonia, causing metabolic activation, a good differentiation between tumor and atelectasis can be achieved using FDG-PET (Fig. 19.1). With this information, the GTV can be defined more precisely and the exposed lung volume at risk can be minimized. Another example is the identification of tumor-affected mediastinal lymph nodes. This can be achieved by FDG-PET with high sensitivity and a high negative predictive value. However, false-positive lymph nodes are sometimes found [11]. Criteria for differentiation between inflammatory and tumor-associated lymphadenopathy have already been defined. Before a curative concept is omitted because of a metabolically active lymph node, a histological examination should be considered. FDG-PET sensitivity and specificity for the detection of mediastinal lymph nodes is superior to conventional noninvasive staging. CT is important in the acquisition of the physical attenuation matrix as the basis for dose calculations as well as for characterization of the anatomical relation of the tumor to pleura, mediastinal structures, and the tracheobronchial system, which is relevant for correct staging. Approximately one-third of the target volumes have to be changed based on FDG-PET findings [3].

In patients with head and neck tumors, the surgical options are limited because of the high density of vital structures. Arguments against a decision for surgery can be the preservation of natural feeding and protection of the upper airways. In radiotherapy planning, structures at risk such as the salivary glands and the spinal cord, and in nasopharyngeal cancer structures such as the chiasm, optical nerves, eyes,

lenses, and lachrymal glands must be taken into consideration. Several studies have demonstrated that FDG-PET optimized the staging for lymph nodes compared to conventional staging. The incremental diagnostic value of FDG-PET is still a matter of discussion. A cost–benefit analysis was presented in 2001 and showed that FDG-PET is effective in view of costs in case of CT nodal-negative patients. However, an 8%–10% improvement in accuracy was found by other authors and was not considered relevant [14, 27]. It has to be taken into account that undetected lymph node metastases in CT-based planning will lead to inadequate radiation. This may be the reason for local failure of therapy and may therefore compromise the curative therapy objective. An example of a modified PTV based on the FDG-PET/CT information, resulting in a modification of radiation therapy field is provided in Figure 19.2 for a patient with inoperable head and neck cancer.

Another field of interest of FDG-PET in patients with clinically apparent lymph node manifestation is the search of the unknown primary (CUP). Moreover, FDG-PET plays an important role in the diagnosis of relapse although data for specificity vary [23, 30]. Inflammatory complications, which occur often after surgery of head and neck cancer, may cause false-positive FDG-PET findings and thus reduce specificity [15, 30]. In a study with a limited number of patients with head and neck tumors, retrospective image fusion

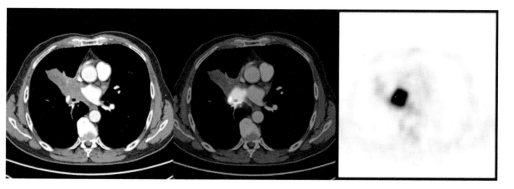

Fig. 19.1. A 59-year-old patient with a central lung cancer (non-small cell lung cancer). Differentiation between atelectasis and tumor-based on FDG-PET

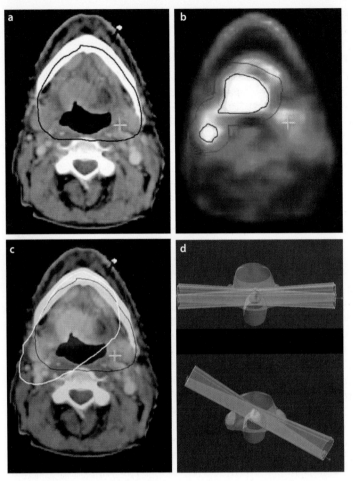

Fig. 19.2a–d. CT and PET/CT-based radiotherapy planning in a patient with inoperable nodal-positive head and neck cancer. A modification of the gross tumor volume (GTV), the planning target volume (PTV), and the physical parameters of radiation fields was observed. **a** PTV-CT; **b** GTV and clinical target volume PET; **c** comparison of CT PTV and PET/CT PTV in the fusion image; **d** modification of radiation fields

of FDG-PET, CT, and MRT was performed in order to optimize PTV. The authors found that when using image fusion, the possibility to preserve the parotid gland was better, although they observed modifications in the PTV in only 11% of the patients studied [22]. In a series of 44 patients, another author described a change in PTV in nearly half of the patients [24]. The reason was the detection of unsuspected tumor manifestations.

Recently another study using FDG-PET/CT for radiotherapy planning was presented [5]. Patients with head and neck tumor, lung cancer, and pelvic tumors were examined. In 56%, a change in gross tumor volume (GTV) was observed, which resulted in a modification of the PTV in 46%. A remarkable result was the reduction of interobserver variability in target volume definition when using the additional FDG-PET information. The difference between the defined volumes was a mean 25.7 cm³ based on CT information; using the additional FDG-PET information this difference was reduced to a mean 9.2 cm³. Moreover, phantom studies were used to validate the volume based on the PET activity, which has very interesting practical implications because deviations in PET activity and real tumor volume can be caused by partial volume effect and spillover of PET activity. In sum, these aspects show that in addition to the correct identification of the primary and its lymph node metastases, the differentiation of tumor and normal tissue is highly relevant in PET-based radiotherapy planning.

In some cancers, FDG is not suitable for the identification and delineation of tumor borders. For these cases, new radiopharmaceuticals have been developed and are currently being evaluated. FDG-PET is not useful for identifying brain tumors because of the high physiological background of glucose metabolism of normal grey matter. In these cases, labeled amino acids are candidates for tumor characterization and delineation [12, 16]. Most of the studies were conducted with C-11-labeled methionine. The disadvantage of this carbon isotope is its short radioactive half-life of 20 min. This precludes tracer application in medical centers located far from the C-11 production site. Lately, fluorine-18-labeled amino acids have been developed for brain tumor diagnostics. The clinical evaluation of these probes in radiotherapy planning is in progress.

FDG-PET is rarely of diagnostic use in prostate cancer and identification of its metastasis. This can both be explained by the topographical relation to the bladder, owing to urine excretion of FDG and by low glucose metabolism of mainly highly differentiated prostate cancer cells. Innovative, predominantly C-11-labeled substances are in use that show a sufficient organ uptake and a lower urinary elimination compared to FDG. In most studies, C-11 or F-18-labeled choline or C-11-labeled acetate are used. Choline is rapidly transported into prostate cancer cells and trapped by phosphorylation. The tracer is probably used to synthesize phosphatidylcholine, which is part of the phospholipids of the cell membrane. Cell proliferation and an increased cell membrane construction is discussed in the process of choline uptake of tumor cells. A correlation of choline uptake intensity with tumor aggressiveness, as represented by grading, has not been shown to date. Furthermore, a differentiation of benign hyperplasia of the prostate and prostate cancer is not possible in all cases. As a one-shop-stop staging and restaging procedure, however, PET and PET-CT with choline has shown promising results so far. Systematic studies in the field of radiotherapy planning are ongoing.

19.3 Prediction of Therapy Response

The radiopharmaceutical used most frequently in oncology is FDG, which characterizes marker cells with enhanced glucose metabolism or at least with enhanced activity of the glucose transporter (Glut-1) and the enzyme hexokinase. It would be desirable to assess the individual radiosensitivity of the tumor by the intensity of glucose metabolism. In this context, it should be mentioned that a correlation of FDG uptake and proliferation activity was already shown for a variety of tumors [28]. It is assumed that tissues with high metabolism and therefore with high mitotic activity will show a good response to radiotherapy. On the other hand, the intensity of glucose metabolism is not a particular marker for characterization of tumor proliferation. Although most studies show a significant correlation between metabolic intensity and histopathological parameters of proliferation, the observed heterogeneity is relatively high. Moreover, benign tumors may sometimes show increased glucose metabolism. An inverse relation between glucose metabolism intensity and individual prognosis was demonstrated for many tumors. In a study with 63 patients with head and neck cancer, a high initial standard uptake value (SUV) correlated in a multivariate analysis with decreased tumor control and disease-specific survival [1]. Furthermore, it must be considered that radiosensitivity also depends on other factors such as tumor oxygenic status. Based on these theoretical aspects, a direct correlation between initial metabolism and therapy response is not to be expected in all cases. Focusing on parameters associated with mechanisms of therapy resistance provides a better chance of characterizing tumors. Probes that correlate more precisely with proliferation or hypoxia are of potentially higher interest than FDG. These developments will be described in Section 19.7.

19.4 Monitoring Therapy Response

In the context of increasingly individualized radiotherapeutic strategies, the definition of early parameters for therapeutic response is increasingly relevant. As outlined above, some factors may predict poor response even before radiation therapy. A prerequisite for the definition of high risk patients is the evaluation of these informative parameters either before or shortly after the initiation of radiotherapy since a regional dose increment has to be discussed for patients who are at high risk for therapy failure or relapse.

The tumor oxygenation parameter, measured invasively, is an example of a prognostically relevant parameter. Moreover, the proportion of vital tumor cells can be examined by biopsies during therapy. These two methods suffer from at least two drawbacks: a multiple sequential characterization is not possible and only a small potentially noninformative part of the tumor can be examined (sampling error). Furthermore, these invasive methods are associated with complications.

In principle, antiproliferative therapy leads to a reduction in glucose metabolism [29, 32]. The detection of early functional deactivation of tumor cells is one of the major strengths of this method. Reductions in glucose metabolism after the first cycle of chemotherapy have been observed in lymphomas. Furthermore, this reduction has been shown to be predictive of good outcome. In view of radiotherapeutic concepts, it would be desirable to characterize the regional response of the tumor already during therapy and to detect potential heterogeneity within the individual tumor. The characterization of these individual factors is necessary for intensification or modification of therapy. Several issues have to be addressed before this concept can be generally recommended. One question in this context is the optimal time to use PET. This time point should be assessed for each tumor separately, since squamous cell cancer has a different radiosensitivity when compared to lymphoma. Furthermore, the body region investigated may play a substantial role. False-positive findings can be caused by the inflammatory reaction of normal tissue (postactinic pneumonitis, mucositis), which might be interpreted as activity of vital tumor cells. In this case, these findings might be interpreted as the resistance of tumor cells to therapy. PET/CT may help to overcome these potential limitations, since identifying landmarks may help to attribute foci of increased glucose metabolism to physiological structures. A second issue is microscopic residual disease. Single therapy-resistant cells can cause a local relapse, but are below PET's detection threshold. Therefore, reducing the dose during therapy should not be recommended lightly. Large prospective trials are needed to justify recommendations on FDG-PET during therapy. Restaging after completion of radiotherapy, however, is a different matter. This has most intensively been studied in lymphoma. The prediction of a potential relapse is very accurate 6 weeks after radiotherapy. High metabolic activity in a residual mass is an indicator of poor prognosis and should either be followed by more aggressive therapy or at least by histological sampling of the PET-positive focus.

19.5 Hybrid Scanners Optimize Time Management and Human Resource Efficiency

The diagnostic improvement offered by hybrid scanners in comparison to sequential image acquisition and fusion is still being discussed [25]. In radiotherapy, several specific advantages can be obtained by using integrated PET/CT scanners. If PET and CT are acquired separately for therapy planning, the radiotherapy team should be present on two occasions to ensure adequate patient positioning. Since patient positioning can be quite time-consuming in individual cases, the use of PET/CT is attractive. Furthermore, hardware alignment of the images leads to optimal image fusion and the time-consuming process of sequential image fusion is no longer necessary.

This modality also provides a much shorter acquisition time. Using PET, transmission images have to be acquired for attenuation correction. For this purpose, the radioactive line or point sources rotate around the patient, and a CT analog transmission image is generated. Given the higher energy of the sources and the far inferior image statistics, these images cannot be used for morphologic diagnosis. The acquisition of a transmission image at 511 keV is not necessary in integrated PET/CT devices, since the CT matrix is used for attenuation correction. Depending on the type of transmission source, the age of the source, and the number of bed positions, approx. 15–30 min of acquisition time can be saved by the simultaneously acquired CT information. This allows for a much better utilization of the PET scanners. The individual patient also benefits from the decreased examination time, since the position of the body during radiation and the immobilization devices are often uncomfortable. The hybrid scanners of the newer generation scanners have a larger gantry diameter than conventional PET scanners. Since the positioning devices and the patient positions, especially of adipose patients, require a large examination space, this aspect is very helpful in daily routine.

19.6 Practical Aspects

The integration of PET or combined PET/CT in radio-oncology requires close cooperation between the nuclear medicine and radiotherapy departments. Only a physician experienced in PET analysis can interpret PET images and consequently can help define GTV and PTV. The PET interpretation depends on tumor type and the location of the tumor. Moreover, experienced radio-oncologists and technicians, who are familiar with patient positioning, are mandatory. Immobilization aids such as thermoplastic masks, which are used for radiation therapy, should be implemented during PET/CT planning. Special patient positioning equipment, such as the belly board used in the prone position should also be available for PET/CT planning. An example is shown in Figure 19.3. In addition, the laser positioning system should be compatible with radiation therapy. A

sufficient PET/CT gantry diameter should also be taken into consideration. Conventional PET scanners have an average diameter of 60 cm. Scanners of the newer generation have gantry diameters up to 70 cm, which is an important advantage for radiotherapy patients because of the use of patient positioning devices.

In defining planning target volumes, it should be remembered that even after optimal examination conditions, inaccuracies can occur during image fusion. In thoracic lesions, this effect can be due to respiratory movements. Even when using identical respiration protocols, shifts between the techniques can be observed, since CT data is collected at the beginning of the examination and is acquired much faster than PET. In such cases, a respiration-triggered recording technique would be ideal, yet this technique is not generally available today.

Image fusion inaccuracies can occur in the abdomen as well: first, upper abdominal organ movement is dependent on respiration; second, intestinal movement, as well as changes in bladder filling, can be responsible for shifts in organ positions that occur during the interval between CT and PET acquisition.

The simultaneous evaluation of PET and CT is obligatory to detect inadequate image fusion. Finally, this can be advantageous when defining planning target volumes, since shifts that arise during the interval between CT and PET acquisition can also occur during each fraction of radiation therapy. These aspects can be kept in mind when defining the PTV by also defining individualized safety margins.

19.7 Innovative Radiopharmaceuticals

The full potential of PET has not been exploited thus far. Imaging of glucose metabolism has turned out to be a very sensitive and clinically helpful method. In principle, many other biochemical processes can be visualized if appropriate ligands and radioactive markers are used. Some of these methods have already been discussed in the previous sections.

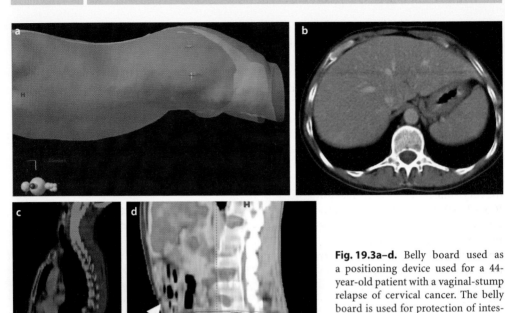

Fig. 19.3a–d. Belly board used as a positioning device used for a 44-year-old patient with a vaginal-stump relapse of cervical cancer. The belly board is used for protection of intestine, which is moved in the cranial ventral direction (*arrow*). An optimal image fusion is only obtained if PET and CT are acquired in the same position. **a** Surface reconstruction in the prone position using the CT information; **b** ventral movement of the organs in the upper abdomen; **c** fusion image (*arrow* shows the vaginal tumor); **d** fusion image transferred into the radiation therapy planning program and calculated dose distribution

A central mechanism for radiation-induced cell elimination is apoptosis. Apoptosis is a genetically controlled energy-consuming process of cell death that is not associated with inflammation as can occur in necrotic cell death. The process of apoptosis is initiated by the cell itself in the case of irreparable damage. However, cell death does not occur as an immediate final step. The different steps of apoptosis offer targets for radiopharmacological targeting in vivo and in vitro. Most studies so far have been conducted with annexin V. This protein binds to phosphatidylserine, which is externalized during the apoptosis process. Deviates or analogs of annexin V and other markers associated with apoptosis are of potential value in view of tumor response to radiation therapy [18].

The in vivo characterization of cell proliferation by PET is also possible. The evaluation of 3-desoxy-18F-fluorothymidine (FLT) is underway. FLT is phosphorylated by the enzyme thymidine kinase after internalization in the cell; after phosphorylation it accumulates in the cell depending on the concentration of the kinase, which is expressed depending on the proliferation process. FLT uptake shows a much better correlation to the immunohistochemically determined proliferation rate when compared to FDG. The disadvantages of FLT in comparison with FDG are the lower intensity of tumor uptake in most cases and the poor delineation of skeletal metastasis because of the high physiological signal of normal bone marrow [4]. In this situation, PET-CT offers the advantage of evaluating structures with a low PET signal, because the co-registered CT matrix is also available.

The use of hypoxia-associated markers in radiation oncology is very promising as well. Hypoxia in tumors is associated with resistance to radiotherapy. For imaging hypoxia, markers retained in the hypoxic milieu of cells are appropriate. Several methods are being evaluated. The most common markers are F-18-labeled misonidazole (FMISO) or ^{60}Cu-diacetyl-bis(N(^{4})-methylthiosemicarbozon) (Cu-ATSM). Preliminary results indicate that retention of these markers is associated with inferior radiation therapy response [8, 9]. These methods to characterize hypoxia seem to be independent of the intensity of glucose metabolism. However, contrast of tumor activity is not as high as FDG uptake in most cases. Again, in this situation PET/CT imaging has advantages in the identification of tumors.

19.8 Focus on Future Research

The data presented herein show that PET offers solutions for many radiation therapy-associated problems. In prospective studies, it remains to be shown that therapy concepts, based on FDG-PET/CT are validated in view of the generally accepted parameters for therapy outcome. It has to be shown that the use of PET/CT improves local tumor control as well as relapse-free survival and total survival. A second aspect is the improvement of quality of life by reducing acute and late toxicity. This can be achieved by an optimized process of indication definition and by protection of normal tissue at risk. Innovative radiotherapy methods such as intensity modulated radiotherapy (IMRT) make it possible to define individualized therapy strategies based on the functional information given by PET. It remains be shown whether diagnosis is improved and fewer therapy-associated side effects can be obtained. In case of positive FDG-PET findings during follow-up after therapy, the consequences for these patient groups will have to be evaluated.

The use of PET/CT is very helpful to evaluate radiopharmaceuticals with low tumor contrast. The example of the hypoxia marker FMISO shows that biologically relevant and prognostically significant metabolic tumor information can be obtained, although the marker itself is suboptimal in tumor imaging. The possibility of a co-registered CT image can be helpful in developing new tracers.

19.9 Consequences for Clinical Practice

Imaging of glucose metabolism is a well-established method in oncology. Optimized staging will have a major influence on the definition of radiotherapy concepts in clearly defined patient groups. Many publications show the great potential of this method in view of optimization of target volumes and follow-up after therapy. In particular, hybrid scanners offer several advantages in view of radiation therapy planning because of optimized image fusion and employee time management. Interdisciplinary guidelines need to be defined that integrate PET and especially PET/CT in the process of radiotherapy planning.

References

1. Allal AS, Dulguerov P, Allaoua M, Haenggeli CA, El-Ghazi el A, Lehmann W, Slosman DO (2002) Standardized uptake value of 2-[(^{18})F] fluoro-2-deoxy-D-glucose in predicting outcome in head and neck carcinomas treated by radiotherapy with or without chemotherapy. J Clin Oncol 20:1398–1404
2. Antoch G, Stattaus J, Nemat AT, Marnitz S, Beyer T, Kuehl H, Bockisch A, Debatin JF, Freudenberg LS (2003) Non-small cell lung cancer: dual-modality PET/CT in preoperative staging. Radiology 229:526–533
3. Bradley J, Thorstad WL, Mutic S, Miller TR, Dehdashti F, Siegel BA, Bosch W, Bertrand RJ (2004) Impact of FDG-PET on radiation therapy volume delineation in non-small-cell lung cancer. Int J Radiat Oncol Biol Phys 59:78–86
4. Buck AK, Halter G, Schirrmeister H, Kotzerke J, Wurziger I, Glatting G, Mattfeldt T, Neumaier B, Reske SN, Hetzel M (2003) Imaging proliferation in

lung tumors with PET: ^{18}F-FLT versus ^{18}F-FDG. J Nucl Med 44:1426–1431

5. Ciernik IF, Dizendorf E, Baumert BG, Reiner B, Burger C, Davis JB, Lutolf UM, Steinert HC, Von Schulthess GK (2003) Radiation treatment planning with an integrated positron emission and computer tomography (PET/CT): a feasibility study. Int J Radiat Oncol Biol Phys 57:853–863

6. Coleman RE (2002) Value of FDG-PET scanning in management of lung cancer. Lancet 359:1361–1362

7. De Jong IJ, Pruim J, Elsinga PH, Vaalburg W, Mensink HJ (2003) Preoperative staging of pelvic lymph nodes in prostate cancer by 11C-choline PET. J Nucl Med 44:331–335

8. Dehdashti F, Mintun MA, Lewis JS, Bradley J, Govindan R, Laforest R, Welch MJ, Siegel BA (2003) In vivo assessment of tumor hypoxia in lung cancer with 60Cu-ATSM. Eur J Nucl Med Mol Imaging 30:844–850

9. Eschmann SM, Paulsen F, Reimold M, Machulla HJ, Bares R (2004) Prognostic impact of ^{18}F-Misonidazole-PET in non small cell lung cancer and head-and neck-cancer prior to radiotherapy. J Nucl Med 45:83P

10. Franzius C (2004) FDG PET: advantages for staging the mediastinum? Lung Cancer 45 [Suppl 2]: S69–S74

11. Graeter TP, Hellwig D, Hoffmann K, Ukena D, Kirsch CM, Schafers HJ (2003) Mediastinal lymph node staging in suspected lung cancer: comparison of positron emission tomography with F-18-fluorodeoxyglucose and mediastinoscopy. Ann Thorac Surg 75:231–235

12. Grosu AL, Lachner R, Wiedenmann N, Stark S, Thamm R, Kneschaurek P, Schwaiger M, Molls M, Weber WA (2003) Validation of a method for automatic image fusion (BrainLAB System) of CT data and ^{11}C-methionine-PET data for stereotactic radiotherapy using a LINAC: first clinical experience. Int J Radiat Oncol Biol Phys 56:1450–1463

13. Hellwig D, Ukena D, Paulsen F, Bamberg M, Kirsch CM (2001) Metaanalyse zum Stellenwert der Positronen-Emissions-Tomographie mit F-18-Fluoro-desoxyglukose (FDG-PET) bei Lungentumoren. Diskussionsbasis der deutschen Konsensus-Konferenz Onko-PET 2000. Pneumologie 55:367–77

14. Hollenbeak CS, Lowe VJ, Stack BC Jr (2001) The cost-effectiveness of fluorodeoxyglucose [18]-F positron emission tomography in the N0 neck. Cancer 92:2341–2348

15. Hustinx R, Smith RJ, Benard F, Rosenthal DI, Machtay M, Farber LA, Alavi A (1999) Dual time point fluorine-18 fluorodeoxyglucose positron emission tomography: a potential method to differentiate malignancy from inflammation and normal tissue in the head and neck. Eur J Nucl Med 26:1345–1348

16. Jager PL, Vaalburg W, Pruim J, de Vries EG, Langen KJ, Piers DA (2001) Radiolabeled amino acids: basic aspects and clinical applications in oncology. J Nucl Med 42:432–445

17. Klabbers BM, Lammertsma AA, Slotman BJ (2003) The value of positron emission tomography for mon-

itoring response to radiotherapy in head and neck cancer. Mol Imaging Biol 5:257–270

18. Lahorte CM, Vanderheyden JL, Steinmetz N, Van De Wiele C, Dierckx RA, Slegers G (2004) Apoptosis-detecting radioligands: current state of the art and future perspectives. Eur J Nucl Med Mol Imaging 31:887–919

19. Lardinois D, Weder W, Hany TF, Kamel EM, Korom S, Seifert B, von Schulthess GK, Steinert HC (2003) Staging of non-small-cell lung cancer with integrated positron-emission tomography and computed tomography. N Engl J Med 348:2500–2507

20. MacManus MP, Hicks RJ, Ball DL, Kalff V, Matthews JP, Salminen E, Khaw P, Wirth A, Rischin D, McKenzie A (2001) F-18 fluorodeoxyglucose positron emission tomography staging in radical radiotherapy candidates with non-small cell lung carcinoma: powerful correlation with survival and high impact on treatment. Cancer 92:886–895

21. Nestle U, Hellwig D, Schmidt S, Licht N, Walter K, Ukena D, Rübe C, Baumann M, Kirsch CM (2002) 2-deoxy-2-[^{18}F]fluoro-D-glucose positron emission tomography in target volume definition for radiotherapy of patients with non-small-cell lung cancer. Mol Imaging Biol 4:257–263

22. Nishioka T, Shiga T, Shirato H, Tsukamoto E, Tsuchiya K, Kato T, Ohmori K, Yamazaki A, Aoyama H, Hashimoto S, Chang TC, Miyasaka K (2002) Image fusion between [18]FDG-PET and MRI/CT for radiotherapy planning of oropharyngeal and nasopharyngeal carcinomas. Int J Radiat Oncol Biol Phys 53:1051–1057

23. Pöpperl G, Lang S, Dagdelen O, Jager L, Tiling R, Hahn K, Tatsch K (2002) Correlation of FDG-PET and MRI/CT with histopathology in primary diagnosis, lymph node staging and diagnosis of recurrency of head and neck cancer Röfo Fortschr Geb Röntgenstr Neuen Bildgeb Verfahr 174:714–720

24. Rahn AN, Baum RP, Adamietz IA, Adams S, Sengupta S, Mose S, Bormeth SB, Hor G, Bottcher HD (1998) Value of ^{18}F fluorodeoxyglucose positron emission tomography in radiotherapy planning of head-neck tumors. Strahlenther Onkol 174:358–364

25. Reinartz P, Wieres FJ, Schneider W, Schur A, Buell U (2004) Side-by-side reading of PET and CT scans in oncology: which patients might profit from integrated PET/CT? Eur J Nucl Med Mol Imaging 31:1456–1461

26. Reske SN, Kotzerke J (2001) FDG-PET for clinical use. Results of the 3rd German Interdisciplinary Consensus Conference, "Onko-PET III", 21 July and 19 September 2000. Eur J Nucl Med 28:1707–1723

27. Schechter NR, Gillenwater AM, Byers RM, Garden AS, Morrison WH, Nguyen LN, Podoloff DA, Ang KK (2001) Can positron emission tomography improve the quality of care for head-and-neck cancer patients? Int J Radiat Oncol Biol Phys 51:4–9

28. Smith TA (1998) FDG uptake, tumor characteristics and response to therapy: a review. Nucl Med Commun 19:97–105

29. Stokkel MP, Draisma A, Pauwels EK (2001) Positron emission tomography with 2-[^{18}F]-fluoro-2-deoxy-D-glucose in oncology. Part IIIb: therapy response monitoring in colorectal and lung tumors, head and neck cancer, hepatocellular carcinoma and sarcoma. J Cancer Res Clin Oncol 127:278–285

30. Terhaard CH, Bongers V, van Rijk PP, Hordijk GJ (2001) F-18-fluoro-deoxy-glucose positron-emission tomography scanning in detection of local recurrence after radiotherapy for laryngeal/ pharyngeal cancer. Head Neck 23:933–941

31. Toloza EM, Harpole L, Detterbeck F, McCrory DC (2003) Invasive staging of non-small cell lung cancer: a review of the current evidence. Chest 123:157S–166S

32. van der Hiel B, Pauwels EK, Stokkel MP (2001) Positron emission tomography with 2-[^{18}F]-fluoro-2-deoxy-D-glucose in oncology. Part IIIa: Therapy response monitoring in breast cancer, lymphoma and gliomas. J Cancer Res Clin Oncol 127:269–277

33. Informationszentrum für Standards in der Onkologie (ISTO), Deutsche Krebsgesellschaft, www.krebsgesellschaft.de. Cited 21 May 2007

Printing: Krips bv, Meppel
Binding: Stürtz, Würzburg